Instructions
for Pediatric
Patients

Instructions for Pediatric Patients

2nd Edition

BARTON D. SCHMITT, MD

Professor of Pediatrics
University of Colorado School of Medicine
Director of General Pediatric Consultative Services
The Children's Hospital
Denver, Colorado

With a Contribution by:
J. Todd Jacobs (deceased)

W.B. SAUNDERS COMPANY
A Division of Harcourt Brace & Company
Philadelphia • London • Toronto • Montreal • Sydney • Tokyo

W.B. SAUNDERS COMPANY
A Division of Harcourt Brace & Company

The Curtis Center
Independence Square West
Philadelphia, Pennsylvania 19106

Library of Congress Cataloging-in-Publication Data

Schmitt, Barton D.
Instructions for pediatric patients / Barton D. Schmitt.—2nd ed.

p.   cm.

ISBN 0–7216–7885–8

1. Child care—Popular works.   I. Title.

RJ61.S363   1999

618.92—dc21

DLC   97-48246

INSTRUCTIONS FOR PEDIATRIC PATIENTS   ISBN 0–7216–7885–8

Printed in the United States of America.

Last digit is the print number: 9   8   7   6   5   4   3   2

This book contains printed instructions written for parents and other caretakers covering the most common health problems occurring in infants, children, and adolescents. The content comes from mainstream pediatrics and has undergone peer review. Because the guidelines are printed on durable paper, you can use the master copy to make multiple office handouts without further permission. The instructions are written for use in pediatric offices, family practice offices, and other clinics where children are seen. These handouts can become the cornerstone of your parent education program.

INFORMATION SHARING

The following is the philosophy behind educating parents about pediatric illnesses and conditions.

1. **Parents are a part of the medical care team.** They know their child better than anyone else. We need them as active participants in the child's treatment program.
2. **Informed parents become better parents.** The more they know about their child's health condition (e.g., asthma or encopresis), the better team members they can be. Smart, informed parents are easier to work with. Also, the quality of decisions made by parents depends on the quality of information they have available (e.g., the pros and cons of tonsillectomy and adenoidectomy). When we give parents the facts, they will usually make the right decision.
3. **Parents already read about medical problems.** We can't provide all health information one-on-one. Parents receive ongoing health advice from friends, relatives, newspapers, magazines, radio, television, and the Internet. Unfortunately, information from the media or nonprofessionals may be confusing, conflicting, or even alarming. Parents' fears and concerns usually can be allayed by the type of accurate, up-to-date, straightforward health advice found in these guidelines.
4. **Medical information should be shared.** There should be no barriers to public disclosure of accurate health information. Access to information is one of our basic freedoms (see the First Amendment).

BENEFITS OF PARENT HANDOUTS FOR PHYSICIANS AND PARENTS

Printed materials are the mainstay of any parent education program (Schmitt et al., 1997). They offer the following advantages:

1. **Increase the amount of information that can be transmitted to the parent.** Most parents would like to have in-depth information about their child's condition. If a child has a chronic disease, it is critical that the family have a complete understanding of how to manage the disease. Most physicians want to be the primary educator, but time constraints in the office limit the amount of information the physician can discuss with parents in the time available. Handouts remove any limits on health education (e.g., our Asthma Center has more than 20 different handouts available to patients). The physician can highlight the more crucial aspects of home treatment and rest assured that the instruction sheets will cover the details. The information sheets supplement the physician's counseling and teaching. In a sense, these information sheets serve as a "physician extender" that expands the physician's counseling and teaching time.
2. **Increase the number of people who receive this information.** The patient instructions can be read by other caretakers who are not present during the office visit. These caretakers may include the spouse, noncustodial parent, grandmother, child care provider, babysitter, or school staff. Giving an extra copy for the grandmother with her name on it may gain her support for a treatment program that she presently opposes (e.g., for thumb sucking). Giving a copy both to the teenager and the parent clarifies the active role the teenager needs to play in the child's health care (e.g., nocturnal enuresis).

3. **Counteract parent forgetfulness.** Normally, people forget 50% of what was said durng an office visit within 5 minutes after leaving the office. At times of crisis (e.g., during an emergency department visit for a febrile seizure), people remember even less. Handouts acknowledge that parents can't memorize everything we tell them. Written instructions become the resource parents can turn to for answers to their questions, although the handout may not improve parental recall. (Isaacman et al., 1992).

4. **Improve parent compliance with treatment regimens.** Forgetfulness (not a dysfunctional family) is the most common cause of poor compliance. Most people can remember only two or three instructions. Studies have shown that compliance is increased if specific recommendations and the reasons behind them are written out (Finney et al., 1985). Written instructions are essential for complex or multistep treatment programs (as with most chronic diseases). To achieve a true understanding of such conditions, the parent needs to reread and rethink the information. Printed instructions can also increase the parents' accountability by making it impossible for them to say that they were not instructed to provide a specific type of care. The printed instructions can serve as a form of contract if the physician requests that the parent or teenager read it, ask questions, and then sign it before leaving the office.

5. **Increase self-care and self-triage.** Handouts encourage parent reading, thinking, and learning. For those who are ready to learn, handouts become their homework assignment. Some parents have "doctor dependency" (i.e., they turn to their child's physician for all medical questions). They don't treat minor symptoms (e.g., mild diarrhea) or give an over-the-counter medicine (e.g., acetaminophen) without first contacting the doctor. Handouts help to clarify the appropriate parent role in common illnesses and provide the study guide for change.

6. **Decrease the use of medications.** Some parents believe that every symptom needs a drug. Some physicians support the "prescription dependency" habit because it's an efficient way to provide medical care. Writing a prescription is an easy answer, but for most symptoms it's not the best answer. The intervention of choice is usually a program that requires more time to explain. The availability of handouts that cover a treatment program helps physicians turn to the better option (e.g., alarms for enuresis, holding techniques for colic, or exercises for backaches).

7. **Help with endless questions.** Some parents, especially "first timers," have endless questions. Some (e.g., neurotic parents) need constant teaching. Others want to review all the pros and cons of a procedure with you (e.g., tympanostomy tubes). All of the parents can be helped with reading materials and a follow-up visit.

8. **Increase parent satisfaction.** Most parents appreciate leaving the physician's office with printed materials. Giving parents something tangible is one way to show we care. This may account for the overuse of prescriptions by some physicians. Information sharing also shows that we consider them partners in health care and that we respect their thinking and common sense. Given in the waiting room, information sheets can show that we value the parent's waiting time.

9. **Expand physician expertise.** Most physicians are good at detecting and categorizing a patient's problems (i.e., the active problem list). Treating some of these problems, however, may be outside our area of expertise. If the problem is not progressive or serious, rather than an automatic referral to a subspecialist, some of these parents can be given a subspecialty handout (e.g., on migraine headache, lactose intolerance, sleep problems, or coughing tic). A follow-up visit can determine whether the child has responded to this intervention (called bibliotherapy) or whether a referral is needed.

10. **Improve self-education.** Handouts are bieducational and therefore especially helpful in resident education. If a resident identifies a problem but doesn't know how to treat it, he can read the handout before discussing it with the parent (e.g., breast-feeding or behavioral problems). Even most experienced physicians have a few weak areas. Handouts can help nurse practitioners and physician assistants expand their roles (Guandolo, 1985).

11. **Save physician time.** Most important, the physician saves the time required to write out separate instructions for each patient. The time required for verbal presentation of the complete treatment plan is reduced. Instead of trying to cover everything, the physician can address the parents' main agenda. The physician can limit verbal instructions to two or three main points, circle them on the handout, and allow the parents to read the remaining information at home. If the handout (e.g., on fever) is read in the waiting room, the physician can use his or her time to address more complex issues rather than answering routine questions. Telephone calls about forgotten instructions (e.g., how to make saline nose drops) can also be avoided.

12. **Help the physician get back on schedule.** A common source of office stress is falling behind in the appointment schedule. Sometimes physicians feel that if they try to answer all of each

parent's questions, they won't have any time left to see more patients. Written information can improve office efficiency and get the physician back on schedule. Some physicians have found that after they make a diagnosis, they can give the parent something to read, see another patient, and then return to discuss specific questions with the previous parent for a few minutes. Another option after diagnosis is to delegate discussion of home care advice to the office nurse. Using the pertinent handout, she can debrief the parent.

13. **Reduce unnecessary telephone callbacks.** Parent handouts encourage appropriate calls and discourage inappropriate ones. The handouts clarify for each topic when to call the physician—immediately, during office hours, or not at all (i.e., when it is safe to continue to treat a child at home). Written instructions prevent unnecessary calls about minor changes. More importantly, they help the parent recognize serious symptoms (e.g., a lethargic newborn, drooling, signs of dehydration, stiff neck, purpura, or petechiae). The handouts on a specific illness (e.g., asthma) prevent callbacks about drug dosages. If parents read handouts the next time their child has a similar illness (e.g., cough, cold, diarrhea), the number of calls for "information only" should decrease. A corollary of good parent education is that as the total number of calls goes down, the percentage of calls about children who need to be seen goes up.

14. **Reduce physician repetition and boredom.** Physicians need handouts that cover diseases that swamp their office. During epidemics of rotavirus or influenza, physicians may have difficulty remembering whether they have already given the parent currently in the office their routine spiel on that condition. Routine information can be transmitted with printed instructions, often before the patient is examined.

15. **Reduce malpractice risk.** If a serious complication develops, the physician who initially saw the child could be sued for providing substandard advice and follow-up instructions. Printed instructions document the exact treatment instructions, drug dosages, and follow-up plan. For example, one of the more common ways for partially treated meningitis to present is in a child who is receiving antibiotics for an ear infection. If a handout on ear infections states clearly to call immediately if the child becomes worse or if fever or earache persists for more than 48 hours while the child is receiving antibiotics, the physician would not be liable if parents did not follow these instructions. Clarification of the indications for recontacting the physician is essential in providing quality medical care (other examples: croup and head trauma). For liability protection, document in the chart the specific handouts that were given and the fact the material was reviewed with the parent. For hospitals, the Joint Commission on Accreditation of Hospitals (JCAHO) requires documentation of the health education process in the chart (Hartmann and Kochmar, 1994). In some emergency departments, parents are asked to sign on the encounter form that they have received specific handouts.

16. **Increase physician satisfaction.** Meeting all of a family's needs during a 15-minute office visit is a challenge. Handouts can help physicians meet some of these needs and reach a greater sense of completion at the end of the visit. Physician satisfaction is also enhanced by some of the benefits previously discussed: eliminating need to write out instructions, expanding the subjects we can cover, decreasing routine questions, decreasing repetitious advice, and being helped to stay on schedule on very busy days.

LIMITATIONS OF PARENT HANDOUTS

We all love the parent who is well educated and devours any handouts we give them, but handouts aren't for everyone. For a handout to be effective, the parent must be able to read, comprehend, and transform the information into action. Knowledge is the foundation of action, but taking the final step requires more motivation than some parents have. Of those parents who implement recommendations within a handout while their child is sick, it is a minority who will refer back to the same handout with questions when their child is sick again.

Low literacy skills can interfere with medical treatment (Miles and Davis, 1995). More than 20% of adults are illiterate or have poor reading skills. They respond best to simple verbal instructions, often with repetition of those instructions. Calling the family by telephone 2 days after the initial visit is also helpful. Medical messages on a telephone advice line are also useful for nonreaders (Schmitt, 1996). Fortunately, many illiterate parents have a close friend or relative who serves as their "assigned reader."

Some parents are "emotional" nonreaders. They throw away the handouts as they leave the clinic area. Many of these parents feel overwhelmed or preoccupied with life's stresses. Often their expectation was to have the child's condition rapidly cured with an antibiotic. Fortunately, this is a small group.

A larger group are parents who read the handout but don't implement the suggestions (Bartlett,

1984). Their follow-through is better if their child is quite sick and they easily perceive the need for intervention. Compliance is also increased when the parent's name is written on the handout and the health care provider directly gives it to the parent. Finally, the lack of translation of handouts into other languages greatly limits their use and efficacy in some communities.

THEORETICAL RISKS OF HANDOUTS

Handouts that list all of the complications of a particular disease cause undue fear and anxiety. Parents want to know the typical prognosis, not the worst-case scenario prognosis. Some of the drug handouts that list all of the potential side effects or the immunization handouts that go into detail about how people acquire the disease (e.g., hepatitis B) lead to more questions rather than fewer. A handout on urinary tract infections stating that renal failure might develop and that the child might need a kidney transplantation if all the dosages of antibiotic are not given causes an inappropriate level of alarm in the parents.

Some handouts may cause unnecessary guilt if they seem to blame the parent for the child's behavior or learning disability. Some handouts cause confusion by contradicting the personal physician's medical decisions. In general, handouts shouldn't speculate about what laboratory studies, imaging studies, or surgery might be needed for a particular condition. In rare instances, a handout has contained inaccurate advice that has led to harm (e.g., fluid replacement that leads to hyponatremia or hypernatremia).

Finally, if the physician starts to replace verbal instructions with handouts, the parent will feel neglected. The parent will complain that their doctor "doesn't have time to talk with me any more." Live communication remains the fundamental medium for conveying information. Handouts must remain a supplemental or backup system.

COST-EFFECTIVENESS OF HANDOUTS

Handouts are an inexpensive form of intervention and will be of increasing importance in a system of managed care and capitation. Handouts cost $.02 to $.05 per copy, depending on whether one uses an office copy machine or an outside copy center. Pediatricians cost about $60 per hour, nurse practitioners about $30 per hour, and Registered Nurses about $15 to $20 per hour. Handouts cut office expenses primarily by saving physician and nurse time (e.g., fewer telephone calls and fewer and briefer office visits).

If parents read handouts, incoming phone calls about forgotten information are reduced. Using a parent handout, Casey and colleagues (1984) produced a 54% decrease in inappropriate calls about fever. Casey reduced unnecessary office visits regarding fever by 74%. Roberts and associates (1983) reduced unnecessary visits for upper respiratory infections by 44%. If the physician uses handouts to back up focused verbal instructions, office or emergency department visits can be shorter. If parents need to make fewer visits to the office, they have fewer co-payments to meet.

Handouts can also reduce costs by decreasing expensive treatment interventions. If parents can be educated on how to care for complex conditions (such as nocturnal enuresis with enuresis alarms), the rate of prescribing expensive drugs can also be decreased. When parents are encouraged to read about the pros and cons of a particular surgical procedure (e.g., tonsillectomy and adenoidectomy) unnecessary surgery can be reduced. By reinforcing the parent's education about bicycle helmets, hot water heater temperature, and car safety seats, we can reduce the hospitalization rate for head injuries, burns, and more serious motor vehicle accidents.

The greatest potential for handouts may be in preventing behavioral problems. It costs less to intervene early. Psychologic counseling is expensive and usually has limited or no coverage in managed care plans. An intervention for sleep problems using a handout was equally effective to direct counseling. A 10-page handout on behavioral modification skills decreased oppositional behavior at home and school in children with attention deficit with hyperactivity disorder precluding the need for expensive counseling (Seymour et al., 1989).

Finally, a book can be the ultimate compendium of handouts. It can be given out in the newborn nursery or at the first office visit. The advantage of a book over single-topic handouts is that it can be read in advance. It also saves the time and cost of copying handouts. A recent study comparing 500 families who received a child care book and 500 who did not showed that it decreased telephone calls, office sick child visits, and pharmacy prescriptions (France et al., in press).

CONTENT OF THESE PARENT HANDOUTS

Each topic is covered in depth so that parents will have the majority of their questions answered after reading it. The home treatment instructions are detailed so that parents should be able to reduce their child's symptoms and improve the comfort level. The names of specific drugs are not listed unless one main drug is prescribed for that particular disease (e.g., penicillin for strep throat or scarlet fever). For most diseases requiring a prescription drug, the physician who gives out the instruction sheet will need to fill in several blanks with the name of the drug, the dosage, the dosing interval, and the number of days of total therapy (e.g., sinus infection, ear infection, urinary tract infection, strep throat, scarlet fever, asthma, scabies). Behavioral topics (e.g., tantrums, toilet training, biting) and health promotion topics (e.g, cholesterol, passive smoking, frequent infections) have been highlighted because they are in demand by families. The preventive approach to various topics (e.g., prevention of sleep problems, toilet training problems, "spoiled" children, sunburn, and tooth decay) is also stressed.

Some of these handouts are identical to those found in my book for parents, *Your Child's Health* (Bantam Books, 1998). Most, however, have been rewritten into an "after-the-office-visit" format. Some handouts describe diseases (e.g., pneumonia or mononucleosis) not covered in the parent book. The writing has been tested for clarity. The reading level is sixth to eighth grade (Davis et al., 1994; Klingbeil et al., 1995). The information has been reviewed by many parents, and it contains no medical or psychiatric jargon.

MAKING CHANGES IN CONTENT (CUSTOMIZING HANDOUTS)

Before distributing a handout, read the material to be sure that there are no major differences in philosophy. For most topics, diagnostic criteria, etiology, and outcomes are factual material on which physicians do not differ. It is in the area of treatment that we see variations in approach, especially in the choice of drugs.

It would be surprising if you agreed with more than 95% of what is contained in these guidelines. Feel free to make changes directly in your master copy. If you disagree with a sentence or a paragraph, cross it out. You could also put a bracket around it and in the margin write "disagree." If you wish to replace a paragraph, type up your changes and tape the new paragraph over the existing one. If you think the guideline is incomplete, type up additional special instructions and add them at the bottom of the page.

Any changes you make, of course, are your legal responsibility. Add your name and date next to all changes, so that anyone who reads the handout will be aware of the source of information. Keep in mind that prescription drugs are not listed, and it is your role to fill in the current drug of choice for your patient's condition.

DUPLICATING PARENT HANDOUTS

These guidelines are printed on durable paper and distributed in a book with perforated pages. You can selectively tear out the master copies, make multiple copies for use in your office setting, and preserve the originals in a loose-leaf binder for future use. The acknowledgment of the author and the publisher is listed as a footer on each page of each handout. Permission to duplicate (photocopy) handouts for noncommercial purposes (to give to your patients) is hereby granted. No special or additional permission is needed to distribute these parent handouts for this purpose. In granting this permission, the author and publisher expect that the practices involving multiple physicians and offices will maintain one set of original master copies in each office setting. We also encourage you to add your name and office telephone number to these handouts.

DESIGNING AN OFFICE HANDOUT SYSTEM

Most physicians intellectually agree with the benefits of a handout system. Implementing handouts in their office, however, often triggers physician reluctance. Some will say, "My office sees 40 patients a day, and no one has time to do this." In truth, once a handout system is in place, this office will be less busy. An office can initiate handouts if it starts small.

Small Handout System. Select the 10 most common illnesses you see. The topics may change somewhat by season (e.g., hay fever versus frostbite). Keep copies of these acute illness topics in each examination room so that you can easily locate them and quickly give them out. Handouts can be kept in manila folders in a desk drawer or in an accordion-type file box.

Select the 20 most common preventive topics and behavioral topics that parents ask about.

Keep copies of these in a display rack in the waiting room so that parents can help themselves. Self-service is the most efficient and inexpensive system.

Large Handout System.   Some physicians want a handout for every subject within the field of pediatrics. They continually collect handouts from various sources. It's impossible to make all of these directly available to parents from display racks. A better system is to provide a menu of available handouts on a bulletin board. A parent can then request particular topics from the receptionist. If a copy machine is available and if selected topics are in a three-ring binder, parents might be permitted to print their own copy. Copies of large numbers of handouts are best stored in a centralized filing cabinet or in a computer.

Protecting Master Copies.   The most common crisis occurs when the office suddenly runs out of copies and the master (original) copy cannot be located for duplication. Put one person in charge of protecting and keeping master copies in a safe place. Keep the masters separate from the copies to be made from them. If copies of certain handouts need to be ordered from an outside source, keep the order forms in a separate established place. Limit the number of people who have access to master copies. Put one person in charge of restocking the display racks and the physician handout drawer on a regular basis.

WHEN TO GIVE HANDOUTS TO PARENTS

Everyone on the office team should become involved with helping parents obtain appropriate handouts. The office staff can use handouts to better utilize waiting time both in the waiting room and in the examination rooms. Opportunities for introducing a handout are many.

In the Waiting Room.   Just as toys are essential for children in the waiting room, so is reading material for the parents. Common, standard topics should be available in racks. Symptoms (e.g., fever or diarrhea) and behavior (e.g., tantrums or thumbsucking) can be "diagnosed" by parents. Parent-driven reading can make the upcoming office visit more efficient. During epidemics (e.g., croup or influenza) or seasonal illness (e.g., sunburn or insect bites), copies of relevant handouts can be placed in the waiting room.

After Nurse Contact.   After the nurse processes the patient and puts her into the examining room, she can provide one or two handouts that are appropriate for the child's illness (e.g., probable chickenpox). The parent can then read the handout while waiting for the physician. A benefit of this procedure is that it reduces the number of routine questions the parent will have for the physician.

After Physician Contact.   After the physician has examined the patient and has made a specific diagnosis, she can hand the parent the related handout. Another option is to write down or mark on a checklist the handout (e.g., asthma, bronchiolitis, pneumonia or infectious mononucleosis) that she wants the parents to receive. The handouts can be given to the parent at the checkout desk from the central file or after it is printed from the computer.

After the First Visit.   Some of the instruction sheets cover universal minor illnesses that every child acquires on multiple occasions. These include cough, sore throat, diarrhea, fever, and others. These parent handouts can be given out as a packet on the first office visit. Thereafter, the handouts can be referred to for home treatment and can save the health care provider considerable telephone time in discussing them.

After Talks to Parent Groups.   Some physicians give parenting classes in their offices. Others give talks to local day care parent groups or parent teacher organizations. Parent handouts are useful to underscore the subject and to give the attendee a take-home message for the partner. Helpful subjects include discipline problems, homework, television, movies, and so on.

After Telephone Requests.   When parents call in to request information about particular topics (e.g., Lyme disease, cholesterol testing, attention deficit disorders, or bedwetting) that would be time-consuming to cover in person, often handouts can be mailed out or sent by Fax machine to the parent.

SUMMARY

Every office visit and patient contact is an opportunity to teach the parent. Optimally, no parent should leave an office without an appropriate handout.

Although a variety of health education options are available, parent handouts remain the most utilized and cost-effective educational tools in primary care. Handouts increase the amount and quality of information that can be provided to patients, enhance compliance with treatment recommendations, and offer appropriate self-care and self triage. They decrease unnecessary telephone calls and visits, malpractice risks, and unnecessary therapies and procedures. Handouts also increase physician satisfaction by expanding physician expertise and allowing the physician to reach a sense of closure with each visit.

Best wishes in all your efforts to enhance parent education in our practice.

REFERENCES

Bartlett EE: Effective approaches to patient education for the busy pediatrician. Pediatrics (Suppl) 1984; 920–923.

Casey R, McMahon F, McCormick MC, et al: Fever therapy: Educational intervention for parents. Pediatrics 1984; 73:600.

Davis TC, Mayeaux EJ, Fredrickson D, et al: Reading ability of parents compared with reading level of pediatric patient education materials. Pediatrics 1994; 93:460.

Finney JW, Friman PC, Rapoff MA, et al: Improving compliance with antibiotic regimens for otitis media: Randomized clinical trial in a pediatric clinic. Am J Dis Child 1985; 139:89.

France EK, Selna MJ, Lyons EE, Beck AL, Calonge BN: Effect of a pediatric self-care book on utilization of services in a group model HMO. In press.

Guandolo VL: We've made our office practice a CME center. Contemp Pediatr 1985; 2:34.

Hartmann RA, Kochar MS: The provision of patient and family education. Parent Ed Counseling 1994; 24:101–108.

Isaacman DJ, Purvis K, Gyuro J, et al: Standardized Instructions: Do they improve communication of discharge information from the emergency department? Pediatrics 1992; 89:1204.

Klingbeil C, Speece MW, Schubiner H: Readability of pediatric patient education materials. Clin Pediar 1995; 34:96–102.

Long N, Rickert VI, Ashcraft EW: Bibliotherapy as an adjunct to stimulant medication in the treatment of attention-deficit hyperactivity disorder. J Pediatr Health Care 1993; 7:82–88.

Miles S, Davis T: Patients who can't read: Implications for the health care system. JAMA 1995; 274:1719–1720.

Roberts CR, Imrey PB, Turner JD, Hosokawa MC, Alster JM: Reducing physician visits for colds through consumer education. JAMA 1983; 250:1986–1989.

Schmitt BD: Parent Advice Line. Phoenix, National Health Enhancement Systems, 1996. [For information, call 1-800-345-3342.]

Schmitt BD, Brayden RM, Kempe A: Parent handouts: Cornerstone of a health education program. Contemp Pediatr 1997; 14:120–143.

Seymour FW, Brock FW, Brock P, et al: Reducing sleep disruptions in young children. Evaluation of therapist-guided and written information approaches: A brief report. J Child Psychol Psychiatry 1989; 30:913.

BARTON D. SCHMITT, M.D., F.A.A.P.

Acknowledgments

I am immeasurably indebted to my original pediatric reviewers for their careful examination of my text for accuracy, safety, objectivity, clarity, and completeness. Their efforts were extraordinary and their feedback invaluable.

Pediatric Review Board
Joseph H. Banks, M.D., Columbus, Ohio
John M. Benbow, M.D., Concord, North Carolina
Daniel D. Broughton, M.D., Rochester, Minnesota
Rosemary D. Casey, M.D., Philadelphia, Pennsylvania
David M. Christopher, M.D., Renton, Washington
Jessie R. Groothuis, M.D., Denver, Colorado
Robin L. Hansen, M.D., Sacramento, California
David L. Kerns, M.D., San Jose, California
Bruce J. McIntosh, M.D., Jacksonville, Florida
Robert D. Mauro, M.D., Denver, Colorado
Cajsa J. Schumacher, M.D., Albany, New York
Daniel R. Terwelp, M.D., Austin, Texas
Wallace C. White, M.D., Denver, Colorado

My appreciation and admiration to the following pediatric subspecialists and pediatric surgeons who have graciously helped me with specific topics and ongoing questions in their areas of expertise:

General Pediatrics:	Drs. Robert Mauro, Steven Poole, Richard Krugman, Stephen Berman, Richard Shiffman, and Burris Duncan
Adolescent Medicine:	Drs. David Kaplan, J. Todd Jacobs, Kathleen Mammel, Ida Nakashima, and Henry Cooper
Emergency Pediatrics:	Drs. Joan Bothner, Keith Battan, and Michael Clemmens
Infectious Disease:	Drs. James Todd, Mary Glode, Mark Abzug, and Brian Lauer
Dermatology:	Drs. William Weston and Joseph Morelli
Allergy:	Drs. James Shira, James Lustig, Allen Bock, David Pearlman, and Fred Leffert
Psychology:	Drs. Edward Christophersen, Jeffrey Dolgan, and Andrea Van Steenhouse
Neonatology:	Drs. Jacinto Hernandez, Susan Niermeyer, Elizabeth Thilo, and Gerald Merenstein
Breast-Feeding:	Drs. Marianne Neifert, Joy Seacat, Lisbeth Gabrielski, and Jack Newman
Cardiology:	Drs. James Wiggins, Robert Wolfe, Henry Sondheimer, and Reginald Washington
Pulmonology:	Drs. Leland Fan, Jeffrey Wagener, and Frank Accurso
Gastroenterology:	Drs. Arnold Silverman, Ronald Sokol, Judy Sondheimer, Nancy Krebs, Michael Narkewicz, and Sharon Taylor
Neurology:	Drs. Paul Moe and Alan Seay
Ear, Nose and Throat:	Drs. Kenny Chan and Ray Wood
Ophthalmology:	Drs. Robert King and Robert Sargent
Dentistry:	Drs. William Mueller and Richard Abrams
Urology:	Dr. Martin Koyle
Orthopedics:	Drs. Robert Eilert, Frank Chang, and Gerard Glancy

My special thanks to the good people at W.B. Saunders Company who helped me complete this project: Lisette Bralow and Judith Fletcher, my editors; Jonel Sofian, the designer; and Ethel Cathers, in marketing.

Contents

PART 5

PEDIATRIC DERMATOLOGY

PART 6

MISCELLANEOUS PHYSICAL PROBLEMS

PART 7

BEHAVIOR PROBLEMS

A. Sleep Problems

B. Discipline Problems

PART 1

NEW BABY CARE

Before the baby is born, most parents prepare a special room. They buy a layette including clothing, a place to sleep, feeding equipment, bathing equipment, and changing supplies. This preparation is called *nesting behavior*. The most common mistake parents on a limited budget can make during this time is buying something they don't need at all or buying an expensive (often fancy) version of an essential piece of equipment.

ESSENTIAL EQUIPMENT

Safety Car Seat. Child restraint seats are essential for transporting your baby in a car. They are required by law in all 50 states. Consider buying one that is convertible and usable until your child reaches 40 pounds and 40 inches. Until your child weighs more than 20 pounds the car seat faces backward; after that time it is moved to a forward-facing position. Car seats must conform to federal safety standards; also, they are ranked by consumer magazines. Many hospitals have a rental program for car seats that can save you money unless you are going to have several children.

Crib. Since your baby will spend so much unattended time in the crib, make certain it is a safe one. Federal safety standards require that all cribs built after 1974 have spaces between the crib bars of 2⅜ inches or less. This restriction is to prevent a child from getting the head or body stuck between the bars. If you have an older crib, be sure to check this distance, which is approximately the width of three fingers. Also, check for any defective crib bars. The mattress should be the same size as the crib so that your baby's head can't get caught in the gap. It should also be waterproof. Bumper pads are unnecessary because infants rarely strike their heads on the railings. The pads have the disadvantage of keeping your baby from seeing out of the crib; they are also something to climb on at a later stage. During the first 2 or 3 months of life it may be more convenient for feeding during the night to have your baby sleep next to your bed in a bassinet, a drawer, a cardboard box, or a basket with a firm pad on the bottom.

Bathtub. Small plastic bathtubs with sponge linings are available. A large plastic dishpan will also suffice for the purpose. A molded sponge lining can be purchased separately. As a compromise, a kitchen sink works well if you are careful about preventing your child from falling against hard edges or turning on the hot water, thereby causing a burn. Until the umbilical cord falls off, keep the water level below the navel. Most children can be bathed in a standard bathtub by 1 year of age.

Bottles and Nipples. If you are feeding your baby formula, you will need about ten 8-ounce bottles. Although clear plastic bottles cost twice as much as glass ones, you will be glad you bought the unbreakable type the first time you or your baby drops one. If you use disposable bottle liners, you probably will need only five bottles. You will also need a corresponding number of nipples. If you prepare more than one bottle at a time, you will need a 1-quart measuring cup and a funnel for mixing a batch of formula.

Diapers: Reusable vs. Disposable. Let's compare disposable diapers with cloth diapers. The rate of diaper rashes is about the same. If you're concerned about using safety pins, worry not. Modern diaper covers come with Velcro straps. The main advantage of disposable diapers is that they are very convenient, freeing the family to travel easily and day care centers to operate efficiently. The diapers made with super absorbent gel have the advantage of not letting urine leak. The main disadvantage of disposable diapers is that they cost more. Disposable diapers average about 20 cents per diaper vs. 12 cents per diaper from the diaper service or 3 cents per diaper if you wash your own (after their initial purchase).

Because of the ecological ramifications of disposable diapers, which type of diaper to use is a controversial issue. Why not take advantage of both options? Use cloth diapers when you are home. Use disposable diapers when you are traveling or as a back-up if you are out of the home. Use disposables when your child has diarrhea because they prevent leakage of watery stools. (Some parents also prefer disposable diapers at night because they are leakproof.) During the first 2 or 3 months of life, when most mothers are exhausted by new baby care, consider a diaper service rather than washing the diapers yourself. You will find that modern diaper services are very efficient, provide excellent sterilized diapers, and pick them up weekly.

Pacifier. A pacifier is useful in soothing many babies. To prevent choking, the pacifier's shield should be at least 1½ inches in diameter and the pacifier should be one single piece. Some of the newer ones are made of silicone (instead of rubber), which lasts longer because it doesn't dry out. The orthodontic-shaped pacifiers are accepted by some babies but not by others.

Nasal Suction Bulb. A suction bulb is essential for helping young babies with breathing difficulties caused by sticky or dried nasal secretions. A suction bulb with a blunt tip is more effective and less likely to irritate the nasal lining than the ones with long, tapered tips (which are used for irrigating ears). The best ones on the market have a small, clear plastic tip (mucus trap) that can be removed from the rubber suction bulb for cleaning.

Thermometer. A rectal thermometer is most helpful if your baby becomes sick. The digital thermometers that display the temperature in 30 seconds are worth the extra few dollars. If you buy a glass thermometer, the ones with four color zones are easier to read.

Diaper and Bottle Bag. For traveling outside the home with your baby you will need an all-purpose backpack to carry the items that allow you to feed your baby and change diapers. Packs often fit on the back of strollers. Backpacks are more comfortable and convenient than shoulder bags.

High Chair. During the first 6 months of life your baby can be held when being fed. Once your child can sit unsupported and take solid foods, a high chair is needed. The most important feature is a wide base that prevents tipping. The tray needs to have a good safety latch. The tray should also have adjustable positions to adapt to your infant's growth. A safety strap is critical. Plastic or metal chairs are easier to clean than wooden chairs. Small, portable, hook-on high chairs that attach directly to the tabletop are gaining in popularity. They are convenient and reasonably priced. The ones with a special clamp that keeps your child from pushing the chair off the tabletop with his feet have a good safety record. By 2 years of age, most toddlers can sit in a youth chair.

Training Cup. By the time your child is 1 year old, she will want to hold her own cup. Buy a spill-proof one with a weighted base, a lid, and a spout. By 2 years of age, most children can use a regular cup.

Bib. To keep food off your baby's clothes, find a molded plastic bib with an open scoop on the bottom to catch the mess.

Safety Gadgets. Once your child is crawling, you will need electric-outlet safety plugs, cabinet door safety locks, bathtub spout protectors, toilet clamps and plastic corner guards for sharp table edges.

HELPFUL EQUIPMENT

The following items mainly provide your child with forms of transportation or special places to play.

Changing Table. Diapers need to be changed 10 to 15 times daily. Although a bed can be used for changing, performing this task without bending over prevents back strain. A regular table or buffet covered with a changing pad can work as well as a special changing table.

Automatic Swing. Although swings are entertaining to most babies, they are especially helpful for crying babies. They come in windup-spring, pendulum-driven, or battery-powered models. The latter two have quieter mechanisms. Again, a sturdy base and crossbars are important for safety.

Front Carrier or Sling. Front packs or slings are great for new babies. They give your child a sense of physical contact and warmth. The slings are helpful during breast-feeding. They allow you freedom to use your hands. Buy one with head support. Carrying a baby in front after 5 or 6 months of age can cause a backache for the parent.

Backpack. Backpacks are useful for carrying babies who are 5 or 6 months old and have good head support. They are an inexpensive way to carry your baby outside when you go shopping, hiking, or walking anywhere. The inner seat can usually be adjusted to different levels.

Stroller. Another way to transport a baby who has outgrown the front pack is in a baby stroller. The most convenient ones are the umbrella type, which fold up and have at least one reclining position. A safety belt is important to keep your baby from standing up and falling. A sunshade is also great for inspiring an afternoon snooze.

Infant Seat or Bouncer Seat. An infant seat is a good place to keep a young baby who is not eating or sleeping. A bouncer seat has the added advantage that your baby can self-initiate movement. Infants prefer this inclined position so they can see what is going on around them. Buy one with a safety strap, but don't substitute it for a car seat. Once children reach 3 to 4 months of age, they can usually tip the infant seat over, so discontinue using it.

Playpen. A playpen is a handy and safe place to leave your baby when you need uninterrupted time to cook a meal or do the wash. Babies like playpens because the slatted or mesh sides afford a good view of the environment. Playpens can be used both indoors and outdoors. As with cribs, the slats should be less than 2⅜ inches apart. The playpens with a fine-weave netting are also acceptable, although sometimes older infants can climb out of them. Bottomless playpens are gaining in popularity. Your baby should be introduced to the playpen by 4 months of age in order to build up positive associations with it. It is very difficult to introduce a playpen after a baby has learned to crawl. Avoid stringing any objects on a cord across the playpen, because your baby could become entangled in them and strangle.

Gates. A gate is essential if your house has stairways that your baby must be protected from. A gate also helps to keep a child in a specific room with you and out of the rest of the house, as when you are working in the kitchen. Many rooms can be closed off with doors. All gates should be climb resistant. The strongest gates are spring loaded.

Humidifier. A humidifier will be helpful in dry climates or areas with cold winters. The new ultrasonic humidifiers are quieter and have other advantages. Do not buy a vaporizer (a gadget that produces steam) because it can cause burns in children and doesn't deliver humidity at as fast a rate as a humidifier.

Food Grinder. The time comes when your baby must make the transition from baby foods to table foods. A baby-food grinder takes the work out of mashing up table foods. It's as effective as a blender, easier to clean, and less expensive. Food processors have the advantage of allowing you to make larger quantities faster than in a grinder. If you buy all your baby food in jars, this item is not necessary.

Teethers. During teething, many infants like to chew on something. Teethers are available in many shapes, sizes, and colors to help comfort your baby.

HARMFUL EQUIPMENT: WALKERS

Over 40% of children who use walkers have an accident requiring medical attention. They suffer fractures, concussions, dental injuries, and lacerations. There have even been some deaths. Don't buy a walker.

Instructions for Pediatric Patients, **2nd Edition,** ©1999 by WB Saunders Company.
Written by Barton D. Schmitt, MD, pediatrician and author of *Your Child's Health,* Bantam Books, a book for parents.

NEWBORN APPEARANCE

Even after your child's physician assures you that your baby is normal, you may find that she looks a bit odd. Your baby does not have the perfect body you have seen in baby books. Be patient. Most newborns have some peculiar characteristics. Fortunately they are temporary. Your baby will begin to look normal by 1 to 2 weeks of age.

This discussion of these transient newborn characteristics is arranged by parts of the body. A few minor congenital defects that are harmless but permanent are also included. Call our office if you have questions about your baby's appearance that this list does not address.

Head

Molding. Molding refers to the long, narrow, cone-shaped head that results from passage through a tight birth canal. This compression of the head can temporarily hide the fontanel. The head returns to a normal shape in a few days.

Caput. This refers to swelling on top of the head or throughout the scalp caused by fluid squeezed into the scalp during the birth process. Caput is present at birth and clears in a few days.

Cephalohematoma. This is a collection of blood on the outer surface of the skull. It is due to friction between the infant's skull and the mother's pelvic bones during the birth process. The lump is usually confined to one side of the head. It first appears on the second day of life and may grow larger for up to 5 days. It doesn't resolve completely until the baby is 2 or 3 months of age.

Anterior Fontanel. The "soft spot" is found in the top front part of the skull. It is diamond shaped and covered by a thick fibrous layer. Touching this area is quite safe. The purpose of the soft spot is to allow rapid growth of the brain. The spot will normally pulsate with each beat of the heart. It normally closes with bone when the baby is between 12 and 18 months of age.

Eyes

Swollen Eyelids. The eyes may be puffy because of pressure on the face during delivery. They may also be puffy and reddened if silver nitrate eye drops are used. This irritation should clear in 3 days.

Subconjunctival Hemorrhage. A flame-shaped hemorrhage on the white of the eye (sclera) is not uncommon. It is caused by birth trauma and is harmless. The blood is reabsorbed in 2 to 3 weeks.

Iris Color. The iris is usually blue, green, gray, or brown or variations of these colors. The permanent color of the iris is often uncertain until your baby reaches 6 months of age. White babies are usually born with blue-gray eyes. Black babies are usually born with brown-gray eyes. Children who will have dark irises often change eye color by 2 months of age; children who will have light-colored irises usually change by 5 or 6 months of age.

Blocked Tear Duct. If your baby's eye is continuously watery, he may have a blocked tear duct. This means that the channel that normally carries tears from the eye to the nose is blocked. It is a common condition, and more than 90% of blocked tear ducts open up by the time the child is 12 months old.

Ears

Folded Over. The ears of newborns are commonly soft and floppy. Sometimes one of the edges is folded over. The outer ear will assume normal shape as the cartilage hardens over the first few weeks.

Flattened Nose

The nose can become misshapen during the birth process. It may be flattened or pushed to one side. It will look normal by 1 week of age.

Mouth

Sucking Callus (or Blister). A sucking callus occurs in the center of the upper lip from constant friction at this point during bottle- or breast-feeding. It will disappear when your child begins cup feedings. A sucking callus on the thumb or wrist may also develop.

Tongue-Tie. The normal tongue in newborns has a short tight band that connects it to the floor of the mouth. This band normally stretches with time, movement, and growth. Babies with symptoms from tongue-tie are rare.

Epithelial Pearls. Little cysts (containing clear fluid) or shallow white ulcers can occur along the gum line or on the hard palate. These are a result of blockage of normal mucous glands. They disappear after 1 to 2 months.

Teeth. The presence of a tooth at birth is rare. Approximately 10% are extra teeth without a root structure. The other 90% are prematurely erupted normal teeth. The distinction can be made with an x-ray. The extra teeth must be removed by a dentist. The normal teeth need to be removed only if they become loose (with a danger of choking) or if they cause sores on your baby's tongue.

Breast Engorgement

Swollen breasts are present during the first week of life in many female and male babies. They are caused by the passage of female hormones across the mother's placenta. Breasts are generally swollen for 2 to 4 weeks, but they may stay swollen longer in breast-fed babies. One breast may lose its swelling before the other one by a month or more. Never squeeze the breast because this can cause infection. Be sure to call our office if a swollen breast develops any redness, streaking, or tenderness.

Female Genitals

Swollen Labia. The labia minora can be quite swollen in newborn girls because of the passage of female hormones across the placenta. The swelling will resolve in 2 to 4 weeks.

Hymenal Tags. The hymen can also be swollen because of maternal estrogen and can have smooth ½-inch projections of pink tissue. These normal tags occur in 10% of newborn girls and slowly shrink over 2 to 4 weeks.

Vaginal Discharge. As the maternal hormones decline in the baby's blood, a clear or white discharge can flow from the vagina during the latter part of the first week of life. Occasionally the discharge will become pink or blood tinged (false menstruation). This normal discharge should not last more than 2 or 3 days.

Male Genitals

Hydrocele. The newborn scrotum can be filled with clear fluid. The fluid is squeezed into the scrotum during the birth process. This painless collection of clear fluid is called a *hydrocele*. It is common in newborn males. A hydrocele may take 6 to 12 months to clear completely. It is harmless but can be rechecked during regular visits. If the swelling frequently changes size, a hernia may also be present and you should call our office during office hours for an appointment.

Undescended Testicle. The testicle is not in the scrotum in about 4% of full-term newborn boys. Many of these testicles gradually descend into the normal position during the following months. In 1-year-old boys only 0.7% of all testicles are undescended; these need to be brought down surgically.

Tight Foreskin. Most uncircumcised infant boys have a tight foreskin that doesn't allow you to see the head of the penis. This is normal and the foreskin should not be retracted.

Erections. Erections occur commonly in a newborn boy, as they do at all ages. They are usually triggered by a full bladder. Erections demonstrate that the nerves to the penis are normal.

Bones and Joints

Tight Hips. Your child's physician will test how far your child's legs can be spread apart to be certain the hips are not too tight. Outward bending of the upper legs until they are horizontal is called *90 degrees of spread*. (Less than 50% of normal newborn hips permit this much spreading.) As long as the upper legs can be bent outward to 60 degrees and are the same on each side, they are fine. The most common cause of a tight hip is a dislocation.

Tibial Torsion. The lower legs (tibia) normally curve in because of the cross-legged posture your baby was confined to while in the womb. If you stand your baby up, you will also notice that the legs are bowed.

Both of these curves are normal and will straighten out after your child has been walking for 6 to 12 months.

Feet Turned Up, In, or Out. Feet may be turned in any direction inside the cramped quarters of the womb. As long as your child's feet are flexible and can be easily moved to a normal position, they are normal. The direction of the feet will become more normal between 6 and 12 months of age.

"Ingrown" Toenails. Many newborns have soft nails that easily bend and curve. However, they are not truly ingrown because they don't curve into the flesh.

Hair

Scalp Hair. Most hair at birth is dark. This hair is temporary and begins to be shed by 1 month of age. Some babies lose it gradually while the permanent hair is coming in; others lose it rapidly and temporarily become bald. The permanent hair will appear by 6 months. It may be an entirely different color from the newborn hair.

Body Hair (Lanugo). Lanugo is the fine downy hair sometimes present on the back and shoulders. It is more common in premature infants. It is rubbed off with normal friction by 2 to 4 weeks of age.

NEWBORN REFLEXES AND BEHAVIOR

Some findings in newborns that concern parents are not signs of illness. Most of these harmless reflexes are due to an immature nervous system and disappear in 3 or 4 months:

- Chin trembling
- Lower lip quivering
- Hiccups
- Irregular breathing. Any irregular breathing pattern is normal if your baby is content, the rate is less than 60 breaths per minute, a pause is less than 10 seconds, and your baby doesn't turn blue; occasionally infants take rapid, progressively deeper, stepwise breaths to completely expand the lungs.
- Passing gas (not a temporary behavior)
- Sleep noise from breathing and moving
- Sneezing
- Spitting up or belching
- Startle reflex or brief stiffening of the body (also called the *Moro* or *embrace reflex*) after noise or abrupt movement
- Straining with bowel movements
- Throat clearing (or gurgling sounds of secretions in the throat)
- Trembling or jitteriness of arms and legs: common during crying. Convulsions are rare (during convulsions babies also jerk, blink their eyes, rhythmically suck with their mouths, and don't cry). If your baby is trembling and not crying, give her something to suck on. If the trembling doesn't stop during sucking, call our office immediately, because your infant may be having a convulsion.
- Yawning

Instructions for Pediatric Patients, **2nd Edition,** ©1999 by WB Saunders Company.
Written by Barton D. Schmitt, MD, pediatrician and author of *Your Child's Health,* Bantam Books, a book for parents.

After the first bath, your newborn will normally have a ruddy complexion from the extra high count of red blood cells. He can quickly change to a pale- or mottled-blue color if he becomes cold, so keep him warm. During the second week of life, the skin normally becomes dry and flaky. This guideline covers seven rashes and birthmarks. Save time by going directly to the one that pertains to your baby.

ACNE OF NEWBORN

More than 30% of newborns develop acne of the face, mainly small red bumps. This neonatal acne begins at 3 to 4 weeks of age and lasts until 4 to 6 months of age. The cause appears to be the transfer of maternal androgens (hormones) just before birth. Since it is temporary, no treatment is necessary. Baby oil or ointments will just make it worse.

DROOLING RASH

Most babies have a rash on the chin or cheeks that comes and goes. This is often due to contact with food and acid that has been spat up from the stomach. Rinse the baby's face with water after all feedings or spittings up.

Other temporary rashes on the face are heat rashes in areas held against the mother's skin during nursing (especially in the summertime). Change your baby's position more frequently and put a cool washcloth on the area. No baby has perfect skin. The babies in advertisements wear makeup.

ERYTHEMA TOXICUM

More than 50% of babies get a rash called erythema toxicum on the second or third day of life. The rash is composed of ½- to 1-inch red blotches with a small white lump in the center. They look like insect bites. They can be numerous, keep occurring, and be anywhere on the body surface. Their cause is unknown; they are harmless and resolve themselves by 2 weeks of age (rarely 4 weeks).

FORCEPS OR BIRTH CANAL TRAUMA

If delivery was difficult, a forceps may have been used to help the baby through the birth canal. The pressure of the forceps on the skin can leave bruises or scrapes or can even damage fat tissue anywhere on the head or face. Skin overlying bony prominences (such as the sides of the skull bone) can become damaged even without a forceps delivery by pressure from the birth canal. Fetal monitors can also cause scrapes and scabs on the scalp. The bruises and scrapes will be noted on day 1 or 2 and disappear by 1 to 2 weeks. The fat tissue injury won't be apparent until day 5 to 10. A thickened lump of skin with an overlying scab is the usual finding. This may take 3 or 4 weeks to resolve. For any breaks in the skin, apply an antibiotic ointment (over-the-counter) four times a day until healed. If it becomes tender to the touch or soft in the center or shows other signs of infection, call our office.

MILIA

Milia are tiny white bumps that occur on the faces of 40% of newborn babies. The nose and cheeks are most often involved, but milia are also seen on the forehead and chin. Although they look like pimples, they are smaller and not infected. They are blocked-off skin pores and will open up and disappear by 1 to 2 months of age. No ointments or creams should be applied to them.

Any true blisters (little bumps containing clear fluid) or pimples (especially of the scalp) that occur during the first month of life must be examined and diagnosed quickly. If they are caused by the herpes virus, treatment is urgent. If you suspect blisters or pimples, call our office immediately.

MONGOLIAN SPOTS

A mongolian spot is a bluish-gray flat birthmark found in more than 90% of Native American, Asian, Hispanic, and black babies. Mongolian spots occur most commonly over the back and buttocks, although they can be present on any part of the body. They vary greatly in size and shape. Most fade away by 2 or 3 years of age, although a trace may persist into adult life.

STORK BITES (PINK BIRTHMARKS)

Flat pink birthmarks (also called *capillary hemangiomas*) occur over the bridge of the nose, the eyelids, or the back of the neck in more than 50% of newborns. The birthmarks on the bridge of the nose and eyelids clear completely by 1 to 2 years of age. Most birthmarks on the nape of the neck also clear, but 25% can persist into adult life. Those on the forehead that run from the bridge of the nose up to the hairline usually persist into adult life. Laser treatment during infancy should be considered.

BATHING

Bathe your baby daily in hot weather and once or twice each week in cool weather. Keep the water level below the navel or give sponge baths until a few days after the cord has fallen off. Submerging the cord could cause infection or interfere with its drying out and falling off. Getting it a little wet doesn't matter. Use tap water without any soap or a nondrying soap such as Dove. Don't forget to wash the face; otherwise, chemicals from milk or various foods build up and cause an irritated rash. Also, rinse off the eyelids with water.

Don't forget to wash the genital area. However, when you wash the inside of the female genital area (the vulva), never use soap. Rinse the area with plain water and wipe from front to back to prevent irritation. This practice and the avoidance of any bubble baths before puberty may prevent many urinary tract infections and vaginal irritations. At the end of the bath, rinse your baby well; soap residue can be irritating.

CHANGING DIAPERS

After wet diapers are removed, just rinse your baby's bottom off with a wet washcloth. After removing soiled diapers, rinse the bottom under running warm water or in a basin of warm water. After you finish the rear area, cleanse the genital area by wiping front to back with a wet cloth. In boys, carefully clean the scrotum; in girls, the creases of the vaginal lips (labia).

SHAMPOO

Wash your baby's hair once or twice weekly with a special baby shampoo that doesn't sting the eyes.

Don't be concerned about hurting the anterior fontanel (soft spot). It is well protected.

LOTIONS, CREAMS, AND OINTMENTS

Newborn skin normally does not require any ointments or creams. Especially avoid the application of any oil, ointment, or greasy substance, since this will almost always block the small sweat glands and lead to pimples or a heat rash. If the skin starts to become dry and cracked, use a baby lotion, hand lotion, or moisturizing cream twice daily. Cornstarch powder can be helpful for preventing rashes in areas of friction. Avoid talcum powder because it can cause a serious chemical pneumonia if inhaled into the lungs.

UMBILICAL CORD

Try to keep the cord dry. Apply rubbing alcohol to the base of the cord (where it attaches to the skin) twice each day (including after the bath) until 1 week after it falls off. Air exposure also helps with drying and separation, so keep the diaper folded down below the cord area or use a scissors to cut away a wedge of the diaper in front.

FINGERNAILS AND TOENAILS

Cut the toenails straight across to prevent ingrown toenails, but round off the corners of the fingernails to prevent unintentional scratches to your baby and others. Trim them weekly after a bath when the nails are softened. Use clippers or special baby scissors. This job usually takes two people unless you do it while your child is asleep.

Instructions for Pediatric Patients, 2nd Edition, ©1999 by WB Saunders Company.
Written by Barton D. Schmitt, MD, pediatrician and author of *Your Child's Health*, Bantam Books, a book for parents.

DEFINITION

Circumcision means cutting off the foreskin or ring of tissue that covers the head (glans) of the penis. This surgical procedure is usually performed on the day of discharge from the hospital.

Fewer children in the United States are being circumcised now than several years ago. Approximately 60% of American newborn males are circumcised now, in contrast to 90% in the 1950s and 60s.

The following information should help you decide what is best for your son.

CULTURAL ASPECTS

Followers of the Jewish and Moslem faiths perform circumcision for religious reasons. Nonreligious circumcision became popular in English-speaking countries between 1920 and 1950 because it was thought that circumcision might help prevent sexually transmitted diseases. Circumcision never became a common practice in Asia, South America, Central America, or most of Europe. Over 80% of the world's male population is not circumcised. Circumcision rates have fallen to 1% of newborn males in Britain, 10% in New Zealand, and 30% in Canada.

PURPOSE OF THE FORESKIN

The presence of the foreskin is not some cosmic error. The foreskin protects the glans against urine, feces, and other types of irritation. Although rare events, infection of the urinary opening (meatitis) and scarring of the opening (meatal stenosis) occur almost exclusively in a circumcised penis. The foreskin may also serve a sexual function, namely, protecting the sensitivity of the glans.

BENEFITS OF CIRCUMCISION

In 1989 the American Academy of Pediatrics issued a new statement on circumcision, clarifying that the procedure carried small potential risks and benefits that parents needed to consider. According to a study by Dr. T. E. Wiswell, circumcision may protect against urinary tract infections during the first year of life. However, there is only a 1% chance that an uncircumcised infant will get a urinary tract infection. Should we circumcise all infants to prevent such a small percentage of urinary tract infections (which are treatable)? Probably not.

Removal of the foreskin prevents infections under the foreskin (posthitis) and persistent tight foreskin (phimosis). However, both of these conditions are uncommon and usually due to excessive and forceful attempts to retract the normal foreskin.

Circumcision does not prevent sexually transmitted diseases later in life, but it does decrease the risk for some of them. Although it does protect against cancer of the penis, good hygiene offers equal protection against this rare condition.

The best argument for circumcision may be so the boy will look "like other boys in his school" or "like his father." The psychological harm of being different from the father has never been documented. Boys may not mind looking different from other males in their family. However, they do mind being harassed in the locker room or shower about their foreskin, which may occur if most of their buddies are circumcised. It can be emotionally painful to be a trailblazer about the appearance of one's genitals.

In the final analysis, nonreligious circumcision is mainly cosmetic surgery.

RISKS OF CIRCUMCISION

Like any surgical procedure, circumcision may cause complications (in less than 1 per 100 circumcisions). Complications that might occur are skin infections, bloodstream infections, bleeding, gangrene, scarring, and various surgical accidents. One study showed that 1 of every 500 circumcised newborns suffered a serious side effect.

In addition, the procedure itself causes some pain. However, this pain can be minimized if physicians use a local anesthetic to block the nerves of the foreskin.

Delaying the decision also carries a risk. If you initially decide not to have a circumcision, and then change your mind after your son is 2 months old, the procedure will require general anesthesia. So try to make your final decision during the first month of the baby's life.

RECOMMENDATIONS

Circumcision of boys for religious purposes will continue. The need to circumcise other boys is open to question. Just because a father was circumcised doesn't mean that this optional procedure must be performed on the son. Because the foreskin comes as standard equipment, you might consider leaving it intact, unless your son will be attending a school where everyone else is likely to be circumcised. The risks and benefits are too small to swing the vote either way. This is a parental decision, not a medical decision.

Instructions for Pediatric Patients, 2nd Edition, ©1999 by WB Saunders Company.

Written by Barton D. Schmitt, MD, pediatrician and author of *Your Child's Health*, Bantam Books, a book for parents.

9

FORESKIN CARE

DEFINITION

At birth the foreskin is normally attached to the head of the penis (glans) by a layer of cells. Over the next 5 to 10 years the foreskin will naturally separate from the head of the penis without any help from us. It gradually loosens up (retracts) a little at a time. Normal erections during childhood probably cause most of the change by stretching the foreskin.

The foreskin generally causes no problems. However, overzealous retraction before the foreskin has fully loosened can cause it to get stuck behind the head of the penis, resulting in severe pain and swelling. If retraction causes bleeding, scar tissue may form and interfere with natural retraction. Occasionally, the space under the foreskin becomes infected. Most of these problems can be prevented.

NORMAL FORESKIN RETRACTION

Some physicians feel that parents should not engage in any attempts at retraction, but this runs the risk of smegma collection and infection. In general, the foreskin requires minimal care. The following suggestions will help maintain good hygiene.

During the first year of life, clean only the outside of the foreskin. Don't engage in any attempts at retraction. Don't put any cotton swabs in the opening.

Begin gentle partial retraction at 1 or 2 years of age. It can be done once each week during bathing. Perform retraction by gently pulling the skin on the shaft of the penis downward toward the abdomen. This will make the foreskin open up, revealing the end of the glans.

During retraction, the exposed part of the glans should be cleansed with water. Wipe away any whitish material (smegma) that you find there. Smegma is simply the accumulation of dead skin cells that are normally shed from the glans and lining of the foreskin throughout life. Do not use soap or leave soapy water under the foreskin because this can cause irritation

and swelling. After cleansing, always pull the foreskin forward to its normal position. *(Note:* A collection of smegma that is seen or felt through the foreskin but that lies beyond the point to which the foreskin is retractable should be left alone until normal separation exposes it.)

Avoid vigorous retraction because this can cause the foreskin to become stuck behind the head of the penis (called *paraphimosis*). Retraction is excessive if it causes any discomfort or crying.

By the time your son is 5 or 6 years old, teach him to retract his own foreskin and clean beneath it once each week during baths to prevent poor hygiene and infection. Gentle reminders are necessary in the early years.

In summary, foreskin retraction is overdone in our society. Keep in mind that any degree of foreskin movement is normal as long as your boy has a normal urine stream. There should be no rush to achieve full retraction. Full retraction always occurs naturally by puberty. As the foreskin becomes retractable on its own, your son should cleanse beneath it to prevent infections.

 CALL OUR OFFICE

IMMEDIATELY if
- The foreskin is pulled back and stuck behind the head of the penis.
- Your child can't pass any urine.
- It looks infected (yellow pus, spreading redness, red streaks).
- Your child starts acting very sick.

During regular hours if
- The urine stream is weak or dribbly.
- You have other concerns or questions.

Instructions for Pediatric Patients, 2nd Edition, ©1999 by WB Saunders Company.
Written by Barton D. Schmitt, MD, pediatrician and author of *Your Child's Health,* Bantam Books, a book for parents.

PREVENTING FATIGUE AND EXHAUSTION

For most mothers the first weeks at home with a new baby are often the hardest in their lives. You will probably feel overworked, even overwhelmed. Inadequate sleep will leave you fatigued. Caring for a baby can be a lonely and stressful responsibility. You may wonder if you will ever catch up on your rest or work. The solution lies in asking for help. No one should be expected to care for a young baby alone.

Every baby awakens one or more times each night. The way to avoid sleep deprivation is to know the total amount of sleep you need per day and to get that sleep in bits and pieces. Go to bed earlier in the evening. When your baby naps you must also nap. Your baby doesn't need you hovering while he sleeps. If sick, your baby will show symptoms. While you are napping take the telephone off the hook and put up a sign on the door saying "Mother and baby sleeping." If your total sleep remains inadequate, hire a babysitter or bring in a relative. If you don't take care of yourself, you won't be able to take care of your baby.

THE POSTPARTUM BLUES

More than 50% of women experience postpartum blues on the third or fourth day after delivery. The symptoms include tearfulness, tiredness, sadness, and difficulty in thinking clearly. The main cause of this temporary reaction is probably the sudden decrease of maternal hormones. Since the symptoms commonly begin on the day the mother comes home from the hospital, the full impact of being totally responsible for a dependent newborn may also be a contributing factor. Many mothers feel let down and guilty about these symptoms because they have been led to believe they should be overjoyed about caring for their newborn. In any event, these symptoms usually clear in 1 to 3 weeks as hormone levels return to normal and the mother develops routines and a sense of control over her life.

There are several ways to cope with the postpartum blues. First, acknowledge your feelings. Discuss them with your husband or a close friend. Also discuss your sense of being trapped and your feeling that these new responsibilities are insurmountable. Don't feel you need to suppress crying or put on a "supermom show" for everyone. Second, get adequate rest. Third, get help with all your work. Fourth, mix with other people, don't become isolated. Get out of the house at least once every week—go to the hairdresser, go shopping, visit a friend, or see a movie. By the third week, setting aside an evening each week for a "date" with your husband is also helpful. If you don't feel better by the time your baby is 1 month old, see your physician about the possibility of needing counseling for depression.

HELPERS: RELATIVES, FRIENDS, SITTERS

As already emphasized, everyone needs extra help during the first few weeks alone with a new baby. Ideally, you were able to make arrangements for help before your baby was born. The best person to help (if you get along with her) is usually your mother or mother-in-law. If not, teenagers or adults can come in several times per week to help with housework or look after your baby while you go out or get a nap. If you have other young children, you will need daily help. Clarify that your role is looking after your baby. Your helper's role is to shop, cook, houseclean, and wash clothes and dishes. If your newborn has a medical problem that requires special care, ask for home visits by a community health nurse.

THE FATHER'S ROLE

The father needs to take time off from work to be with his wife during labor and delivery, as well as on the day she and his child come home from the hospital. If the couple has a relative who will temporarily live in and help, the father can continue to work after the baby comes home. However, when the relative leaves, the father can take saved-up vacation time as paternity leave. At a minimum he needs to work shorter hours until his wife and baby have settled in.

The age of noninvolvement of the father is over. Not only does the mother need the father to help her with household chores, but also the baby needs to develop a close relationship with the father. Today's father helps with feeding, changing diapers, bathing, putting to bed, reading stories, dressing, disciplining, homework, playing games, and calling the physician when the child is sick.

A father may avoid interacting with his baby during the first year of life because he is afraid he will hurt his baby or that he won't be able to calm the child when the baby cries. The longer a father goes without learning parenting skills, the harder it becomes to master them. At a minimum, a father should hold and comfort his baby at least once each day.

VISITORS

Only close friends and relatives should visit you during your first month at home. They should not visit if they are sick. To prevent unannounced visitors, the parents can put up a sign saying "Mother and baby sleeping. No visitors. Please call first." Friends without children may not understand your needs. During visits the visitor should pay special attention to older siblings.

FEEDING YOUR BABY: ACHIEVING WEIGHT GAIN

Your main assignments during the early months of life are loving and feeding your baby. All babies lose a few ounces during the first few days after birth. However, they should never lose more than 7% of their birth weight (usually about 8 ounces). Most bottle-fed babies are back to birth weight by 10 days of age and breast-fed babies by 14 days of age. Infants then gain approximately 1 ounce per day during the early months. If milk is provided liberally, the normal newborn's hunger drive ensures appropriate weight gain.

A breast-feeding mother often wonders if her baby is getting enough calories, since she can't see how many ounces the baby takes. Your baby is doing fine if she demands to nurse every 1½ to 2½ hours, appears satisfied after feedings, takes both breasts at each nursing, wets six or more diapers each day, and passes three or more soft stools per day. Whenever you are worried about your baby's weight gain, bring her to our office for a weight check. Feeding problems detected early are much easier to remedy than those of long standing. A special weight check 1 week after birth is a good idea for infants of a first-time breast-feeding mother or a mother concerned about her milk supply.

DEALING WITH CRYING

Crying babies need to be held. They need someone with a soothing voice and a soothing touch. You can't spoil your baby during the early months of life. Over-sensitive babies may need an even gentler touch. For additional help, request "The Crying Baby" handout.

TAKING YOUR BABY OUTDOORS

You can take your baby outdoors at any age. You already took your baby outside when you left the hospital, and you will be going outside again when you go for the baby's 2-week checkup.

Dress the baby with as many layers of clothing as an adult would wear for the outdoor temperature. A common mistake is overdressing a baby in summer.

In winter a baby needs a hat because there is often not much hair to protect against heat loss. Cold air or winds do not cause ear infections or pneumonia.

The skin of babies is more sensitive to the sun than the skin of older children. Keep sun exposure to small amounts (10 to 15 minutes at a time). Protect your baby's skin from sunburn with longer clothing and a bonnet.

Camping and crowds should probably be avoided during your baby's first month of life. Also, during your baby's first year of life try to avoid close contact with people who have infectious illnesses.

THE THIRD- OR FOURTH-DAY-OF-LIFE MEDICAL CHECKUP

Early discharge from the newborn nursery has become commonplace for full-term babies. Early discharge means going home after 24 to 48 hours of life. In general, this is a safe practice if the baby's hospital stay has been uncomplicated. These newborns need to be rechecked 2 days after discharge for feeding status, urine and stool production, jaundice, breathing status, and general health. In some cases, this special recheck will be provided in your home.

THE 2-WEEK MEDICAL CHECKUP

This checkup is probably the most important medical visit for your baby during the first year of life. By 2 weeks of age your baby will usually have developed symptoms of any physical condition that was not detectable during the hospital stay. Your child's physician will be able to judge how well your baby is growing from height, weight, and head circumference.

This is also the time your family is under the most stress of adapting to a new baby. Try to develop a habit of jotting down questions about your child's health or behavior at home. Bring this list with you to office visits to discuss with your child's physician. We welcome the opportunity to address your agenda, especially if your questions are not easily answered by reading or talking with other mothers.

If at all possible, have your husband join you on these visits. We prefer to get to know the father during a checkup rather than during the crisis of an acute illness.

If you think your newborn is sick between these routine visits, be sure to call our office for help.

Instructions for Pediatric Patients, **2nd Edition,** ©1999 by **WB Saunders Company.**
Written by Barton D. Schmitt, MD, pediatrician and author of *Your Child's Health,* Bantam Books, a book for parents.

DEFINITION

- Yellow scales and crusts attached to the scalp.
- Scales can be greasy or dry.
- Not itchy or painful.
- Begins in the first 2 to 6 weeks of life. Is usually gone by 6 months of age.

Cause

The cause of cradle cap is unknown. It may be caused by maternal hormones that crossed the placenta before birth and stimulated the oil glands. It is not caused by poor hygiene. Cradle cap is not contagious and does not recur. If redness also occurs behind the ears, in body creases (armpit, groin and neck), and in the diaper area, cradle cap is part of a condition called *seborrheic dermatitis*.

Expected Course

Without treatment it can last for months, but it will eventually clear up on its own. With treatment it is usually cleared up in a few weeks.

HOME CARE

1. **Antidandruff shampoo**. Antidandruff shampoos slow down the scaling and flaking of skin. They do not require a prescription.

Your child's antidandruff shampoo is _____.

Be careful to keep it out of the eyes. Wash your baby's hair with it twice a week. While the hair is lathered, massage your baby's scalp with a soft brush or rough washcloth. Don't worry about hurting the soft spot; it's well protected. Once the cradle cap has cleared up, use a regular shampoo twice a week.

2. **Softening thick crusts or scales**. If your child's scalp is very crusty, put some baby oil or olive oil on the scalp 1 hour before washing to soften the crust. Wash all the oil off, however, or it may worsen the cradle cap.

3. **Resistant cradle cap**. If the rash is red and irritated, apply 1% hydrocortisone cream (nonprescription) three times a day for 7 days.

 CALL OUR OFFICE

During regular hours if
- The cradle cap lasts more than 2 weeks with treatment.
- It starts to look infected.
- The rash spreads beyond the scalp.
- You have other concerns or questions.

DEFINITION

Any rash in the skin area covered by a diaper

Causes

Almost every child gets diaper rashes. Most are due to prolonged contact with moisture, bacteria, and ammonia. The skin irritants are made by the action of bacteria from bowel movements on certain chemicals in the urine. Bouts of diarrhea cause rashes in most children. Diaper rashes occur equally with cloth and disposable diapers.

Expected Course

With proper treatment these rashes are usually better in 3 days. If they do not respond, a yeast infection (*Candida*) has probably occurred. Suspect this if the rash becomes bright red and raw, covers a large area, and is surrounded by red dots. You will need a special cream for a yeast infection.

HOME CARE

Change Diapers Frequently. The key to successful treatment is keeping the area dry and clean so that it can heal itself. Check the diapers about every hour, and if they are wet or soiled, change them immediately. Exposure to stools causes most of the skin damage. Make sure that your baby's bottom is completely dry before closing up the fresh diaper.

Increase Air Exposure. Leave your baby's bottom exposed to the air as much as possible each day. Practical times are during naps or after bowel movements. Put a towel or diaper under your baby. When the diaper is on, fasten it loosely so that air can circulate between it and the skin. Avoid airtight plastic pants for a few days. If you use disposable diapers, punch holes in them to let air in.

Rinse the Skin with Warm Water. Washing the skin with soap after every diaper change will damage the skin. Use a mild soap (such as Dove) only after bowel movements. The soap will remove the film of bacteria left on the skin. After using a soap, rinse well. If the diaper rash is quite raw, use warm water soaks for 15 minutes three times every day.

Nighttime Care. At night use the new disposable diapers that are made with materials that lock wetness inside the diaper and away from the skin. Avoid plastic pants at night. Until the rash is better, awaken once during the night to change your baby's diaper.

Creams and Ointments. Most babies don't need any diaper creams or powders. If your baby's skin is dry and cracked, however, apply an ointment to protect the skin after washing off each bowel movement. A barrier ointment is also needed whenever your child has diarrhea.

Your baby's ointment is _____.

Cornstarch reduces friction and can be used to prevent future diaper rashes after this one is healed. Studies show that cornstarch does not encourage yeast infections. Avoid talcum powder because of the risk of pneumonia if your baby inhales it.

Yeast Infections. If the rash is bright red or does not respond to 3 days of warm water cleansing and air exposure, suspect a yeast infection. Apply Lotrimin cream (no prescription necessary) 4 times per day or after each bottom rinse for bowel movements.

Prevention of Diaper Rash. Changing the diaper immediately after your child has a bowel movement and rinsing the skin with warm water are the most effective things you can do to prevent diaper rash.

If you use cloth diapers and wash them yourself, you will need to use bleach (such as Clorox, Borax, or Purex) to sterilize them. During the regular cycle, use any detergent. Then refill the washer with warm water, add 1 cup of bleach, and run a second cycle. Unlike bleach, vinegar is not effective in killing germs.

 ## CALL OUR OFFICE

IMMEDIATELY if
- It looks infected (yellow pus, pimples, blisters, spreading redness, red streaks).
- Your child starts acting very sick.

During regular hours if
- The rash isn't much better in 3 days.
- You have other concerns or questions.

Instructions for Pediatric Patients, 2nd Edition, ©1999 by WB Saunders Company.
Written by Barton D. Schmitt, MD, pediatrician and author of *Your Child's Health*, Bantam Books, a book for parents.

DEFINITION

In jaundice the skin and the whites of the eyes (the sclera) are yellow because of increased amounts of a yellow pigment in the body called *bilirubin*. Bilirubin is produced by the normal breakdown of red blood cells. It accumulates if the liver doesn't excrete it into the intestines at a normal rate.

TYPES OF JAUNDICE

Physiological (Normal) Jaundice

Physiological jaundice occurs in more than 50% of babies. An immaturity of the liver leads to a slower processing of bilirubin. The jaundice first appears at 2 to 3 days of age. It usually disappears by 1 to 2 weeks of age, and the levels reached are harmless.

Breast-feeding Jaundice

Breast-feeding jaundice occurs in 5% to 10% of newborns. It's caused by an insufficient intake of breast milk (calories and fluid). It follows the same pattern as physiological jaundice.

Breast-Milk Jaundice

Breast-milk jaundice occurs in 1% to 2% of breast-fed babies. It is caused by a special substance (inhibitor) that some mothers produce in their milk. This substance (an enzyme) increases the resorption of bilirubin from the intestine. This type of jaundice starts at 4 to 7 days of age and may last 3 to 10 weeks.

Blood Group Incompatibility (Rh or ABO Problems)

If a baby and mother have different blood types, sometimes the mother produces antibodies that destroy the newborn's red blood cells. This causes a sudden buildup in bilirubin in the baby's blood. This type of jaundice usually begins during the first 24 hours of life. Rh problems are now preventable with an injection of RhoGAM to the mother within 72 hours after delivery. This prevents her from forming antibodies that might endanger subsequent babies.

TREATMENT OF SEVERE JAUNDICE

High levels of bilirubin (usually above 20 mg/dl) can cause deafness, cerebral palsy, or brain damage in some babies. High levels usually occur with blood-type problems. These complications can be prevented by lowering the bilirubin by means of phototherapy (blue light that breaks down bilirubin in the skin). In many communities, phototherapy can be used in the home. In rare cases in which the bilirubin reaches dangerous levels, an exchange transfusion may be used.

TREATMENT OF BREAST-FEEDING JAUNDICE

Try to increase breast milk production. Read about breast-feeding or talk with a lactation specialist. Increase the frequency of feedings. Nurse your baby every 1½ to 2½ hours during the day. Don't let your baby sleep more than 4 hours at night without a feeding. If you must supplement, supplement with formula, not glucose water.

TREATMENT OF BREAST-MILK JAUNDICE

The bilirubin level can rise above 20 mg/dL in less than 1% of infants with breast-milk jaundice. Almost always, elevations to this level can be prevented by more frequent feedings. Nurse your baby every 1½ to 2½ hours. Since bilirubin is carried out of the body in the stools, passing frequent bowel movements is helpful. If your baby sleeps more than 4 hours at night, awaken him for a feeding.

Occasionally the bilirubin will not come down with frequent feedings. In this situation the bilirubin level can be reduced by alternating each breast-feeding with formula feeding for 2 or 3 days. Supplementing with glucose water is not as helpful as formula for moving the bilirubin out of the body. Whenever you miss a nursing, be sure to use a breast pump to keep your milk production flowing. Breast-feeding should never be permanently discontinued because of breast-milk jaundice. Once the jaundice clears, you can return to full breast-feeding and you need not worry about the jaundice coming back.

CALLING OUR OFFICE

Newborns often leave the hospital within 24 to 48 hours of birth. Parents therefore have the responsibility to closely observe the degree of jaundice in their newborn. The amount of yellowness is best judged by viewing your baby unclothed in natural light.

 CALL OUR OFFICE

IMMEDIATELY if
- Your baby doesn't pass urine in more than 8 hours.
- Your baby develops a fever over 100.4°F (38°C) measured rectally.
- Your baby starts to look or act sick.

During regular hours if
- Your baby looks deep yellow or orange.
- Your baby has less than 3 BMs per day.
- Jaundice is not gone by day 14.
- You have other questions or concerns.

DEFINITION

Reflux or regurgitation is the spitting up of one or two mouthfuls of stomach contents. It is usually seen during or shortly after feedings. In contrast to vomiting, the milk comes up without any effort or discomfort. Reflux usually begins in the first weeks of life. More than half of all infants have it to some degree.

Cause

Poor closure of the valve (or ring of muscle) at the upper end of the stomach is responsible. This condition is also called *gastroesophageal reflux* (GER) or *chalasia*. Reflux is harmless as long as your infant doesn't spit up large amounts that interfere with normal weight gain.

Expected Course

Spitting up improves with age. By 7 months of age, most reflux has decreased or resolved. The reasons for this are probably the ability to sit up and the introduction of solid foods. By the time your baby has been walking for 3 months, even severe reflux should be totally cleared up.

HOME CARE

Feed Smaller Amounts. Overfeeding always makes spitting up worse. If the stomach is filled to capacity, spitting up is more likely. Give your baby smaller amounts (at least 1 ounce less than you have been giving). Your baby doesn't have to finish a bottle. Wait at least 2½ hours between feedings because it takes that long for the stomach to empty itself.

Avoid Pressure on the Abdomen. Avoid tight diapers. They put added pressure on the stomach. Don't double your child up during diaper changes. Don't let people hug your child or play vigorously right after meals.

Burp Your Child to Reduce Spitting Up. Burp your baby two or three times during each feeding. Do it when she pauses and looks around. Don't interrupt her feeding rhythm in order to burp her. Keep in mind that burping is less important than giving smaller feedings and avoiding tight diapers.

Keep in a Vertical Position After Meals. After meals, try to hold your baby in an upright position using a front pack, backpack, or swing for 30 minutes. When your infant is in an infant seat, keep him from getting scrunched up by putting a pad under his buttocks so that he's more stretched out. After your child is 6 months old, a jumpy seat or walker can be helpful for maintaining an upright posture. To make the walker safe, buy one without wheels or remove the wheels. The best sleeping position for severe reflux is on the baby's side with the right side down. If the esophagus becomes irritated (esophagitis), talk to your doctor about sleeping prone (face down).

Cleaning Up. One of the worst aspects of spitting up in the past was the odor. This was caused by the effect of stomach acid on the butterfat in cow's milk. The odor is not present with commercial formulas because they contain vegetable oils. A more common concern is clothing stains from milk spots. Use the powdered formulas, which stain the least. Also, don't pick up your child when you have your best clothes on. Try to confine your baby to areas without rugs (for example, the kitchen).

 CALL OUR OFFICE

IMMEDIATELY if
- There is blood in the spit-up material.
- The spitting up causes your child to choke or cough.

During regular hours if
- Your baby doesn't seem to improve with this approach. (We can discuss how to thicken feedings with cereal.)
- Your baby is not gaining weight normally.
- You have other concerns or questions.

Instructions for Pediatric Patients, 2nd Edition, ©1999 by WB Saunders Company.
Written by Barton D. Schmitt, MD, pediatrician and author of *Your Child's Health*, Bantam Books, a book for parents.

DEFINITION

- Continuously watery eye
- Tears running down the face even without crying
- During crying, nostril on blocked side remains dry
- Onset before 1 month of age
- Eye not red and eyelid not swollen (unless the soggy tissues become infected)
- This diagnosis must be confirmed by a physician.

Cause

Your child probably has a blocked tear duct on that side. This means that the channel that normally carries tears from the eye to the nose is blocked. Although the obstruction is present at birth, the delay in onset of symptoms can be explained by the occasional delay in tear production until the age of 3 or 4 weeks in some babies.

Expected Course

This is a common condition, affecting 6% of newborns. Both sides are blocked 30% of the time. Over 90% of blocked tear ducts open up spontaneously by the time the child is 12 months of age. If the obstruction persists beyond 12 months of age, an ophthalmologist (eye specialist) can open it with a special probe.

HOME CARE FOR PREVENTING EYE INFECTION

Because of poor drainage, eyes with blocked tear ducts become easily infected. The infected eye produces a yellow discharge. To keep the eye free of infection, massage the lacrimal sac (where tears collect) twice daily to empty it of old fluids. A small amount of clear fluid should come out. Always wash your hands carefully before doing this. The lacrimal sac is located in the inner lower corner of the eye. Start at the inner corner of the eye and press *upward* using a cotton swab. The massage technique is somewhat controversial. Some physicians recommend massaging downward in hopes of washing out the plug that blocks the lower duct. If the eye becomes infected, it is very important to begin antibiotic eye drops. Some physicians recommend not massaging the sac at all. Massage in either direction must be done gently, since it may irritate the eyelid tissue and contribute to infection.

 ## CALL OUR OFFICE

IMMEDIATELY if
- The eyelids are red or swollen.
- A red lump appears at the inner lower corner of the eyelid.

During regular hours if
- Lots of yellow discharge is present.
- Your child reaches 12 months of age and the eye is still watering.
- You have other concerns or questions.

DEFINITION

Teething is the normal process of new teeth working their way through the gums. Your baby's first tooth may appear any time between the ages of 3 months and 1 year. Most children have completely painless teething. The only symptoms are increased saliva, drooling, and a desire to chew on things. It occasionally causes some mild gum pain, but it doesn't interfere with sleep. The degree of discomfort varies from child to child, but your child won't be miserable. When the back teeth (molars) come through (age 6 to 12 years), the overlying gum may become bruised and swollen. This is harmless and temporary.

Since teeth erupt continuously from 6 months to 2 years of age, many unrelated illnesses are blamed on teething. Fevers are also common during this time because after 6 months infants lose the natural protection provided by their mother's antibodies.

DEVELOPMENT OF BABY TEETH

Your baby's teeth will usually erupt in the following order:

1. Two lower incisors
2. Four upper incisors
3. Two lower incisors and all four first molars
4. Four canines
5. Four second molars

HOME CARE

Gum Massage. Find the irritated or swollen gum. Vigorously massage it with your finger for 2 minutes. Do this as often as necessary. If you wish, you may use a piece of ice to massage the gum.

Teething Rings. Your baby's way of massaging her gums is to chew on a smooth, hard object. Solid teething rings and ones with liquid in the center (as long as it's purified water) are fine. Most children like them cold. Offer a teething ring or wet washcloth that has been chilled in the refrigerator but not frozen in the freezer. A piece of chilled banana may help. Avoid ice or Popsicles that could cause frostbite of the gums. Avoid hard foods that your baby might choke on (such as raw carrots), but teething biscuits are fine.

Diet. Avoid salty or acid foods. Your baby probably will enjoy sucking on a nipple, but if he complains, use a cup for fluids temporarily. A few babies may need acetaminophen for pain relief for a few days.

Acetaminophen. If the pain increases, give acetaminophen orally for 1 day. Special teething gels are unnecessary. Many teething gels contain benzocaine, which can cause an allergic reaction. If you want to use a gel, do not apply it more than four times a day.

Common Mistakes in Treating Teething

- Teething does not cause fever, sleep problems, diarrhea, diaper rash, or lowered resistance to any infection. It probably doesn't cause crying. If your baby develops fever while teething, the fever is due to something else.
- Don't tie the teething ring around the neck. It could catch on something and strangle your child. Attach it to clothing with a "catch-it" clip.

 ## CALL OUR OFFICE

During regular hours if
- Your child develops a fever over 101°F (38.3°C).
- Your child develops crying that doesn't have a cause.
- You have other questions or concerns.

Instructions for Pediatric Patients, 2nd Edition, ©1999 by WB Saunders Company.
Written by Barton D. Schmitt, MD, pediatrician and author of *Your Child's Health*, Bantam Books, a book for parents.

DEFINITION

- White, irregularly shaped patches that coat the inside of the mouth and sometimes the tongue, adhere to the mouth, and cannot be washed away or wiped off easily like milk. (If the only symptom is a uniformly white tongue, it's due to a milk diet, not thrush.) Thrush causes mild discomfort.
- Bottle-fed or breast-fed child

Cause

Thrush is caused by a yeast (*Candida*) that grows rapidly on the lining of the mouth in areas abraded by prolonged sucking (as when a baby sleeps with a bottle or pacifier). A large pacifier or nipple can also injure the lining of the mouth. Thrush may also occur when your child has recently been taking a broad-spectrum antibiotic. Thrush is not contagious since it does not invade normal tissue.

HOME CARE

Nystatin Oral Medicine. The drug for clearing this up is nystatin oral suspension. It requires a prescription. Give 1 mL of nystatin four times daily. Place it in the front of the mouth on each side (it doesn't do any good once it's swallowed). If the thrush isn't responding, rub the nystatin directly on the affected areas with a cotton swab or with gauze wrapped around your finger. Apply it after meals, or at least don't feed your baby anything for 30 minutes after application. Do this for at least 7 days or until all the thrush has been gone for 3 days. If you are breast-feeding, apply nystatin to any irritated areas on your nipples.

Decrease Sucking Time to 20 Minutes per Feeding. Prolonged sucking (as when a baby sleeps with a bottle or pacifier) can abrade the lining of the mouth and make it more prone to yeast infection. If sucking on a nipple is painful for your child, temporarily use a cup. If the thrush recurs and your child is bottle-fed, switch to a nipple with a different shape and made from silicone.

Restrict Pacifier Use to Bedtime. Eliminate the pacifier temporarily except when it's really needed for going to sleep. If your infant is using an orthodontic-type pacifier, switch to a smaller, regular one. Soak all nipples in water at 130°F (55°C), the temperature of most hot tap water, for 15 minutes.

Diaper Rash Associated with Thrush. If your child has an associated diaper rash, assume it is due to yeast. Request nystatin cream and apply it four times daily.

 CALL OUR OFFICE

During regular hours if
- Your child refuses to drink.
- The thrush gets worse on treatment.
- The thrush lasts beyond 10 days.
- You have other concerns or questions.

PART 2

FEEDING AND EATING

Babies who are breast-fed have fewer infections and allergies during the first year of life than babies who are fed formula. Breast milk is also inexpensive and served at the perfect temperature. Breast-feeding becomes especially convenient when a mother is traveling with her baby. Overall, breast milk is nature's best food for young babies.

HOW OFTEN TO FEED

The baby should nurse for the first time in the delivery room. The second feeding will usually be at 4 to 6 hours of age, after he awakens from a deep sleep. Until your milk supply is well established (usually 4 weeks), nurse your infant whenever he cries or seems hungry ("demand feeding"). Thereafter, babies can receive adequate breast milk by nursing every 2 to 2½ hours. If your baby cries and less than 2 hours have passed, he can be rocked or carried in a front pack. If the baby is sleeping and more than 3 hours have passed since the last feeding during the day, wake him up. During the night, allow one 5-hour interval if the baby is sleeping. Your baby will not gain adequately unless he nurses eight or more times per day initially. The risks of continuing to nurse at short intervals (less than 1½ hours) are that "grazing" will become a habit, your baby won't be able to sleep through the night, and you won't have much free time.

HOW LONG PER FEEDING

Nurse your baby 10 minutes on the first breast and as long as he wants on the second breast. Your goal is to have your baby nurse for a total of about 30 minutes at each feeding. It's common to need to stimulate your baby before he will take the second breast. Remember to alternate which breast you start with each time. Once your milk supply is well established (about 2 to 3 weeks after birth), 10 minutes of nursing per breast is fine when you are in a hurry (since your child usually gets over 90% of the milk in this time). However, try not to nurse for periods shorter than 20 minutes because it may give inadequate calories and lead to a need for more frequent feedings.

HOW TO KNOW YOUR BABY IS GETTING ENOUGH BREAST MILK

In the first couple weeks, if your baby has three or more good-sized bowel movements per day and six or more wet diapers per day, he is receiving a good supply of breast milk. (*Caution:* Infrequent bowel movements are not normally seen before the second month of life.) In addition, most babies will act satisfied after completing a feeding. Your baby should be back to birth weight by 10 to 14 days of age if breast-feeding is going well. Therefore the 2-week checkup by your baby's physician is very important. The presence of a letdown reflex is another indicator of good milk production.

THE LETDOWN REFLEX

A letdown reflex develops after 2 to 3 weeks of nursing and is indicated by tingling or milk ejection in the breast just before feeding (or when you are thinking about feeding). It also occurs in the opposite breast while your baby is nursing. Letdown is enhanced by adequate sleep, adequate fluids, a relaxed environment, and reduced stress (such as low expectations about how much housework gets done). If your letdown reflex is not present yet, take extra naps and ask your husband and friends for more help. Also consider calling the local chapter of La Leche League, a support group for nursing mothers.

SUPPLEMENTAL BOTTLES

Do not offer your baby any routine bottles during the first 4 to 6 weeks after birth because this is when you establish your milk supply. Good lactation depends on frequent emptying of the breasts. Supplemental bottles take away from sucking time on the breast. If your baby is not gaining well, see your physician or a lactation specialist for a weight check and evaluation.

After your baby is 6 weeks old and nursing is well established, you may want to offer him a bottle of expressed milk or water once a day so that he can become accustomed to the bottle and the artificial nipple. Once your baby accepts bottle feedings, you can occasionally leave your baby with a sitter and go out for the evening or return to work outside the home. You can use pumped breast milk that has been refrigerated or frozen.

EXTRA WATER

Babies do not routinely need extra water. Even when they have a fever or the weather is hot and dry, breast milk provides enough water.

PUMPING THE BREASTS TO RELIEVE PAIN OR COLLECT MILK

Severe engorgement (severe swelling) of the breasts decreases milk production. To prevent engorgement, nurse your baby more often. Also, compress the area around the nipple (the areola) with your fingers at the start of each feeding to soften the areola. For milk release, your baby must be able to grip and suck on the areola as well as the nipple. Every time you miss a feeding (for example, if you return to work outside the home), pump your breasts. Also, whenever your breasts hurt and you are unable to feed your baby, pump your breasts until they are soft. If you don't relieve engorgement, your milk supply can dry up in 2 to 3 days.

A breast pump is usually unnecessary because pumping can be done by hand. Ask someone to teach you the Marmet technique.

Collect the breast milk in plastic containers or plastic bottles because some of the immune factors in the milk stick to glass. Pumped breast milk can be saved for 48 hours in a refrigerator or up to 3 months in a freezer. To thaw frozen breast milk, put the plastic container of breast milk in the refrigerator (it will take a few hours to thaw) or place it in a container of warm water until it has warmed up to the temperature your baby prefers.

SORE NIPPLES

Clean a sore nipple with water after each feeding. Do not use soap or alcohol because they remove natural oils. At the end of each feeding, the nipple can be coated with some breast milk to keep it lubricated. For cracked nipples, apply 100% lanolin (no prescription necessary) after feedings.

Sore nipples are usually due to poor latching on and a feeding position that causes undue friction on the nipple. Position your baby so that he directly faces the nipple without turning his neck. At the start of the feeding, compress the nipple and areola between your thumb and index finger so that your baby can latch on easily. Throughout the feeding, hold your breast from below so that the nipple and areola aren't pulled out of your baby's mouth by the weight of the breast. Slightly rotate your baby's body so that his mouth applies pressure to slightly different parts of the areola and nipple at each feeding.

Start your feedings on the side that is not sore. If one nipple is extremely sore, temporarily limit feedings to 10 minutes on that side.

VITAMINS/FLUORIDE FOR THE BABY

Breast milk contains all the necessary vitamins and minerals except vitamin D and fluoride. Full-term dark-skinned babies and all premature babies need 400 units of vitamin D each day. White babies who have little or no sun exposure (less than 15 minutes twice a week) also need vitamin D supplements. From 6 months to 6 years of age, children need fluoride to prevent tooth decay; 0.25 mg of fluoride drops should be given each day. In the United States this is a prescription item that you can obtain from your child's physician.

VITAMINS FOR THE MOTHER

A nursing mother can take a multivitamin tablet daily if she is not following a well-balanced diet. She especially needs 400 units of vitamin D and 1200 mg of both calcium and phosphorus per day. A quart of milk (or its equivalent in cheese or yogurt) can also meet this requirement.

THE MOTHER'S MEDICATIONS

Almost any drug a breast-feeding mother consumes will be transferred in small amounts into the breast milk. Therefore try to avoid any drug that is not essential, just as you did during pregnancy.

Some commonly used drugs that are safe for you to take while nursing are acetaminophen, ibuprofen, penicillins, erythromycin, cephalosporins, stool softeners, antihistamines, decongestants, mild sedatives, cough drops, nose drops, eye drops, and skin creams. Aspirin and sulfa drugs can be taken if your baby is more than 2 weeks old *and* not jaundiced. Consult your physician about all other drugs. Take drugs that are not harmful immediately after you breast-feed your child so that the level of drugs in the breast milk at the time of the next feeding is low.

BURPING

Burping is optional. Its only benefit is to decrease spitting up. Air in the stomach does not cause pain. If you burp your baby, burping two times during a feeding and for about 1 minute is plenty. Burp your baby when switching from the first breast to the second and at the end of the feeding.

CUP FEEDING

Introduce your child to a cup at approximately 6 months of age. Total weaning to a cup will probably occur somewhere between 9 and 18 months of age, depending on your baby's individual preference. If you discontinue breast-feeding before 9 months of age, switch to bottle-feeding first. If you stop breast-feeding after 9 months of age, you may be able to go directly to cup feeding.

 ## CALL OUR OFFICE

During regular hours if
- Your baby doesn't seem to be gaining adequately.
- Your baby has less than six wet diapers per day.
- During the first month, your baby has less than three bowel movements per day.
- You suspect your baby has a food allergy.
- Your breasts are not full (engorged) before feedings by day 5.
- You have painful engorgement or sore nipples that do not respond to the recommended treatment.
- You have a fever (also call your obstetrician).
- You have other questions or concerns.

Instructions for Pediatric Patients, 2nd Edition, ©1999 by WB Saunders Company.
Written by Barton D. Schmitt, MD, pediatrician and author of *Your Child's Health,* Bantam Books, a book for parents.

Breast milk is best for babies, but breast-feeding isn't always possible. Use an infant formula if

- You decide not to breast-feed.
- You need to discontinue breast-feeding and your infant is less than 1 year of age.
- You need to occasionally supplement your infant after breast-feeding is well established.

Note: If you want to breast-feed but feel your milk supply is insufficient, don't discontinue breast-feeding. Instead seek help from your physician or a lactation nurse.

COMMERCIAL FORMULAS

Infant formulas are a safe alternative to breast milk. They have been designed to resemble breast milk and fulfill the nutritional needs of your infant by providing all known essential nutrients in their proper amounts. Most formulas are derived from cow's milk. A few are derived from soybeans and are for infants who may be allergic to the type of protein in cow's milk. Bottle-feeding can provide your child with all the emotional benefits and many of the health benefits of breast-feeding. Bottle-fed babies grow as rapidly and are as happy as breast-fed babies. A special advantage of bottle-feeding is that the father can participate.

Use a commercial formula that is iron fortified to prevent iron deficiency anemia, as recommended by the American Academy of Pediatrics. The amount of iron in iron-fortified formula is too small to cause any diarrhea or constipation. Don't use the low-iron formulas.

Most commercial infant formulas are available in three forms: powder, concentrated liquid, and ready-to-serve liquid. Powder and ready-to-serve liquids are the most suitable forms when a formula is occasionally used to supplement breast milk.

PREPARING COMMERCIAL FORMULAS

The concentrated formulas are mixed 1:1 with water. Two ounces of water are mixed with each level scoop of powdered formula. Never make the formula more concentrated by adding extra powder or extra concentrated liquid. Never dilute the formula by adding more water than specified. Careful measuring and mixing ensure that your baby is receiving the proper formula.

If you use tap water for preparing formula, use only water from the cold water tap. If the water hasn't been used for several hours, let the water run for 2 minutes before you use it. (Old water pipes may contain lead-based solder, and lead dissolves more in warm water or standing water.) Fresh, cold water is safe. If you make one bottle at a time, you don't need to use boiled water. Just heat cold tap water to the preferred temperature. Most city water supplies are quite safe. If you have well water, either boil it for 10 minutes

(plus one minute for each 1000 feet of elevation) or use distilled water until your child is 6 months of age. If you prefer to prepare a batch of formula, you must use boiled or distilled water and closely follow the directions printed on the side of the formula can. This prepared formula should be stored in the refrigerator and must be used within 48 hours.

HOMEMADE FORMULAS FROM EVAPORATED MILK

If necessary, you can make your own formula temporarily from evaporated milk. Evaporated milk formulas carry some of the same risks as whole cow's milk. This formula needs supplements of vitamins and minerals. It also requires sterilized bottles because it is prepared in a batch. If you must use it in a pinch, mix 13 ounces of evaporated milk with 19 ounces of boiled water and 2 tablespoons of corn syrup. Place this mixture in sterilized bottles and keep them refrigerated until used.

WHOLE COW'S MILK

Whole cow's milk should not be given to babies before 12 months of age because of increased risks of iron deficiency anemia and allergies. The ability to drink from a cup doesn't mean you should switch to cow's milk. While it used to be acceptable to introduce whole cow's milk after 6 months of age, studies have shown that infant formula is the best food during the first year of life for babies who are not breast-fed. Skim milk or 2% milk should not be given to babies before 2 years of age because the fat content of regular milk (approximately 3.5% butterfat) is needed for rapid brain growth.

TRAVELING

When traveling, use powdered formula for convenience. Put the required number of scoops in a bottle, add cold tap water, and shake. A more expensive alternative is to use throwaway bottles of ready-to-use formula. This product avoids problems with contaminated water.

FORMULA TEMPERATURE

In summer many children prefer cold formula. In winter most prefer warm formula. By trying various temperatures, you can find out which your child prefers. If you do warm the formula, be certain to check the temperature before giving it to your baby. If it is too hot, it could burn your baby's mouth.

AMOUNTS AND SCHEDULES

Newborns usually start with 1 ounce per feeding, but by 7 days they can take 3 ounces. The amount of formula that most babies take per feeding (in ounces) can be calculated by dividing your baby's weight (in pounds) in half. Another way to calculate the ounces per feeding is to add 3 to your baby's age (in months) with a maximum of 8 ounces per feeding at 5 or 6 months of age. The average ounces of formula a baby needs in 24 hours is the baby's weight in pounds multiplied by 2. The maximal amount recommended per day is 32 ounces. Overfeeding can cause vomiting, diarrhea, or excessive weight gain. If your baby needs more than this and is not overweight, consider starting solids.

In general, your baby will need six to eight feedings per day for the first month, five to six feedings per day from 1 to 3 months, four to five feedings per day from 3 to 7 months, and three to four feedings per day thereafter. If your baby is not hungry at some of the feedings, the feeding interval should be increased.

LENGTH OF FEEDING

A feeding shouldn't take more than 20 minutes. If it does, you are overfeeding your baby or the nipple is clogged. A clean nipple should drip about 1 drop per second when the bottle of formula is inverted.

Formula Storage. Prepared formula should be stored in the refrigerator and must be used within 48 hours. Prepared formula left at room temperature for more than 1 hour should be discarded. At the end of each feeding, discard any formula left in the bottle, because it is no longer sterile.

EXTRA WATER

Babies do not routinely need extra water. They should be offered a bottle of water twice daily, however, when they have a fever or when the weather is hot and dry.

BURPING

Burping is optional. It doesn't decrease crying. Although it may decrease spitting up, air in the stomach does not cause pain. Burping two times during a feeding and for about 1 minute is plenty.

VITAMINS/IRON/FLUORIDE

Commercial formulas with iron contain all your baby's vitamin and mineral requirements except fluoride. (*Note:* All soy-based formulas are iron fortified.) In the United States the most common cause of anemia in children under 2 years old is iron deficiency (largely because iron is not present in cow's milk). Iron can also be provided at 4 months of age by adding iron-fortified cereals to the diet.

From 6 months to 16 years of age, children need fluoride to prevent dental caries. If the municipal water supply contains fluoride and your child drinks at least 1 pint each day, this should be adequate. Otherwise, fluoride drops or tablets (without vitamins) should be given separately. This is a prescription item that can be obtained from your child's physician. Added vitamins are unnecessary after your child has reached 1 year of age and is on a regular balanced diet, but continue the fluoride.

CUP FEEDING

Introduce your child to a cup at approximately 4 to 6 months of age. Total weaning to a cup will probably occur somewhere between 9 and 18 months of age, depending on your baby's individual preference.

BABY-BOTTLE TOOTH DECAY: PREVENTION

Sleeping with a bottle of milk, juice, or any sweetened liquid in the mouth can cause severe decay of the newly erupting teeth. Prevent this tragedy by not using the bottle as a pacifier or allowing your child to take it to bed.

Instructions for Pediatric Patients, 2nd Edition, ©1999 by WB Saunders Company.
Written by Barton D. Schmitt, MD, pediatrician and author of *Your Child's Health*, Bantam Books, a book for parents.

DEFINITION

Breast- or bottle-feeding can be considered prolonged after about 18 months of age, but delayed weaning is not always a problem. The older toddler who only occasionally nurses or drinks from a bottle doesn't necessarily need to be pressured into giving up the bottle or breast. Delayed weaning should be considered a problem only if it is causing one or more of the following types of harm:

- Refusal to eat any solids after 6 months of age
- Anemia confirmed by a routine screening test at 1 year of age
- Tooth decay or baby-bottle caries
- Obesity from overeating
- Daytime withdrawal and lack of interest in play because the child is always carrying a bottle around
- Frequent awakening at night for refills of a bottle
- Inability to stay with a babysitter because the child is exclusively breast-fed and refuses a bottle or cup

If any of these criteria apply to your baby, proceed to the following section. Otherwise, continue to breast- or bottle-feed your baby when she wants to be fed (but less than four times each day) and don't worry about complete weaning at this time.

HOW TO ELIMINATE EXCESSIVE BREAST OR BOTTLE FEEDINGS

To decrease breast- or bottle-feedings to a level that won't cause any of the preceding side effects, take the following steps:

1. **Reduce milk feedings to three or four per day.** When your child comes to you for additional feedings, give him extra holding and attention instead. Get your child on a schedule of three main meals per day plus two or three nutritious snacks.
2. **Introduce cup feedings if this was not done at 6 months of age.** Cup feedings are needed as substitutes for breast- or bottle-feedings regardless of the age at which weaning occurs. The longer the infant goes without using a cup, the less willing he will be to try it. Starting daily cup feedings by 5 or 6 months of age is a natural way to keep breast- or bottle-feedings from becoming too important.
3. **Immediately stop allowing your child to carry a bottle around during the day.** The companion bottle can interfere with normal development that requires speech or two-handed play. It can also contribute to problems with tooth decay. You can explain to your child that "it's not good for you" or "you're too old for that."
4. **Immediately stop allowing your child to take a bottle to bed.** Besides causing sleep problems, taking a bottle to bed carries the risk of causing tooth decay. You can offer the same explanations as in the above paragraph.
5. Once you have made these changes, you need not proceed further unless you wish to eliminate breast- or bottle-feedings completely. Attempt total weaning only if your family is not under stress (such as might be caused by moving or some other major change) and your child is not in crisis (from illness or trying to achieve bladder control, for example). Weaning from breast or bottle to cup should always be done gradually and with love. The "cold turkey," or abrupt withdrawal, approach will only make your child angry, clingy, and miserable. Although there is no consensus about the best time to wean, there is agreement about the appropriate technique.

HOW TO ELIMINATE BREAST-FEEDING COMPLETELY

1. **Offer formula in a cup before each breast-feeding.** If your child refuses formula, offer expressed breast milk. If that fails, add some flavoring he likes to the formula. If your child is older than 12 months, you can use whole milk. Some infants won't accept a cup until they've nursed for several minutes.
2. **Gradually eliminate breast-feedings.** First, eliminate the feeding that is least important to your child (usually the midday one). Replace it with a complete cup feeding. About once every week drop one more breast feeding. The bedtime nursing is usually the last to be given up, and there's no reason why you can't continue it for months if that's what you and your child want. Some mothers prefer to wean by decreasing the length of feedings. Shorten all feedings by 2 minutes each week until they are 5 minutes long. Then eliminate them one at a time.
3. **Relieve breast engorgement.** Since the breast operates on the principle of supply and demand, reduced sucking time eventually reduces milk production. In the meantime, express just enough milk to relieve breast pain resulting from engorgement. (This is better than putting your baby to the breast for a minute, because she probably won't want to stop nursing.) Remember that complete emptying of the breast increases milk production. An acetaminophen product may also help relieve discomfort.
4. **If your child asks to nurse after you have finished weaning, respond by holding her instead.** You can explain that the milk is all gone. If she has a strong sucking drive, more pacifier time may help.

HOW TO ELIMINATE BOTTLE-FEEDING COMPLETELY

1. **Offer formula in a cup before each bottle-feeding.** Use whole milk if your child is 1 year of age or older.

2. **Make the weaning process gradual.** Eliminate one bottle-feeding every 3 or 4 days, depending on your child's reaction. Replace each bottle-feeding with a cup-feeding and extra holding.

3. **Eliminate bottle-feedings in the following order: midday, late afternoon, morning, and bedtime.** The last feeding of the day is usually the most important one to the child. When it is time to give up this feeding, gradually reduce the amount of milk each day over the course of a week.

4. **After you have completed the weaning process, respond to requests for a bottle by holding your child.** You can explain that bottles are for little babies. You may even want to have your child help you carry the bottles to a neighbor's house. If your child has a strong need to suck, offer a pacifier.

 CALL OUR OFFICE

During regular hours if

- Your child is over 6 months of age and won't eat any food except milk and won't drink from a cup.
- Your child has tooth decay.
- You think your child has anemia.
- This approach to weaning has not been successful after trying it for 1 month.
- Your child is over 3 years old.
- You have other questions or concerns.

Instructions for Pediatric Patients, 2nd Edition, ©1999 by WB Saunders Company.
Written by Barton D. Schmitt, MD, pediatrician and author of *Your Child's Health,* Bantam Books, a book for parents.

DEFINITION

Weaning is the replacement of bottle- or breast-feedings (nipple feedings) with drinking from a cup and eating solid foods. Weaning occurs easily and smoothly unless the breast or bottle has become overly important to the child.

HOW TO PREVENT WEANING PROBLEMS

Children normally develop a reduced interest in breast- and bottle-feedings between 6 and 12 months of age if they are also taking cup- and spoon-feedings. If a child hasn't weaned by the age of 12 to 18 months, the parent often has to initiate it, but the child is still receptive. After 18 months of age, the child usually resists weaning because he has become too attached to the breast or bottle. If your child shows a lack of interest in the breast or bottle at any time after 6 months of age, start to phase out these nipple feedings.

You can tell that your baby is ready to begin weaning when he throws the bottle down, takes only a few ounces of milk and then stops, chews on the nipple rather than sucking it, refuses the breast, or nurses for only a few minutes and then wants to play. The following steps encourage early natural weaning at 9 to 12 months:

1. **Keep formula feedings to four times per day or fewer after your child reaches 6 months of age.** Some breast-fed babies may need five feedings per day until 9 months of age. Even at birth, feedings should be kept to eight times daily or fewer.

2. **Give older infants their daytime milk at mealtime with solids.** Once your child is having just four milk feedings each day, be sure three of them are given at mealtime with solids rather than as part of the ritual before naps. Your child can have the fourth feeding before going to bed at night.

3. **After your baby is 4 to 6 weeks old and breast-feeding is well established, offer a bottle of expressed breast milk or water daily.** This experience will help your baby become accustomed to a bottle so that you can occasionally leave him with a sitter. This step is especially important if you will be returning to work or school. The longer after 2 months you wait to introduce the bottle, the more strongly your infant will initially reject it. If you wait until 4 months of age, the transition period may take up to 1 week.

Once bottle feedings are accepted, you will need to continue them at least three times weekly.

4. **Hold your child for discomfort or stress instead of nursing him.** You can comfort your child and foster a strong sense of security and trust without nursing every time he is upset. If you always nurse your child in such situations, your child will learn to eat whenever upset. He will also be unable to separate being held from nursing, and you may become an "indispensable mother."

5. **Don't let the bottle or breast substitute for a pacifier.** Learn to recognize when your baby needs non-nutritive sucking. At these times, instead of offering your child food, encourage him to suck on a pacifier or thumb. Feeding your baby every time he needs to suck can lead to obesity.

6. **Don't let the bottle or breast become a security object at bedtime.** Your child should be able to go to sleep at night without having a breast or bottle in his mouth. He needs to learn how to put himself to sleep. If he doesn't, he will develop sleep problems that require the parents' presence during the night.

7. **Don't let a bottle become a daytime toy.** Don't let your child carry a bottle around as a companion during the day. This habit may keep him from engaging in more stimulating activities.

8. **Don't let your child hold the bottle or take it to bed.** Your child should think of the bottle as something that belongs to you; hence, he won't protest giving it up, since it never belonged to him in the first place.

9. **Offer your child formula or breast milk in a cup by 6 months of age.** For the first few months your child will probably accept the cup only after he has drunk some from the bottle or breast. However, by 9 months of age your child should be offered some formula or breast milk from a cup before breast- or bottle-feedings.

10. **Help your baby become interested in foods other than milk by 4 months of age.** Introduce solids with a spoon by 4 months of age to formula-fed babies and by 6 months to breast-fed infants. Introduce finger foods between 8 and 10 months of age, when he develops a pincer grip. As soon as your child is able to eat finger foods, include him at the table with the family during mealtime. He will probably become interested in the foods that he sees you eating and will ask for them. Consequently, his interest in exclusive milk feedings will diminish.

Instructions for Pediatric Patients, 2nd Edition, ©1999 by WB Saunders Company.
Written by Barton D. Schmitt, MD, pediatrician and author of *Your Child's Health,* Bantam Books, a book for parents.

SOLID (STRAINED) FOODS

AGE FOR STARTING SOLID FOODS

The best time to begin using a spoon to feed your child is when he can sit with some support and voluntarily move his head to engage in the feeding process. This time is usually between 4 and 6 months of age. Breast milk and commercial formulas meet all your baby's nutritional needs until 4 to 6 months of age. Introducing strained foods earlier just makes feeding more complicated. Research has shown that it won't help your baby sleep through the night.

TYPES OF SOLID FOODS

Cereals are usually the first solid food introduced into your baby's diet. Generally these are introduced at 4 months of age in formula-fed infants and 6 months of age in breast-fed infants.

Start with rice cereal, which is less likely to cause allergies than other cereals. Barley and oatmeal may be tried 1 or 2 weeks later. A mixed cereal should be added to your baby's diet only after each kind of cereal in the mixed cereal has been separately introduced.

Strained or pureed vegetables and fruits are the next solid foods introduced to your baby. Although the order of foods is not important, introduce only one new food at a time and no more than three per week. If your infant doesn't seem to like the taste of cereals, start with a fruit (such as bananas).

Between 8 and 12 months of age, introduce your baby to mashed table foods or junior foods (although the latter are probably unnecessary). If you make your own baby foods in a baby-food grinder or electric blender, be sure to add enough water to get a consistency that your baby can easily swallow.

Although there is controversy about them, egg whites, wheat, peanut butter, fish, and orange juice may be more likely to cause allergies than other solids and should be avoided until 1 year of age (especially in infants with allergies).

SPOON-FEEDING

Spoon-feeding is begun at 4 to 6 months of age. By 8 to 10 months of age, most children want to try to feed themselves and can do so with finger foods. By 15 to 18 months of age, most children can use a spoon independently for foods they can't pick up with their fingers, and the parent is no longer needed in the feeding process.

Place food on the middle of the tongue. If you place it in front, your child will probably push it back at you. Some infants get off to a better start if you place the spoon between their lips and let them suck off the food. Some children constantly bat at the spoon or try to get a grip on it during feedings. These children need to be distracted with finger foods or by having a spoon of their own to play with.

FINGER FOODS

Finger foods are small bite-sized pieces of soft foods. Most babies love to feed themselves. Finger foods can be introduced between 9 and 10 months of age or whenever your child develops a pincer grip. Since most babies will not be able to feed themselves with a spoon until 15 months of age, finger foods keep them actively involved in the feeding process. Good finger foods are dry cereals (such as Cheerios or Rice Krispies), slices of cheese, pieces of scrambled eggs, slices of canned fruit (peaches, pears, or pineapple) or soft fresh fruits, slices of banana, crackers, cookies, and breads.

SNACKS

Once your baby starts eating three meals a day or at 5-hour intervals, small snacks will often be necessary to tide him over to the next meal. Most babies go to this pattern between 6 and 9 months of age. The midmorning and midafternoon snack should be a nutritious, nonmilk food. Fruits and dry cereals are recommended. If your child is not hungry at mealtime, the snacks should be made smaller or eliminated.

TABLE FOODS

Your child should be eating the same meals that you do by approximately 1 year of age. This assumes that your diet is well balanced and that you carefully dice any foods that would be difficult for your baby to chew. Avoid foods such as raw carrots that could be choked on.

IRON-RICH FOODS

Throughout our lives we need iron in our diets to prevent anemia. Certain foods are especially good sources of iron. Red meats, fish, and poultry are best. Some young children will eat only lunch meats, and the low-fat ones are fine. Adequate iron is also found in iron-enriched cereals, beans of all types, egg yolks, peanut butter, raisins, prune juice, sweet potatoes, and spinach.

VITAMINS

Added vitamins are unnecessary after your child has reached 1 year of age and is on a regular balanced diet. If he's a picky eater, give him one chewable vitamin pill per week.

Instructions for Pediatric Patients, 2nd Edition, ©1999 by WB Saunders Company. Written by Barton D. Schmitt, MD, pediatrician and author of *Your Child's Health,* Bantam Books, a book for parents.

DEFINITION

Characteristics of a child with a normal decline in appetite:

- It seems to you that your child doesn't eat enough, is never hungry, or won't eat unless you spoon feed her yourself.
- Your child is between 1 and 5 years old.
- Your child's energy level remains normal.
- Your child is growing normally.

Cause

Between 1 and 5 years of age many children normally gain only 4 or 5 pounds each year even though they probably gained 15 pounds during their first year. Children in this age range can normally go 3 or 4 months without any weight gain. Because they are not growing as fast, they need less calories and they seem to have a poorer appetite (this is called *physiological anorexia*). How much a child chooses to eat is governed by the appetite center in the brain. Kids eat as much as they need for growth and energy. Many parents try to force their children to eat more than they need because they fear that poor appetite might cause poor health or a nutritional deficiency. This is not true, however; forced feedings interfere with the normal pleasure of eating and actually decrease a child's appetite.

Expected Course

Once you allow your child to be in charge of how much is eaten, the unpleasantness at mealtime and your concerns about her health should disappear in 2 to 4 weeks. Your child's appetite will improve when she becomes older and needs to eat more.

HELPING A POOR EATER REDISCOVER HER APPETITE

1. **Put your child in charge of how much she eats.** Trust your child's appetite center. The most common reason for some children never appearing hungry is that they have so many snacks and meals that they never become truly hungry. Offer your child no more than two small snacks of nutritious food each day, and provide them only if your child requests them. If your child is thirsty between meals, offer water. Limit the amount of juice your child drinks to less than 6 ounces each day. Let your child miss one or two meals if she chooses and then watch her appetite return. Skipping a meal is harmless.
2. **Never feed your child if she is capable of feeding herself.** The greatest tendency of parents of a child with a poor appetite is to pick up the spoon, fill it with food, smile, and try to trick the child into taking it. Once your child is old enough to use a spoon independently (usually 15 to 18 months), never again pick it up for her. If your child is hungry, she will feed herself.
3. **Offer finger foods.** Finger foods can be started at 8 to 10 months of age. Such foods allow your child to feed herself at least some of the time, even if she is not yet able to use a spoon.
4. **Limit milk to less than 16 ounces each day.** Milk contains as many calories as most solid foods. Drinking too much milk can fill kids up and dull their appetites.
5. **Serve small portions of food—less than you think your child will eat.** A child's appetite is decreased if she is served more food than she could possibly eat. If you serve your child a small amount on a large plate, she is more likely to finish it and gain a sense of accomplishment. If your child seems to want more, wait for her to ask for it. Avoid serving your child any foods that she strongly dislikes (such as some vegetables).
6. **Consider giving your child daily vitamins.** Although vitamins are probably unnecessary, they are not harmful in normal dosages and may allow you to relax about your child's eating patterns.
7. **Make mealtimes pleasant.** Draw your children into the conversation. Avoid making mealtimes a time for criticism or struggle over control.
8. **Avoid conversation about eating.** Don't discuss how little your child eats in her presence. Trust your child's appetite center to look after her food needs. Also, don't praise your child for eating a lot. Children should eat to please themselves.
9. **Don't extend mealtime.** Don't make your child sit at the dinner table after the rest of the family is done eating. This will only cause your child to develop unpleasant associations with mealtime.
10. **Prevention.** By the time your child is 8 to 10 months old, start giving her finger foods. By 12 months of age, your child will begin to use a spoon, and she should be able to feed herself completely by 15 months of age.

 CALL OUR OFFICE

During regular hours if
- Your child is losing weight.
- Your child has not gained any weight in 6 months.
- Your child has associated symptoms of illness (such as diarrhea, fever).
- Your child gags on or vomits some foods.
- Someone is punishing your child for not eating.
- This approach has not improved mealtimes in your house within 1 month.
- You have other questions or concerns.

PICKY EATERS

DEFINITION

- The child complains about or refuses specific foods, especially vegetables and meats.
- The child pushes these foods around the plate.
- The child hides these foods or gives them to a pet under the table.
- Peak age for this behavior is toddler or preschool years.
- The child eats enough total foods and calories per day.

Cause

Children of all ages (and adults) commonly have a few food dislikes. Sometimes these foods are disliked because of their color, but more commonly it's because they are difficult to chew. Tender meats are better accepted than tough ones, as are well-cooked vegetables. Some children are repulsed by foods with a bitter taste. Occasionally in a child who gags on large pieces of all foods, large tonsils are the cause.

Expected Outcome

Most children who are picky eaters try new foods in the school years because of peer pressure. The voracious appetite during the adolescent growth years also increases their willingness to experiment. If the parent tries to force the child to eat a food he doesn't like, the child may gag or even vomit. Forced feedings always interfere with the normal pleasure of eating and eventually decrease the appetite.

LIVING WITH A PICKY OR FINICKY EATER

1. **Try to prepare a main dish that everyone likes.** Try to avoid any unusual main dish that your child strongly dislikes. Some children don't like foods that are mixed together, such as casseroles. These can be reintroduced at a later time.
2. **Allow occasional substitutes for the main dish.** If your child refuses to eat the main dish and this is an unusual request, a substitute dish can be allowed. An acceptable substitute would be breakfast cereal or simple sandwich the child prepares for himself. A parent should never become a short-order cook and prepare any extra foods for mealtime. The child should know that we expect him to learn to eat the main dish that has been prepared for the family.
3. **Respect any strong food dislikes.** If your child has a few strong food dislikes (especially any food that makes him gag), he should not be served that food when it's prepared as part of the family meal. Never pressure your child to eat all foods. It will only lead to a power struggle, gagging, or even vomiting.
4. **Don't worry about vegetables, just encourage more fruits.** Because vegetables tend to be hard to chew and some of them are bitter, they are commonly rejected by children and even by many adults. Keep in mind that fruits and vegetables are from the same food group. There are no essential vegetables. Vegetables can be entirely replaced by fruits without any nutritional harm to your child. This is not a health issue. Don't make your child feel guilty about avoiding some vegetables.
5. **Don't allow complaining about food at mealtimes.** Have a rule that it's OK to decline a serving of a particular food or to push it to the side of the plate, but complaining about it is unacceptable.
6. **Ask your child to taste new foods.** Many tastes are acquired. He may eventually learn that he likes a food he initially refuses. For some picky eaters, it may take seeing other people eat a certain food 10 times before they're even willing to taste it, and another 10 times of tasting it before they develop a liking for it. Don't try to rush this normal process of adapting to new foods. Trying to force a child to eat one bite of a food per year of age is not helpful with most picky eaters. Instead, it's better to trust them when they say that they have tasted the food in question.
7. **Don't argue about dessert.** An unnecessary area of friction for picky eaters is a rule that if you don't clean your plate, you can't have any dessert. Since desserts are not harmful, a better approach is to allow your child one serving of dessert regardless of what he eats. However, there are no seconds on dessert for children who don't eat an adequate amount of the main course. Desserts don't have to be sweets—they can be nutritious desserts such as fruit.
8. **Don't extend mealtime.** Don't keep your child sitting at the dinner table after the rest of the family is done. This will only cause your child to develop unpleasant associations with mealtime.
9. **Keep mealtimes pleasant.** Make it an important family event. Draw your children into friendly conversation. Tell them what's happened to you today and ask about their day. Talk about fun subjects unrelated to food. Avoid making it a time for criticism or struggle over control.
10. **Avoid conversation about eating at any time.** Don't discuss food intake in your child's presence. Trust the appetite center to look after your child's caloric needs. Also, don't provide praise for appropriate eating. Don't give bribes or rewards for meeting your eating expectations. Children should eat to satisfy their appetite, not to please the parent. Occasionally the child can be praised for trying a new food although he does not like its taste or texture.
11. **Consider giving your child a daily vitamin-mineral supplement.** Although vitamins are probably unnecessary for most of us, they are not harmful in normal amounts and may allow you to relax more about your child's eating patterns.

Instructions for Pediatric Patients, 2nd Edition, ©1999 by WB Saunders Company.
Written by Barton D. Schmitt, MD, pediatrician and author of *Your Child's Health,* Bantam Books, a book for parents.

Cholesterol is the normal way fat is carried in the bloodstream. It has become a health issue because high cholesterol levels carry an increased risk of coronary heart disease (CHD). A 1% decrease in blood cholesterol leads to a 2% decrease in risk of CHD in adults. Societies with low serum cholesterol usually have a low incidence of CHD. The amount of cholesterol and saturated fats we eat contributes to the level of cholesterol in our bloodstreams. The level of cholesterol in childhood tends to persist (track) into adulthood in about 50% of children. This ability of the child's level of cholesterol to predict the adult level increases with each passing year. Further, reducing the cholesterol and saturated fat in the diet does reduce the level of cholesterol in the bloodstream. One major goal of preventive medicine is to lower cholesterol to healthy levels.

TYPES OF CHOLESTEROL

Cholesterol is composed of high-density lipoprotein (HDL), low-density lipoprotein (LDL), and triglycerides. The HDL is called the "good" cholesterol because it carries cholesterol away from the arteries and to the liver for elimination. LDL is referred to as the "bad" cholesterol. An excess of LDL deposits cholesterol on the inner walls of the arteries over time. In addition to reducing total cholesterol levels, we would like to see you increase your HDL and decrease your LDL. A 1% rise in HDL may give a 3% reduction in CHD in adults.

NORMAL AND ABNORMAL CHOLESTEROL LEVELS

Normal cholesterol levels remain rather constant between 120 and 170 throughout childhood. After 18 years of age they tend to rise about 1 point per year of age. For total cholesterol and LDL, a healthy or desirable level is below the 75th percentile. A borderline high level is between the 75th and 95th percentiles. A high or abnormal level is above the 95th percentile. In general, levels above the 75th percentile should be lowered because the normal values in the United States are considerably higher than normal values in countries with a low incidence of CHD.

		Children	Adults
Total Cholesterol	>95th Percentile	>200	>240
	>75th	>170	>200
	Desirable	<170	<200
LDL	>95th	>130	>160
	>75th	>110	>130
	Desirable	<110	<130

The desired level for HDL, which we want to be high since it is protective, is above the 25th percentile. A borderline low value is between the 5th and 25th percentiles. A low or abnormal value is below the 5th percentile.

		Children	Adults
HDL	<5th	<35	<30
	<25th	<45	<40
	Desirable	>45	>40

HIGH-RISK CHILDREN: WHAT AGE TO TEST?

The American Academy of Pediatrics and the American Heart Association are in complete agreement that all children who have risk factors for CHD should be screened soon after 2 years of age. The reason children aren't tested before 2 years is that during this period of rapid growth and development the diet needs to be high in fat. Two main risk factors should be considered: (1) a family history of high blood cholesterol and (2) a family history of CHD. The latter includes an early (less than 50 years of age in men or less than 60 years of age in women) history of heart attack, angina, stroke, or bypass surgery. The family history is considered positive if these diseases have occurred in parents, grandparents, aunts, or uncles. Information must be obtained about the grandparents since the parents are often too young to have entered the high-risk age group for CHD. Over 50% of children with high cholesterol levels are identified by screening these high-risk children.

ALL OTHER CHILDREN: WHAT AGE TO TEST?

The practice of performing cholesterol testing on all children is controversial. The main reason for universal testing is to identify all children with high cholesterol levels. Eating and exercise patterns in children need to be established early if they are to be followed throughout life. The main arguments against testing all children are that testing is costly, high cholesterol levels do not persist into adulthood 50% to 60% of the time, and healthy diets can be started in all children without knowing cholesterol levels. If routine testing is done, it's usually performed between 2 and 5 years of age, often on school entry.

RETESTING CHILDREN WITH HIGH CHOLESTEROL LEVELS

If your child's cholesterol value is borderline high or high, the test will be repeated in 1 to 2 weeks to confirm that the value is high. There is some normal day-to-day variation in cholesterol levels. If the level remains high, it's assumed to be accurate. Children with confirmed high total cholesterol levels (greater than the 95th percentile) will then have blood drawn for a lipid profile or panel. This test measures not only total cholesterol, but also LDL, HDL, and triglycerides. Depending on the results, diet and exercise treatment will be initiated and the level repeated in approximately 2 to 4 months. If your child has a high-normal total cholesterol level (greater than the 75th percentile), treatment can be started without additional tests. The test for total cholesterol will probably be repeated yearly. The reason we don't obtain routine lipid panels in all children is that they cost approximately $70, in contrast to $25 for a total cholesterol test. In addition, the lipid panel requires blood drawn from a vein (which can be a more difficult procedure in a child) rather than a simple finger stick.

RETESTING CHILDREN WITH NORMAL CHOLESTEROL LEVELS

Children with cholesterol levels below the 75th percentile do not need their cholesterol rechecked until they become adolescents. Most physicians who treat adults repeat cholesterol levels every 5 years as long as they remain within normal range.

TESTING FAMILY MEMBERS

If your child's value is high (greater than the 95th percentile), we recommend that you have everyone else in your family tested for total cholesterol. A child with a high level is a good indication for parents or siblings with high levels. In over 80% of cases, other family members also have high values. This will provide you with additional reasons to start your family on a healthier diet and exercise program. If your child's cholesterol level is high or high-normal, see the information sheet entitled "Treating High Cholesterol Levels."

Instructions for Pediatric Patients, 2nd Edition, ©1999 by WB Saunders Company.
Written by Barton D. Schmitt, MD, pediatrician and author of *Your Child's Health,* Bantam Books, a book for parents.

If your child's cholesterol level is high or borderline high, start the programs listed in this information sheet. (If your child's cholesterol level is normal, it would still be a good idea to place your family on the same programs.) High cholesterol levels are not the only risk factor for coronary heart disease (CHD). The following risk factors are just as harmful as being on a high-cholesterol diet: physical inactivity, obesity, and smoking. The more risk factors that you and your child have, the higher is the risk of CHD. Living a long and healthy life requires healthy eating and exercise patterns. It is easier to start these habits as a child than to have to adopt them as an adult. Review with your family the following ways to reduce cholesterol levels. If you are already carrying out most of these recommendations, you are protecting your child's heart and blood vessels.

A LOW-FAT DIET

The American Heart Association recommends that all children over 2 years of age be on a low-cholesterol, low–saturated fat diet. Currently, most Americans take in 40% of their daily calories as fat. A healthy (prudent) diet keeps fat to 30% of total calories. The goal is to eat fat in moderation, not to eliminate fat entirely. Lowering your child's fat intake to 30% of daily calories carries no risk for children over 2 years old. (None of the following recommendations apply to children under 2 years of age.) Foods of plant origin, such as fruits, vegetables, and grains, do not contain cholesterol. Foods of animal origin, such as meats, eggs, and milk products, do contain cholesterol. Our blood cholesterol is raised by consuming cholesterol itself or by eating saturated fats that stimulate the production of cholesterol. Even without any fat intake, the liver produces a small amount of cholesterol each day. Therefore we will always have a blood cholesterol level. Serving a low-fat diet in your house is quite easy:

- Serve more fish, turkey, and chicken since they have less fat than red meats. Buy lean ground beef for hamburgers. Use lean ham or turkey for sandwiches.
- Trim the fat from meats and remove the skin from poultry before eating.
- Avoid the meats with the highest fat content, such as bacon, sausages, salami, pepperoni, and hot dogs.
- Limit the number of eggs eaten to three or four per week.
- Limit the amount of all meats to portions of moderate size.
- Use 1% or skim (0.5%) milk instead of whole milk (which is 3.5% fat).
- Use a margarine product instead of butter.
- Avoid deep-fat fried food or food fried in butter or fat. If you prefer to fry meats, use margarine or nonstick cooking sprays.
- Increase your child's fiber intake. Fiber is found in most grains, vegetables, and fruits.

FAMILY EXERCISE PROGRAM

Exercise is the best way to raise your HDL level. Your goal should be 20 to 30 minutes of vigorous exercise three times a week. Vigorous exercise must involve the large muscles of the legs and cause your heart to beat faster (aerobic exercise). Vigorous exercise also improves your heart's response to work. A child is much more likely to exercise if you exercise with him. Encourage your child to try the following forms of exercise:

- Walk or bike instead of riding in a car.
- Use stairs instead of elevators.
- Take the dog for a walk, jump rope, or play ball if bored.
- Join a team (such as soccer) or learn a new sport (such as roller skating) that requires vigorous (aerobic) activity. Swimming and jogging are sports that burn lots of calories. Sports such as baseball and football do not exercise the heart.
- Exercise to a videotape or music.
- Limit television and video game time to 2 hours or less per day. These sitting activities interfere with physical fitness.
- Use an exercise bike, dance, or run in place while watching television.
- Support better physical education programs and aerobics classes in your schools.

IDEAL BODY WEIGHT

Children who are overweight tend to have a low HDL level and a high LDL level. Helping your child return to ideal body weight will improve the blood cholesterol levels. Decreasing fat in a person's diet automatically decreases the calories consumed, because fat has twice as much calories as the same amount of protein or carbohydrates. A low-fat diet *and* exercise are the key ingredients for losing weight. If your child is overweight, also request the guideline entitled "Overweight."

SMOKE-FREE HOME

A good way to raise your HDL level is to stop smoking. Also avoid exposing your child to passive smoking. If someone in your home has a problem with smoking, request the guideline "Passive Smoking."

SETTING A GOOD EXAMPLE

If your child needs to lower his cholesterol level, he will need help from his family. You cannot put him on a special diet without putting the entire family on it. You cannot put him on a special exercise program without having other family members participate. Eat healthy foods and snacks, so your child will eat similarly. Play more sports and watch fewer television sports shows—as you would like your child to do.

SUGAR AND SWEETS

A popular misconception suggests that eating sugar is harmful or at least a weakness. Many well-educated parents worry needlessly about sugar, candy, and desserts. For purposes of discussion, sweets can be identified as any food in which sucrose, fructose, glucose, corn syrup, honey, or other sugars are listed as the first ingredient on the packaging. Sweets are not bad. The body needs sugar to function and the brain needs glucose to think. Sweets just need to be eaten in moderation. If you want to protect your child's health, get after the Cholesterol Monster, not the Sugar Monster and the Cookie Monster.

THE NORMAL SWEET TOOTH

Soon after birth, infants show a preference for sweet solutions (such as breast milk) over unsweetened solutions. Many humans are born with a "sweet tooth," probably on a genetic basis. Most adults also naturally seek out and enjoy sweets. Giving candy as a gift for holidays or birthdays is a common symbol of affection. Many members of the animal kingdom also show a craving for sweets.

People forget that the recommended daily amount of calories from carbohydrates (sugar and starches) is 55%. The amount from refined sugars (sucrose) should not exceed 10% of the daily calories. Sugar is present naturally in most foods except the meat group. Lactose is the sugar present in milk, fructose is the sugar present in fruits, and maltose is the sugar present in grain products. Sucrose, the sugar found in sugar cane and sugar beets, has no greater adverse effect on body functioning than any of the other sugars.

SIDE EFFECTS OF SUGAR

The main risk of sugar is its ability to increase tooth decay. Tooth decay is also the only permanent harm from consuming too much sugar. This risk can be greatly reduced by brushing the teeth after sugar-containing foods are eaten and drinking fluoridated water. The foods causing the most dental cavities (caries) are those that stick to the teeth (for example, raisins). The greatest risk factor for severe dental caries is falling asleep or walking around with a bottle of sugar solution in the mouth. The solution can be fruit juice, Kool-Aid, or milk. This type of tooth decay is called "baby-bottle caries."

A temporary side effect may be seen 2 to 4 hours after excessive sugar consumption. The reaction is probably due to a rapid fall in blood glucose and consists of sweating, hunger, dizziness, tiredness, or sleepiness. This reaction to a sugar binge is brief and harmless and can be relieved by the passage of time and eating a food containing some sugar, such as a fruit juice. These symptoms do not occur after eating a normal amount of sweets, and they do not occur in everyone.

MYTHS ABOUT SUGAR

Eating sugar is basically not harmful. Candy does not cause cancer, heart disease, or diabetes mellitus. The following are some common overconcerns:

1. **Obesity.** Obesity is due to overeating in general and not specifically to eating sugars. Fatty foods have twice the calories per amount as sugary foods and are much more related to obesity. Studies have shown that lean people tend to eat more sugar than overweight people.
2. **Hyperactivity.** Extensive research has shown that sugar does not cause or worsen hyperactivity. In fact, a high intake of refined sugar may cause a relaxed state or even drowsiness.
3. **Junk food.** The term *junk food* has led to considerable confusion in the United States. Some people define any sweet or dessert as a junk food. Others define fast foods as junk foods. Let's junk this negative term that implies if a food is sweet or purchased from a fast-food chain, it's bad for your health. It's not that simple.

RECOMMENDATIONS FOR THE SAFE USE OF SUGAR

1. **Allow sugar in moderation.** In general, eating foods in moderation is healthy, but eating foods in excess is unhealthy. One precaution is to avoid sweets if possible during the first year of life. If they are introduced too early, they may interfere with a willingness to try new foods that are unsweetened. (*Note:* These guidelines about sugar in moderation may not apply to children with diabetes mellitus.)
2. **Don't try to forbid sugar.** Some parents do this in hopes of preventing a preference for sweet foods. Since this preference is present at birth, we have little influence over it. If we forbid sweets entirely, children may become fascinated with them. With candy and other sweets so readily available in stores and vending machines, a sugar embargo cannot be monitored and becomes unenforceable as a child grows up. If we make an issue of it, this becomes an unnecessary battleground.
3. **Limit the amount of sweets you buy.** The more sweets there are in the house, the more your child will eat. Try to purchase breakfast cereals and cookies in which sugar is not the main ingredient.
4. **Limit how much sweets are eaten.** Whereas one candy bar is fine, eating an entire bag of candy is unacceptable. Try to eliminate bingeing on candy or sweets. Do this mainly by setting a good example. Exceptions of allowing extra candy can be made on Halloween, other holidays, birthdays, and other parties. The worst that could happen is that your child could become extra sleepy or have a mild stomachache.
5. **Allow sweets for desserts.** As stated earlier,

Instructions for Pediatric Patients, 2nd Edition, ©1999 by WB Saunders Company.
Written by Barton D. Schmitt, MD, pediatrician and author of *Your Child's Health,* Bantam Books, a book for parents.

sweets cause symptoms only if they are eaten in excess. As long as they follow a well-balanced meal, they cause no symptoms. An acceptable dessert can therefore be just about anything, including candy.

6. **Discourage sweets for snacks.** Candy, soft drinks, and other sweets are not a good choice for a snack. Since very little else is eaten with the snack, consuming mainly refined sugar may cause some rebound symptoms several hours later. Teach your child that if he does take a soft drink or Kool-Aid as a snack, he should eat something else from the grain or fruit food group along with it. An occasional sweet drink with a sugar substitute is fine. Stock up on nutritious snacks (such as fruit juices, yogurt, graham crackers, oatmeal cookies, and popcorn). In fact, most cookies are not sweets since the main ingredient is flour. Also, set a good example by what you eat for snacks.

7. **Insist that the teeth be brushed after eating sweets.** Encourage your child to rinse his mouth with some water after eating when he's away from home. Unless you encourage this good habit, a "sweet tooth" can become a "decayed tooth."

SPECIAL BENEFITS OF SUGAR

The occasional use of candy as a reward is not habit forming. The joy of eating sweets is a natural preference, not enhanced by this practice. Candy and other sweet treats are a powerful incentive. Whether we like it or not, the best motivators are always items that children crave. In addition, candy is inexpensive and easy to purchase. Because of the many types of candy, the child also has many choices. Candy may bring about a breakthrough with a negative child who has not responded to other approaches. Star charts and praise should be used simultaneously for improved behavior and continued after the candy has been phased out.

Second, sugar can be useful in helping a finicky eater try an essential new food. Some children who have been breast-fed until almost 1 year of age will not accept any milk products. One way of helping them make this transition is by sweetening the cow's milk temporarily with honey or other flavorings. (**Caution:** Avoid giving honey before 1 year of age because of the small risk of botulism for this age group.) After the child is drinking adequate amounts of milk, the sweetener can be gradually phased out.

Third, some children take bitter medicines easier when they are mixed with a sweet flavoring such as Kool-Aid powder, chocolate pudding, or pancake syrup.

OVERVIEW

Let's be honest. Most adults and children enjoy sweets. Most children spend part of their allowance on sweets. Eating sweets in moderation is fine. A well-balanced diet can include some daily sweets.

 CALL OUR OFFICE

During regular hours if
- Your child frequently binges on sweets.
- You find yourself repeatedly reminding your child about sweets.
- You think your child has a problem with sugar.
- You have other questions or concerns.

FOOD ALLERGIES

DEFINITION

Although food allergies tend to be overdiagnosed, about 5% of children have true reactions to foods. Suspect that your child may have a food allergy if the following three characteristics are present:

1. Your child has allergic symptoms within 2 hours after eating certain foods. The most common reactions involve the mouth (for example, swelling), gastrointestinal tract (for example, diarrhea), or skin (for example, hives). Rarely, a child has a severe allergic reaction (anaphylactic reaction) that may be life threatening. Common anaphylactic symptoms are a rapid onset of difficult breathing, difficult swallowing, or a fall in blood pressure (shock).
2. Your child has other allergic conditions, such as eczema, asthma, or hay fever. Children with these conditions have a much higher rate of associated food allergies than nonallergic children.
3. Other family members (parents or siblings) have food allergies. Food allergies are often inherited.

Cause

Allergic children produce antibodies against certain foods. When these antibodies come into contact with the allergic food, the reaction releases numerous chemicals that cause the symptoms. The tendency to be allergic is inherited. If one parent has allergies, about 40% of the children will develop allergies. If both parents have allergies, about 75% will. Sometimes the child is allergic to the same food as the parent.

Expected Course

At least half of the children who develop a food allergy during the first year of life outgrow it by 2 or 3 years of age. Some food reactions (such as to milk) are more commonly outgrown than others. Whereas 3% to 4% of infants have a cow's milk allergy, less than 1% of them develop a lifelong allergy to milk. Allergies to peanuts, tree nuts, fish, and shellfish (shrimp, crab, and lobster) often persist for life.

COMMON SYMPTOMS OF FOOD ALLERGIES

The following symptoms are all commonly seen with food allergies. In some cases the food aggravates the underlying allergic condition.

- Swelling of lips, tongue, or mouth
- Diarrhea or vomiting
- Hives
- Itchy red skin (especially with underlying eczema)

Some less common symptoms are

- Sore throat or throat clearing
- Nasal congestion, runny nose, sneezing, or sniffing (especially with underlying hay fever)

An occasional child with asthma, migraine headaches, colic, or recurrent abdominal pain may have some attacks triggered by food allergies. These children, however, also have some of the typical symptoms (in the preceding lists) that occur with food reactions. Attention deficit disorder and behavioral disorders, as isolated symptoms, have not been scientifically linked to food allergies.

COMMON ALLERGIC FOODS

Overall, the most allergic food is the peanut. In infants, egg and milk products are more common. The following five foods account for over 80% of food reactions: peanuts (and peanut butter), eggs, cow's milk products, soybeans (and soy formula), and wheat. Eight foods (fish, shellfish, tree nuts, and the preceding five foods) account for over 95% of food reactions. Four foods (chocolate, strawberries, corn, and tomatoes) are highly overrated as triggers of symptoms. Although commonly mentioned, they rarely cause any allergic symptoms.

DIAGNOSING A FOOD ALLERGY

1. **Keep a diary of symptoms and recently eaten foods.** If the ingestion of a particular food is clearly the cause of particular symptoms, go directly to step 2. Otherwise, be a good detective and keep a symptom/food diary for 2 weeks. Anytime your child has symptoms, write down the foods eaten during the preceding meal. After 2 weeks, examine the diary for foods that were repeatedly consumed on days your child had symptoms. Expect some inconsistency, depending on the amount of food consumed. Although anaphylactic reactions can be triggered by small amounts of allergic foods, other symptoms (such as diarrhea) usually increase as the amount of the allergic food increases, but not to the point of being serious. Reactions to food may be worse when a child is also reacting to other substances in the environment such as pollens. Therefore, food allergies may flare up during pollen season.
2. **Eliminate the suspected food from the diet for 2 weeks.** Record any symptoms that occur during this time. If you have eliminated the correct food, all symptoms should disappear. Most children improve within 2 days and almost all of them improve after 1 week of avoiding the allergic food.
3. **Rechallenge your child with the suspected food.** (*Caution:* This step should never be carried out if your child has experienced a severe or anaphylactic reaction to a food.) The purpose of rechallenging is to prove that the suspected food is definitely the cause of your child's symptoms. Give your child a small amount of the suspected food. The same symptoms should appear anywhere from 10 minutes to 2 hours after the food is consumed. Call us before doing this.

Instructions for Pediatric Patients, 2nd Edition, ©1999 by WB Saunders Company.
Written by Barton D. Schmitt, MD, pediatrician and author of *Your Child's Health,* Bantam Books, a book for parents.

TREATMENT OF FOOD ALLERGIES

1. **Avoid the allergic food.** This should keep your child free of symptoms. If you are breast-feeding, eliminate the food your child is allergic to from your diet until breast-feeding is discontinued. Food allergens can be absorbed from your diet and enter your breast milk. Talk to a nutritionist if you have questions.

2. **Consider avoiding other foods in that food group.** Some children are allergic to two or more foods. Occasionally the foods belong to the same food group. The most common cross-reaction involves children allergic to ragweed pollen. They commonly react to watermelon, cantaloupe, musk-melon, honeydew melon, or other foods in the gourd family. Children allergic to peanuts may rarely cross-react with soybean, peas, or other beans. Surprisingly, most tree nuts are unrelated to each other and do not cross-react with peanuts.

3. **Provide substitutes for any missing vitamins or minerals.** Eliminating single foods usually does not cause any side effects. If a major food group (such as milk products) is eliminated, however, your child will develop vitamin D and calcium deficiency unless he receives appropriate supplements. Talk to your physician or a nutritionist about this.

4. **Rechallenge your child with the food in about 3 to 6 months.** (*Caution:* Never rechallenge a child who has had a severe or anaphylactic reaction to a food. Such a child should avoid that food for the rest of his life and keep an emergency kit with an epinephrine-loaded syringe at home, at school, and in the car.) Many food allergies are temporary. For children under 3 years of age, challenge them every 6 months until they are 3 years old. If they continue to react each time, have them evaluated by a board-certified allergist before permanently eliminating that food from the diet.

5. **Give Benadryl for hives.** If hives or itching are the only symptom, give Benadryl 4 times a day in the appropriate dosage until the hives have been gone for 12 hours.

PREVENTING FOOD ALLERGIES IN HIGH-RISK CHILDREN

High-risk or allergy-prone children are those who have parents or siblings with asthma, eczema, severe hay fever, or documented food allergies. The risk is highest if both parents are allergic to foods. The onset of allergies in these children may be delayed by being somewhat careful about their diet. If possible they should breast-feed during the first year of life. The mother should avoid milk products, peanuts, and eggs in her diet during this time. If the mother cannot breast-feed, there are two choices: a formula made from protein hydrolysate (known as an elemental formula) or a soy protein formula. The allergy-prone child should avoid all solid foods until 6 months old. Try to avoid milk products, eggs, peanut butter, soy protein, fish, wheat, and citrus fruits during the entire first year of life. Try to avoid the most allergic foods (peanuts and fish) until 2 years of age.

 ## CALL AN EMERGENCY RESCUE SQUAD (911)

IMMEDIATELY if
- Your child develops any serious symptoms such as wheezing, croupy cough, difficult breathing, passing out, or tightness in the chest or throat.

 ## CALL OUR OFFICE

IMMEDIATELY if
- Widespread hives, swelling, or itching occurs.

During regular hours if
- You suspect your child has a food allergy.
- You want to rechallenge your child with a food you suspect.
- You have other questions or concerns.

RECOMMENDED READING

S. Allan Bock: Food Allergy: A Primer for People. Vantage Press, New York, 1988.

The Food Allergy Network (8-page newsletter of practical tips published 6 times a year), 4744 Holly Avenue, Fairfax, VA 22030 or call 703-691-3179.

Instructions for Pediatric Patients, 2nd Edition, ©1999 by WB Saunders Company.

Written by Barton D. Schmitt, MD, pediatrician and author of *Your Child's Health,* Bantam Books, a book for parents.

39

OVERWEIGHT: A WEIGHT-REDUCTION PROGRAM

DEFINITION

- Your child appears overweight to an objective person.
- Your child weighs more than 20% over the ideal weight for her height.
- The skinfold thickness (fat layer) of your child's upper arm is more than 1 inch (25 mm), as measured with a special instrument.
- More than 25% of American children are overweight.

Causes

The tendency to be overweight is usually inherited. If one parent is overweight, half of the children will be overweight. If both parents are overweight, most of their children will be overweight. If neither parent is overweight, the children have a 10% chance of being overweight.

Heredity alone (without overeating) accounts for most mild obesity (defined as less than 30 pounds overweight in an adult). Moderate obesity is usually due to a combination of heredity, overeating, and underexercising. Some overeating is normal in our society, but only those who have the inherited tendency to be overweight will gain significant weight when they overeat. It is therefore not reasonable to blame your child for being overweight.

Less than 1% of obesity has an underlying medical cause. Your physician can easily determine this by a simple physical examination.

Expected Course

Losing weight is very difficult. Keeping the weight off is also a chore. The best time for losing weight is when a child is over 15 years old, that is, when she becomes very concerned with appearance. The self-motivated teenager can follow a diet and lose weight regardless of what the family eats. Helping children lose weight between 5 and 15 years of age is very difficult because they have access to so many foods outside the home and are not easily motivated to lose weight. It is not quite as difficult to help a child less than 5 years old to lose weight because the parents have better control of the foods offered to the child.

HOW TO HELP OLDER CHILDREN AND TEENAGERS LOSE WEIGHT

Readiness and Motivation

Teenagers can increase their motivation by joining a weight-loss club such as TOPS or Weight Watchers. Sometimes schools have classes for helping children lose weight. A child's motivation can often be improved if diet and exercise programs are undertaken by the entire family. A cooperative parent-child weight-loss program with individual goals is usually more helpful than a competitive program focused on who can lose weight faster.

Protecting Your Child's Self-esteem

Self-esteem is more important than an ideal body weight. If your child is overweight, he is probably already disappointed in himself. He needs his family to support him and accept him as he is. Self-esteem can be reduced or destroyed by parents who become overconcerned about their child's weight. Avoid the following pitfalls:

- Don't tell your child he's fat. Don't discuss his weight unless he brings it up.
- Never try to put your child on a strict diet. Diets are unpleasant and should be self-imposed.
- Never deprive your child of food if he says he is hungry. Withholding food eventually leads to overeating.
- Don't nag him about his weight or eating habits.

Setting Weight-Loss Goals

Pick a realistic target weight, depending on your child's bone structure and degree of obesity. The loss of 1 pound per week is an attainable goal, but your child will have to work quite hard to maintain this rate of weight loss for several weeks. Have your child weigh himself no more than once each week; daily weighings generate too much false hope or disappointment. Keeping a record of weekly weights may provide added motivation. When losing weight becomes a strain, have your child take a few weeks off from the weight-loss program. During this time, try to help your child stay at a constant weight.

Once your child has reached the target weight, the long-range goal is to try to stay within 5 pounds of that weight. Staying at a particular weight is possible only through permanent moderation in eating and maintaining a reasonable exercise program. Your child will probably always have the tendency to gain weight easily and it's important that he understand this.

Diet: Decreasing Calorie Consumption

Your child should eat three well-balanced meals of average-size portions every day. There are no forbidden foods; your child can have a serving of anything family or friends are eating. However, there are forbidden portions. While your child is reducing, she must leave the table a bit hungry. Your child cannot lose weight if she eats until full (satiated).

Encourage average portions and discourage seconds. Shortcuts such as fasting, crash dieting, and diet pills rarely work and may be dangerous. Liquid diets are safe only if used according to directions. If you have any questions, consult a dietitian.

Calorie counting is helpful for some people, but it is usually too time consuming. Consider the following guidelines on what to eat and drink:

- Fluids: Mainly use low-calorie drinks such as skim milk, fruit juice diluted in half with water, diet drinks, or flavored mineral water. Because milk has

Instructions for Pediatric Patients, 2nd Edition, ©1999 by WB Saunders Company.
Written by Barton D. Schmitt, MD, pediatrician and author of *Your Child's Health*, Bantam Books, a book for parents.

lots of calories, your child should drink no more than 16 ounces of skim or low-fat milk each day. Since fruit juices and 2% milk have similar calories per ounce, keep juice consumption to 8 ounces or less per day. All other drinks should be either water or diet drinks. Encourage your child to drink six glasses of water each day.

- Meals: Serve fewer fatty foods (for example, eggs, bacon, sausage, butter). A portion of fat has twice as many calories as the same portion of protein or carbohydrate. Trim the fat off meats. Serve more baked, broiled, boiled, or steamed foods and fewer fried foods. Serve more fruits, vegetables, salads, and grains.
- Desserts: Encourage smaller-than-average portions. Encourage more gelatin and fresh fruits as desserts. Avoid rich desserts. Do not serve seconds.
- Snacks: Serve only low-calorie foods such as raw vegetables (carrot sticks, celery sticks, raw potato sticks, pickles), raw fruits (apples, oranges, cantaloupe), popcorn, or diet soft drinks. Limit snacks to two each day.
- Vitamins: Give your child one multivitamin tablet daily during the weight-loss program.

Eating Habits

To counteract the tendency to gain weight, your youngster must be taught eating habits that will last for a lifetime. You can help your child lose and keep off unwanted pounds by doing the following:

- Discourage skipping any of the three basic meals.
- Encourage drinking a glass of water before meals.
- Serve smaller portions.
- Suggest chewing the food slowly.
- Offer second servings only if your child has waited for 10 minutes after finishing the first serving.
- Don't purchase high-calorie snack foods such as potato chips, candy, or regular soft drinks.
- Do purchase and keep available diet soft drinks and fresh fruits and vegetables.
- Leave only low-calorie snacks out on the counter—fruit, for example. Put away the cookie jar.
- Store food only in the kitchen. Keep it out of other rooms.
- Offer no more than two snacks each day. Discourage your child from continual snacking ("grazing") throughout the day.
- Allow eating in your home only at the kitchen or dining-room table. Discourage eating while watching television, studying, riding in a car, or shopping. Once eating becomes associated with these activities, the body learns to expect it.

- Discourage eating alone.
- Help your child reward herself for hard work or studying with a movie, television, music, or a book rather than food.
- Put up reminder cards on the refrigerator and bathroom mirror that state: *Eat less.*

Exercise: Increasing Calorie Expenditure

Daily exercise can increase the rate of weight loss as well as the sense of physical well-being. The combination of diet and exercise is the most effective way to lose weight. Try the following forms of exercise:

- Walk or bike instead of riding in a car.
- Use stairs instead of elevators.
- Learn new sports. Swimming and jogging are the sports that burn the most calories. Your child's school may have an aerobic class.
- Take the dog for a long walk.
- Spend 30 minutes daily exercising or dancing to records or music on television.
- Use an exercise bike or Hula-Hoop while watching television. (Limit television sitting time to 2 hours or less each day.)

Social Activities: Keeping the Mind Off Food

The more outside activities your child participates in, the easier it will be for her to lose weight. Spare time fosters nibbling. Most snacking occurs between 3 and 6 PM. Help your child fill after-school time with activities such as music, drama, sports, or scouts. A part-time job after school may help. If nothing else, encourage your child to call or visit friends. An active social life almost always leads to weight reduction.

 CALL OUR OFFICE

During regular hours if
- Your child has not improved his eating and exercise habits after trying this program for 2 months.
- Your child is a compulsive overeater.
- You find yourself frequently nagging your child about his eating habits.
- Your child is trying to lose weight and doesn't need to do so.
- You think your child is depressed.
- Your child has no close friends.
- You have other questions or concerns.

OVERWEIGHT: PREVENTION IN INFANTS

DEFINITION

An overweight baby is one with a weight gain far out of proportion to height gain. An overweight baby looks fat. Such a baby is not necessarily a healthy one. The infants who continue to be overweight as children and adults usually have parents, siblings, or grandparents who are overweight. Any infant with a strong family tendency toward obesity needs help. Overfeeding teaches a child to overeat. Some physicians wait until such a child shows signs of being overweight before making any alterations in the diet, but prevention is easier than treatment.

DIETARY PRECAUTIONS TO PREVENT AN EXCESSIVE WEIGHT GAIN IN INFANTS

If someone in your family has a problem with easy weight gain, consider the following dietary precautions to prevent your baby from becoming overweight. If your child is already overweight, these guidelines will also be helpful. The goal for growing children is always slowing the rate of weight gain (not weight loss).

- From the beginning, try to teach your child to stop eating before she reaches a point of satiation. Help her stop before she has a sense of complete fullness and a reluctance to eat another bite. When she closes her mouth, turns her head, or wants to play, she's losing interest in feeding.
- Try to breast-feed. Breast-fed babies tend to be lighter in weight.
- If you are breast-feeding, avoid grazing. Grazing is nursing at frequent intervals, sometimes hourly. Such infants learn to eat when they are upset and to use food as a stress reliever.
- If you are bottle-feeding, don't allow your child to keep a bottle as a companion during the day or night. Children who are allowed to carry a bottle around with them learn to eat frequently and use food as a comforting device.
- Don't feed your baby every time she cries. Most crying babies want to be held and cuddled or may be thirsty and just need some water.
- Also teach your infant to use human contact (rather than food) to relieve stress and discomfort.
- Don't assume a sucking baby is hungry. Your baby may just want a pacifier or help with finding her thumb. Also, don't use teething biscuits or other foods in place of a teething ring.
- Don't insist that your baby finish every bottle. Unless your baby is underweight, she knows how much formula she needs.
- Don't enlarge the hole in the nipple of a baby bottle. The formula will come out of the bottle too fast.
- Feed your infant no more often than every 2 hours at birth and no more often than every 3 hours from 2 to 6 months of age.
- Feed your child slowly rather than rapidly. Don't do anything to hurry your child's pace of eating. It takes 15 to 20 minutes for the sensation of fullness to develop. The rapid-eating habit in adults has been associated with obesity.
- Avoid solids until your child is 4 months old (6 months old in breast-fed babies).
- Change to three meals daily by 6 months of age.
- Don't insist that your child clean her plate or finish a jar of baby food.
- Don't encourage your child to eat more after she signals she is full by turning her head or not opening her mouth.
- Discontinue breast- and bottle-feeding by 12 months of age. A study by Dr. W. S. Agras found that delayed weaning was associated with more obesity.
- Avoid sweets until at least 12 months of age.
- Don't give your child food as a way to distract her or keep her occupied. Instead, give her something to play with when you need some free time.
- Use praise and physical contact instead of food as a reward for good behavior.

Caution: Also don't underfeed your infant. Don't put your baby on low-fat milk or skim milk before 2 years of age. Your baby's brain is growing rapidly and needs the fat content of whole milk. While overfeeding is more common than underfeeding in infancy, underfeeding is more harmful.

 ## CALL OUR OFFICE

During regular hours if
- You are uncertain whether your infant is overweight.
- You are concerned about your infant's weight gain.

Instructions for Pediatric Patients, 2nd Edition, ©1999 by WB Saunders Company.
Written by Barton D. Schmitt, MD, pediatrician and author of *Your Child's Health,* Bantam Books, a book for parents.

PART 3

PREVENTIVE PEDIATRICS

Antibiotics are strong medicines that can kill bacteria. They have saved many lives and prevented many serious complications. However, antibiotics have no impact on viral infections. One of the more important decisions made daily by every physician is whether a child's infection is viral or bacterial. Parents can learn to make some of these decisions themselves.

VIRAL INFECTIONS

Viruses cause most infections in children:

- All colds
- All cases of croup
- Most (99%) coughs
- Most (95%) fevers
- Most (90%) sore throats
- Ninety-nine percent of diarrhea and vomiting

BACTERIAL INFECTIONS

Bacterial infections are much less common than viral infections. Bacteria cause

- Most ear infections
- Most sinus infections
- Ten percent of sore throats (strep throat)
- Whooping cough (pertussis)
- Some pneumonia (lung infection)

Some symptoms are overrated as indicators of a bacterial infection. Yellow nasal discharge is more likely to be a normal part of the recovery from a cold than a clue to a sinus infection. Yellow phlegm (sputum) is a normal part of a viral tracheitis or bronchitis, not a sign of pneumonia. High fevers can be due to a virus or bacteria.

PREVENTION OF BACTERIAL INFECTIONS

Another false belief is that children with colds need antibiotics to prevent ear or sinus infections. In some cases the antibiotic does work, but in most cases the antibiotic just selects out a resistant germ to cause a secondary bacterial infection. It's smarter to save the antibiotic for those children who go on to develop a bacterial infection. After a cold, about 10% of children develop an ear infection (otitis media) and 1% develop a sinus infection (sinusitis). Why give antibiotics to the other 89% who don't need them?

BACTERIAL RESISTANCE

When bacteria become resistant to an antibiotic, that antibiotic can no longer kill that type of bacteria. Excessive use of antibiotics is the number one cause of resistant strains of bacteria, and research shows that 50% of prescriptions for antibiotics are inappropriate (mainly when they are given for coughs and colds). This makes future treatment of bacterial infections more difficult. Many bacteria are now resistant to antibiotics that used to control them. When we turn to newer and more expensive antibiotics, bacteria develop resistance to them as well. In the battle between antibiotics and bacteria, the bacteria seem to be winning.

SIDE EFFECTS OF ANTIBIOTICS

If your child doesn't need an antibiotic, giving him one is a bad idea, because all antibiotics have side effects. Some children taking antibiotics develop diarrhea, nausea, vomiting, or a rash. If a rash occurs, we are left with the difficult question: is it a drug allergy or an unrelated viral rash (such as roseola)? Since it's difficult to be sure, many children are mislabeled as allergic to a family of antibiotics, and a potentially useful antibiotic is not available when the child really needs it.

SUMMARY

Don't wish your child were on an antibiotic unless he or she really needs one. Don't pressure your child's doctor for an antibiotic. If your child has a viral illness, an antibiotic will not shorten the course of the fever or help the other symptoms. Antibiotics will not get your child back to school or you back to work sooner. If your child develops side effects from the antibiotic, he or she will feel worse instead of better.

Let's save antibiotics for ear infections, sinus infections, strep throat, and other bacterial infections. Let's not waste them on yellow nasal discharge, yellow phlegm, high fevers, and other normal symptoms associated with coughs and colds. Treat your child's symptoms with over-the-counter medicines or home remedies. Many just need extra TLC (tender loving care) until they feel better. Call back if your child develops any new signs that suggest a bacterial illness. Usually antibiotics are not the answer when your child becomes sick.

Instructions for Pediatric Patients, 2nd Edition, ©1999 by WB Saunders Company.
Written by Barton D. Schmitt, MD, pediatrician and author of *Your Child's Health*, Bantam Books, a book for parents.

CAR SAFETY SEATS

The major killer as well as the major crippler of children in the United States is motor vehicle crashes. Approximately 700 children under the age of 5 years are killed each year, and about 60,000 are injured. Proper use of car safety seats can reduce traffic fatalities by at least 80%. All 50 states have passed laws that require children to ride in approved safety seats.

A parent cannot protect a child by holding her tightly. In a 30-mph crash, the child will either be crushed between the parent's body and the dashboard or ripped from the parent's arms and possibly thrown from the car. Car safety seats also help to control a child's misbehavior, prevent motion sickness, and reduce the number of accidents caused by a child distracting the driver.

CHOOSING A CAR SAFETY SEAT

Types of Car Safety Seats

There are three types of car safety seats:

- Infant safety seats are installed in a rear-facing position only and can be used from birth until a child weighs approximately 20 pounds.
- Convertible safety seats can be used in both rear- and forward-facing positions.
- Booster safety seats are forward facing.

Matching Car Safety Seats with Your Child's Weight

- Birth to 20 pounds: Use an infant safety seat until your child is over 20 pounds and able to sit up alone. Keep your child facing backward as long as possible because it protects her from neck injuries.
- Over 20 pounds: Use a convertible car seat in the forward-facing position. Keep it rear-facing if the child is less than 1 year of age.
- Over 40 pounds and over 40 inches tall: Use a booster safety seat. A booster seat is needed when your child has outgrown the convertible safety seat but is too small to fit properly into the regular seat belt. This also enables your child to see out the window.
- Over 60 pounds: Use the regular car seat (without a booster seat) and with a lap belt low across the thighs. To add a shoulder strap, your child also needs to be over 4 feet (48 inches) tall. Using a shoulder strap before your child is 4 feet tall can cause neck injuries. If the shoulder strap runs across the neck (rather than the shoulder), your child needs to stay in a booster seat. Never put the shoulder belt under both arms or behind your child's back.

INSTALLATION OF CAR SAFETY SEATS

- Always follow the manufacturer's directions for installation and use of the car seat: improper installation or use will not protect your child.
- Whenever possible and at any age, put the safety seat in the back seat of the car, which is much safer than the front seat.
- For cars with air bags, infants riding in **rear**-facing child safety seats should **never** be placed in the front seat of a car or truck with a passenger-side air bag. They must be in the car's rear seat or they must not ride in that vehicle. Air bags have saved many lives, but they are very hazardous to infants in rear-facing child safety seats. If the air bag opens, the child will be caught in the air bag and could suffocate.
- For cars with air bags, children in **forward**-facing child safety seats should also ride in a car's rear seat. If the vehicle does not have a rear seat, children riding in the front seat should be positioned as far back as possible from the air bag. Move the seat all the way back to maximize the child's distance from the dashboard.

USING A CAR SAFETY SEAT PROPERLY*

If used consistently and properly, your child's safety seat can be a lifesaver. Your attitude toward safety belts and car safety seats is especially important. If you treat buckling up as a necessary, automatic routine, your child will follow your lead and also accept safety seats and seat belts. To keep your child safe and happy, follow these guidelines:

- Always use the safety seat. Use the safety seat on the first ride home from the hospital, and continue using it for every ride.
- Everyone buckles up! Allow *no* exceptions for older kids and adults. If adults ride unprotected, the child quickly decides that safety is just kid stuff.
- Give praise for appropriate behavior in the car.
- A bored child can become disruptive. Keep a supply of favorite soft toys and munchies on hand.
- *Never* let a fussy child out of the car seat or safety belt while the car is in motion. If your child needs a break, *stop* the car. Responding to complaints by allowing your child to ride unprotected is a disastrous decision that will make it harder to keep him in the seat on the next ride.
- If a child tries to get out of the seat, stop the car and firmly but calmly explain that you won't start the car until he is again buckled in the car seat.
- Make a vinyl seat pad more comfortable in hot weather by covering it with a cloth pad or towel.
- When your child travels in another person's car (such as a babysitter's or grandparent's), insist that the driver also place your child in a safety seat.
- For long-distance trips, plan for frequent stops and try to stop before your child becomes restless. Cuddle a young child; let an older child snack and run around for 10 to 15 minutes.

*Adapted from the American Academy of Pediatrics with permission, 1996.

Instructions for Pediatric Patients, 2nd Edition, ©1999 by WB Saunders Company. Written by Barton D. Schmitt, MD, pediatrician and author of *Your Child's Health*, Bantam Books, a book for parents.

DEFINITION

Description

- This tooth decay is in the baby teeth.
- The upper front teeth (incisors) are usually damaged first.
- Although the process starts soon after tooth eruption, it is often not noticed until about 1 year of age.
- White spots on the baby teeth is the earliest sign.
- This is the main type of tooth decay in infants.
- The infant is allowed to have a bottle in the bed (a crib bottle).
- The older infant or toddler is allowed to carry a bottle around during the day (a tote bottle).

Cause

Baby bottle tooth decay (BBTD) is caused by prolonged contact with sugar in liquid. Milk, formula, juice, Kool-Aid, and soft drinks all contain sugar. If your child falls asleep with a bottle in his or her mouth or constantly drinks from a bottle during the day, the sugar coats the upper teeth. The normal bacteria in the mouth change the sugar to an acid. Because the enamel of baby teeth is only half the thickness of an eggshell, the acid gradually dissolves the enamel and allows decay to occur in the underlying tooth structure.

The availability of plastic bottles instead of glass bottles has led many parents to be less concerned about giving their infant a bottle. A bottle of formula or juice is a quick way to help a child go to sleep at night or to deal with middle-of-the-night crying. It also becomes a handy way to deal with fussiness during the daytime. Many parents are unaware of the side effects of allowing a child to sip from a bottle.

Expected Outcome

If BBTD is not detected and treated, decay will eventually destroy the teeth and they will break off at the gumline. The decay will continue to destroy the root of the tooth and cause ongoing pain. Dental repair of BBTD requires general anesthesia. If the problem is detected at an early level, the teeth can be covered with stainless steel caps. If the decay is severe, the teeth will need to be pulled out. The child will then have to chew with the teeth on the side of the mouth and may also be teased about the missing teeth in front. The baby teeth are important because they save the appropriate space for the permanent teeth to fill later. If they are lost too early, the permanent teeth may come in crooked or be crowded.

HOW TO PROTECT YOUR CHILD FROM BABY BOTTLE TOOTH DECAY

1. **Never give your infant a crib bottle.** Don't bottle-feed your baby until she falls asleep. It is the most common cause of bottle dependency and it eventually will cause sleep problems because your child will expect bottle-feeding as a transition into sleep, even following normal awakenings during the night. Separate the last bottle-feeding of the evening from bedtime. Even though baby teeth don't start coming in until 6 months, don't start a bad habit that will later need to be broken. In general, don't allow your infant to ever think that the bottle is her property. You won't voluntarily get it back.
2. **Don't allow your infant to have a tote or companion bottle during the day.** Don't substitute a bottle for a pacifier, security object, toy, or being held. Give a bottle only during mealtimes.
3. **Introduce a cup by 6 months of age.** Introducing a cup is the best way to prevent bottle dependency. Don't expect self-initiated weaning unless a child has been exposed to a cup. Also don't expect weaning to occur in a day or a week. It takes gradual exposure to a cup over 3 months or longer for a child to learn to prefer the cup over the bottle.
4. **If your infant has developed a bottle habit, continue to offer it, but fill it only with water.** Water cannot harm the tooth enamel. Water is also boring and will help your child eventually give up the bottle. The bottle itself is not harmful.

 CALL OUR OFFICE

During regular hours if
- Your child cannot give up the bottle.
- You see white spots on the baby teeth.
- You think your child might have BBTD.
- You have other questions or concerns.

TOOTH DECAY: PREVENTION

Tooth decay causes toothaches, lost teeth, malocclusion, and costly visits to the dentist. Fortunately, modern dentistry can prevent 80% to 90% of tooth decay.

FLUORIDE

Fluoride builds strong, decay-resistant enamel. Fluoride is needed from 6 months to 16 years of age (1995 American Dental Association recommendation). Drinking fluoridated water (containing 0.7 to 1.2 parts per million) or taking a prescription fluoride supplement is the best protection against tooth decay, reducing cavities by 70%.

If fluoride is consumed in drinking water, a child must take at least 1 pint per day (preferably 1 quart per day by school age).

If your city's water supply doesn't have fluoride added or you are breast-feeding, ask your physician for a prescription for fluoride drops or tablets during your next routine visit. The dosage of fluoride required for prevention of tooth decay is 0.25 mg per day in the first 3 years; 0.5 mg from 3 to 6 years of age; and 1.0 mg over age 6. Give fluoride on an empty stomach, because mixing it with milk reduces its absorption to 70%.

Bottled water usually doesn't contain adequate fluoride. Call the producer for information. If your child drinks bottled water containing less than 0.7 parts per million of fluoride, ask your child's physician for a fluoride supplement.

Fluoride is safe. Over half of all Americans drink fluoridated water. Fluoride has been added to water supplies for over 50 years.

One concern about fluoride is white spots or mottling on the teeth (fluorosis). This can occur when a child ingests 2 mg or more per day. The preventive dose is 1 mg or less. Children can ingest excessive fluoride if they receive supplements when it is already present in the city water supply. Occasionally they ingest it by eating toothpaste. A ribbon of toothpaste contains about 1 mg of fluoride. Therefore people of all ages should use only a drop of toothpaste the size of a pea. This precaution and encouraging your child not to swallow the toothpaste will prevent fluorosis.

TOOTHBRUSHING AND FLOSSING

The purpose of toothbrushing is to remove plaque from the teeth. Plaque is an invisible scum that forms on the surface of teeth. Within this plaque, mouth bacteria change sugars to acids, which in turn etches the enamel.

- Toothbrushing should begin before 1 year of age.
- Help your child brush at least until 6 years of age. Most children don't have the coordination to brush their own teeth adequately before then.
- Try to brush after each meal, but especially after the last meal or snack of the day.
- To prevent mouth bacteria from changing food caught in the teeth into acid, brush the teeth within the first 5 to 10 minutes after meals.
- Brush the molars (back teeth) carefully. Decay usually starts in the pits and crevices there.
- If your child is negative about toothbrushing, have him brush your teeth first before you brush his.
- A fluoride toothpaste is beneficial. People of all ages tend to use too much toothpaste; a drop the size of a pea is all that is needed.
- If your child is in a setting where she can't brush her teeth, teach her to rinse her mouth with water after meals instead.
- Dental floss is very useful for cleaning between the teeth where a brush can't reach. Flossing should begin when your child's molars start to touch. In the early years, most of the teeth have spaces between them.

DIET

A healthy diet from a dental standpoint is one that keeps the sugar concentration in the mouth at a low level. The worst foods contain sugar and also stick to the teeth.

- Prevent baby-bottle caries by not letting your infant sleep with a bottle of milk or juice. If your baby, after the teeth erupt, must have a bottle at night, it should contain only water. It is better to put your child to bed after finishing the bottle.
- Discourage prolonged contact with sugar (e.g., hard candy) or any sweets that are sticky (e.g., caramels or raisins).
- Avoid frequent snacks.
- Give sugar-containing foods only with meals.
- Parents worry needlessly about soft drinks. The sugar in these products does not bind to the teeth and is cleared rather rapidly from the mouth.
- Since no one can keep children away from candy completely, try to teach your child to brush after eating it.

DENTIST VISITS

The American Dental Association recommends that dental checkups begin at 3 years of age (sooner for dental symptoms or abnormal-looking teeth).

DENTAL SEALANTS

The latest breakthrough in dental research is dental sealing of the pits and fissures of the biting surfaces of the molars. Fluoride does little to prevent decay on these surfaces. A special plastic seal can be applied to the top surfaces of the permanent molars at about 6 years of age. The seal may protect against decay for 10 to 20 years without needing replacement. Ask your child's dentist about the latest recommendations.

Instructions for Pediatric Patients, 2nd Edition, ©1999 by WB Saunders Company.
Written by Barton D. Schmitt, MD, pediatrician and author of *Your Child's Health,* Bantam Books, a book for parents.

OVERVIEW OF DEVELOPMENT

The most rapid changes in development occur during the first year of life. A baby grows from a helpless little bundle into a walking, talking, unique personality. Almost all parents wonder if their baby is developing at the right pace. There is wide variation in normal development. Although the average child walks at 12 months, the normal age for walking is any time between 9 and 16 months of age. Motor development occurs in an orderly sequence, starting with lifting the head, then rolling over, sitting up, crawling, standing, and walking. Although the sequence is predictable and follows the maturation of the spinal cord downward, the rate at which these stages happen varies. Speech develops from cooing to babbling, to imitating speech sounds, to first words, to using words together. Again, however, the rate can normally vary considerably.

The most reassuring signs that a child is developing normally are an alert facial expression, alert eyes, and curiosity about his surroundings. The main determinant of a child's social, emotional, and language development is the amount of positive contact he has with the parents. The expressions that your baby experiences during the first 3 years of life determine permanent wiring of the brain.

WAYS TO STIMULATE YOUR CHILD'S NORMAL DEVELOPMENT

1. **Hold your baby as much as possible.** Touching and cuddling is good for your baby. Give him lots of eye contact, smiles, and affection. Use feedings as a special opportunity for these warm personal interactions.
2. **Talk to your baby.** Babies of all ages enjoy being talked and sung to. Babies must first hear language before they can use it themselves. You don't need a script—just put into words whatever you are thinking and feeling.
3. **Play with your baby.** If this doesn't come easy for you, try to loosen up and rediscover your free spirit. Respond to your baby's attempts to initiate play. Provide your baby with various objects of interest. Toys need not be expensive, for example, homemade mobiles, rattles, spools, pots and pans, and boxes. Encourage your baby's efforts at discovering how to use his hands and mind.
4. **Read to your baby.** Even 4-month-olds enjoy looking at pictures in a book. Cut out interesting pictures from magazines and put them in a scrapbook for your baby. Look at the family photo album. By 8 months of age, begin reading stories to your child.
5. **Show your baby the world.** Enrich his experi-ence. Point out leaves, clouds, stars, and rainbows. Help your toddler describe what he sees or experiences. Everything we see or do has a name.
6. **Provide your child with social experiences with other children by age 2 years.** If he is not in day care, consider starting or joining a play group. Young children can learn important lessons from each other, especially how to get along with other people.
7. **Avoid formal teaching until age 4 or 5.** Some groups have recently overemphasized academic (cognitive) development of young children. The effort to create "superkids" through special lessons, drills, computer programs, and classes can put undue pressure on young children and may result in an early loss of interest in learning. Old-fashioned creative play and spontaneous learning provide a foundation for later academic efforts and are much more beneficial during the early years.

 CALL OUR OFFICE

During regular hours if your child does not meet the following developmental milestones*

1. **Speech and hearing**
   - Makes gurgling, cooing, or babbling sounds by age 3 months
   - Turns head to quiet sounds or whispers by age 9 months
   - Makes "ma-ma" and "da-da" sounds by age 12 months
   - Uses at least three specific words by age 2 years

2. **Fine motor skills**
   - Plays with hands by touching them together by age 6 months
   - Uses fingers to put pieces of food in mouth by age 12 months
   - Uses a cup without spilling by age 18 months

3. **Gross motor skills**
   - Rolls over by age 6 months
   - Sits without support by age 9 months
   - Supports own weight on legs when held by parent under the arms by age 9 months
   - Walks across a large room without help by age 18 months

*From Milestones, reprinted with permission of William K. Frankenburg, M.D.

Some emergency symptoms are either difficult to recognize or are not considered serious by some parents. Most parents will not overlook or underestimate the importance of a major burn, major bleeding, choking, a convulsion, or a coma. However, if your child has any of the following symptoms, also contact our office immediately.

Sick Newborn. If your baby is less than 1 month old and sick in any way, the problem could be serious.

Severe Lethargy. Fatigue during an illness is normal, but watch to see if your child stares into space, won't smile, won't play, is too weak to cry, is floppy, or is hard to awaken. These are serious symptoms.

Severe Pain. If your child cries when you touch or move her, this can be a symptom of meningitis. A child with meningitis also doesn't want to be held. Constant screaming and inability to sleep also point to severe pain.

Can't Walk. If your child has learned to walk and then loses the ability to stand or walk, he or she probably has a serious injury to the legs or an acute problem with balance. If your child walks bent over, holding his or her abdomen, he or she probably has a serious abdominal problem such as appendicitis.

Tender Abdomen. Press on your child's belly while he or she is sitting in your lap and looking at a book. Normally you should be able to press an inch or so in with your fingers in all parts of the belly without resistance. It is significant if your child pushes your hand away or screams. If the belly is also bloated and hard, the condition is even more dangerous.

Tender Testicle or Scrotum. The sudden onset of pain in the groin can be from twisting (torsion) of the testicle. This requires surgery within 8 hours to save the testicle.

Labored Breathing. You should assess your child's breathing after you have cleaned out the nose and when he or she is not coughing. If your child has difficulty in breathing, tight croup, or obvious wheezing, she needs to be seen immediately. Other signs of respiratory difficulty are a breathing rate of more than 60 breaths/minute, bluish lips, or retractions (pulling in between the ribs).

Bluish Lips. Bluish lips or cyanosis can indicate a reduced amount of oxygen in the bloodstream.

Drooling. The sudden onset of drooling or spitting, especially associated with difficulty in swallowing, can mean that your child has a serious infection of the tonsils, throat, or epiglottis (top part of the windpipe).

Dehydration. Dehydration means that your child's body fluids are low. Dehydration usually follows severe vomiting or diarrhea. Suspect dehydration if your child has not urinated in 8 hours; crying produces no tears; the mouth is dry rather than moist; or the soft spot in the skull is sunken. Dehydration requires immediate fluid replacement by mouth or intravenously.

Bulging Soft Spot. If the anterior fontanel is tense and bulging, the brain is under pressure. Since the fontanel normally bulges with crying, assess it when your child is quiet and in an upright position.

Stiff Neck. To test for a stiff neck, lay your child down, then lift the head until the chin touches the middle of the chest. If he or she is resistant, place a toy or other object of interest on the belly so he or she will have to look down to see it. A stiff neck can be an early sign of meningitis.

Injured Neck. Discuss any injury to the neck, regardless of symptoms, with your child's physician because of the risk of damage to the spinal cord.

Purple Spots. Purple or blood-red spots or dots on the skin can be a sign of a serious bloodstream infection, with the exception of explained bruises, of course.

Fever Over 105°F (40.6°C). All the preceding symptoms are stronger indicators of serious illness than the level of fever. All of them can occur with low fevers as well as high ones.

Fevers become strong indicators of serious infection only when the temperature rises above 105°F (40.6°C). In infants, a rectal temperature less than 97.5°F (36.5°C) can also be serious.

Instructions for Pediatric Patients, 2nd Edition, ©1999 by WB Saunders Company.
Written by Barton D. Schmitt, MD, pediatrician and author of *Your Child's Health*, Bantam Books, a book for parents.

DEFINITION

Your child has a fever if any of the following apply:

- Rectal temperature is over 100.4°F (38.0°C).
- Oral temperature is over 99.5°F (37.5°C).
- Axillary (armpit) temperature is over 99.0°F (37.2°C).
- Ear (tympanic) temperature (taken in the ear) is over 100.4°F (38.0°C) (if set in rectal mode), or > 99.5°F (37.5°C) (if set in oral mode). (*Note*: Not reliable if your child is less than 6 months old.)
- Pacifier temperature is over 99.5°F (37.5°C). (*Note*: Not accurate in general. New digital ones are accurate. This mode is okay for screening if your child is over 3 months old.)
- Tactile fever (the impression that your child has a fever because he or she feels hot to the touch) is evident. Tactile fevers are more accurate than we used to think; however, if you're going to call your child's doctor about a fever, actually take his or her temperature.

The body's average temperature when it is measured orally is 98.6°F (37°C), but it normally fluctuates during the day. Mild elevation (100.4° to 101.3°F or 38° to 38.5°C) can be caused by exercise, excessive clothing, a hot bath, or hot weather. Warm food or drink can also raise the oral temperature. If you suspect such an effect on the temperature of your child, take his or her temperature again in one-half hour.

Causes

Fever is a symptom, not a disease. Fever is the body's normal response to infections and plays a role in fighting them. Fever turns on the body's immune system. The usual fevers (100° to 104°F [37.8° to 40°C]) that all children get are not harmful. Most are caused by viral illnesses; some are caused by bacterial illnesses. Teething does not cause fever.

Expected Course

Most fevers with viral illnesses range between 101° and 104°F (38.3° to 40°C) and last for 2 to 3 days. In general, the height of the fever doesn't relate to the seriousness of the illness. How sick your child acts is what counts. Fever causes no permanent harm until it reaches 107°F (41.7°C). Fortunately, the brain's thermostat keeps untreated fevers below this level.

Although all children get fevers, only 4% develop a brief febrile convulsion. Since this type of seizure is generally harmless, it is not worth worrying excessively about. If your child has had high fevers without seizures, your child is probably safe.

HOME CARE

Treat All Fevers with Extra Fluids and Less Clothing. Encourage your child to drink extra fluids, but do not force him or her to drink. Popsicles and iced drinks are helpful. Body fluids are lost during fevers because of sweating.

Clothing should be kept to a minimum because most heat is lost through the skin. Do not bundle up your child; it will cause a higher fever. During the time your child feels cold or is shivering (the chills), give him or her a light blanket.

Acetaminophen Products for Reducing Fever. Children older than 2 months of age can be given any one of the acetaminophen products. All have the same dosage.

Remember that fever is helping your child fight the infection. Use drugs only if the fever is over 102°F (39°C) and preferably only if your child is also uncomfortable. Give the correct dosage for your child's age every 4 to 6 hours, but no more often.

Two hours after they are given, these drugs will reduce the fever 2° to 3°F (1° to 1.5°C). Medicines do not bring the temperature down to normal unless the temperature was not very elevated before the medicine was given. Repeated dosages of the drugs will be necessary because the fever will go up and down until the illness runs its course. If your child is sleeping, don't awaken him for medicines.

Caution: The dropper that comes with one product should not be used with other brands.

Dosages of Acetaminophen. See accompanying table.

Ibuprofen Products. All ibuprofen products are now available without a prescription. Give the correct dosage for your child's weight every 6 to 8 hours as needed. (See accompanying table.)

Ibuprofen and acetaminophen are similar in their abilities to lower fever, and their safety records are similar. One advantage that ibuprofen has over acetaminophen is a longer-lasting effect (6 to 8 hours instead of 4 to 6 hours). However, acetaminophen is still the drug of choice for controlling fever in most

ACETAMINOPHEN DOSAGE (FOR FEVER AND PAIN)

Child's weight (lb) more than	7	14	21	28	42	56	84	112
Total amount (mg)	40	80	120	160	240	325	458	650
Drops (80 mg per dropper)	½	1	1½	2	3	—	—	—
Syrup 160 mg/5 mL (1 tsp)	—	½	¾	1	1½	2	2½	4
Chewable 80-mg tablets	—	—	1½	2	3	4	5–6	8
Chewable 160-mg tablets	—	—	—	1	1½	2	3	4
Adult 325-mg tablets	—	—	—	—	—	1	1–1½	2

IBUPROFEN DOSAGE (FOR FEVER AND PAIN)								
Child's weight (lb) more than	12	18	24	36	48	60	72	96
Total amount (mg)	50	75	100	150	200	250	300	400
Drops (50 mg per dropper)	1	1½	2	3	4	—	—	—
Liquid 100 mg/5 ml (1 tsp)	½	¾	1	1½	2	2½	3	4
Chewable 50-mg tablets	—	—	2	3	4	5	6	8
Adult 200-mg tablets	—	—	—	—	1	1	1½	2

conditions. Children with special problems requiring a longer period of fever control may do better with ibuprofen.

Avoid Aspirin. The American Academy of Pediatrics has recommended that children (through 21 years of age) not take aspirin if they have chickenpox or influenza (any cold, cough, or sore throat symptoms). This recommendation is based on several studies that have linked aspirin to Reye's syndrome, a severe encephalitis-like illness. Most pediatricians have stopped using aspirin for fevers associated with any illness.

ALTERNATING ACETAMINOPHEN AND IBUPROFEN

We don't recommend combining these medicines for the following reasons:

- No added benefit in reducing fever compared with either product used alone. (Reason: both drugs have the same mechanism of action.)
- Can cause dosage errors and poisoning (especially if you give one product too frequently).
- You don't need to control fever this closely.
- If you are instructed by your physician to alternate both products, do it as follows:
  - Use both if the fever is over 104°F (40°C) and unresponsive to one medicine alone.
  - Give a fever medicine every 4 hours (acetaminophen every 8 hours and ibuprofen every 8 hours).
  - Only alternate medicines for 24 hours or less, then return to a single product.

Sponging. Sponging is usually not necessary to reduce fever. Never sponge your child without giving her acetaminophen first. Sponge immediately only in emergencies such as heatstroke, delirium, a seizure from fever, or any fever over 106°F (41.1°C). In other cases sponge your child only if the fever is over 104°F (40°C), the fever stays that high when you take the temperature again 30 minutes after your child has taken acetaminophen or ibuprofen, and your child is uncomfortable. Until acetaminophen has taken effect (by resetting the body's thermostat to a lower level), sponging will just cause shivering, which is the body's attempt to raise the temperature.

If you do sponge your child, sponge her in lukewarm water (85° to 90°F [29° to 32°C]). (Use slightly cooler water for emergencies.) Sponging works much faster than immersion, so sit your child in 2 inches of water and keep wetting the skin surface. Cooling comes from evaporation of the water. If your child shivers, raise the water temperature or wait for the acetaminophen to take effect. Don't expect to get the temperature below 101°F (38.3°C). Don't add rubbing alcohol to the water; it can be breathed in and cause a coma.

 CALL OUR OFFICE

IMMEDIATELY if
- Your child is less than 3 months old.
- The fever is over 105°F (40.6°C).
- Your child looks or acts very sick.

Within 24 hours if
- Your child is 3 to 6 months old (unless the fever is due to a diphtheria-pertussis-tetanus (DPT) shot).
- The fever is between 104° and 105°F (40° to 40.6°C), especially if your child is less than 2 years old.
- Your child has had a fever more than 24 hours without an obvious cause or location of infection.
- Your child has had a fever more than 3 days.
- The fever went away for more than 24 hours and then returned.
- You have other concerns or questions.

Instructions for Pediatric Patients, 2nd Edition, ©1999 by WB Saunders Company.
Written by Barton D. Schmitt, MD, pediatrician and author of *Your Child's Health,* Bantam Books, a book for parents.

TAKING THE TEMPERATURE

Obtaining an accurate measurement of your child's temperature requires some practice. If you have questions about this procedure, ask a physician or nurse to demonstrate how it's done and then to observe you doing the same.

Shaking a Glass Thermometer. Shake until the mercury line is below 98.6°F (37°C).

Where to Take the Temperature

- Rectal temperatures are the most accurate. Oral or eardrum temperatures are also accurate if done properly. Axillary (armpit) temperatures are the least accurate but are better than no measurement.
- For a child younger than 5 years old, a rectal temperature is preferred. Axillary temperature is adequate for screening if it is taken correctly. If your infant is less than 90 days old (3 months old) *and* axillary temperature is over 99.0°F (37.2°C), check it by taking the rectal temperature. The reason we need a rectal temperature taken for young infants is that if they have a true fever, they need to be evaluated immediately.
- For a child 5 years old or older, take the temperature orally (by mouth).

Taking Rectal Temperatures

- Have your child lie stomach down on your lap.
- Before you insert the thermometer, apply some petroleum jelly to the end of the thermometer and to the opening of the anus.
- Insert the thermometer into the rectum about 1 inch. During the first 6 months of life, gently insert the rectal thermometer ¼ to ½ inch (inserting until the silver tip disappears is about ½ inch). Never try to force it past any resistance. (Reason: it could cause perforation of the bowel.)
- Hold your child still while the thermometer is in.
- Leave the thermometer in your child's rectum for 2 minutes.

Taking Axillary Temperatures

- Place the tip of the thermometer in a dry armpit.
- Close the armpit by holding the elbow against the chest for 4 or 5 minutes. You may miss detecting a fever if the thermometer is removed before 4 minutes.
- If you're uncertain about the result, check it with a rectal temperature.

Taking Oral Temperatures

- Be sure your child has not taken a cold or hot drink within the last 30 minutes.
- Place the tip of the thermometer under one side of the tongue and toward the back. An accurate temperature depends on proper placement. Ask a physician or nurse to show you where it should go.
- Have your child hold it in place with the lips and fingers (not the teeth) and breathe through the nose, keeping the mouth closed.
- Leave it inside for 3 minutes.
- If your child can't keep his or her mouth closed because of nose blockage, suction out the nose.

Reading a Glass Thermometer. Find where the mercury line ends by rotating the thermometer until you can see the mercury.

TYPES OF THERMOMETERS

Glass (with Mercury) Thermometers. Glass thermometers are hard to read for many people but are the least expensive ($5.00). Glass thermometers come in two forms, oral with a thin tip and rectal with a rounder tip. This difference is not too important. If necessary, a rectal thermometer can be used in the mouth and an oral thermometer can be used in the rectum, as long as the thermometer is cleaned with rubbing alcohol and you are extra careful with rectal insertion.

Digital Thermometers. Digital thermometers record temperatures with a heat sensor and run on a button battery. They measure quickly, usually in less than 30 seconds. The temperature is displayed in numbers on a small screen. The same thermometer can be used to take both rectal and oral temperatures. Buy one for your family; they cost about $10.00.

Ear Thermometers. Many hospitals and medical offices now take your child's temperature using an infrared thermometer that reads the temperature of the eardrum. In general, the eardrum temperature provides a measurement that is as accurate as the rectal temperature. The outstanding advantage of this instrument is that it measures temperatures in less than 2 seconds. It also requires no cooperation by the child and causes no discomfort (the thermometer is placed at the ear's opening). An ear thermometer for home use is available, but it's expensive ($60.00).

CONVERSION OF DEGREES FAHRENHEIT (F) TO DEGREES CENTIGRADE (C)

96.8°F = 36.0°C	102.0°F = 38.9°C
98.6°F = 37.0°C	103.0°F = 39.5°C
99.5°F = 37.5°C	104.0°F = 40.0°C
100.0°F = 37.8°C	105.0°F = 40.6°C
100.4°F = 38.0°C	106.0°F = 41.1°C
101.0°F = 38.3°C	107.0°F = 41.7°C

FEVER PHOBIA: UNDERSTANDING THE MYTHS

Misconceptions about the dangers of fever are commonplace. Unwarranted fears about harmful side effects from fever cause lost sleep and unnecessary stress for many parents. Let the following facts help you put fever into perspective.

MYTH: All fevers are bad for children.
FACT: Fevers turn on the body's immune system. Fevers are one of the body's protective mechanisms.

Most fevers are good for children and help the body fight infection. Use the following definitions to help put your child's level of fever into perspective:

100°–102°F (37.8°–38.9°C)	Low-grade fevers are beneficial. Try to keep the fever in this range.
102°–104°F (38.9°–40°C)	Moderate-grade fevers are beneficial.
>104°F (>40°C)	High fevers cause discomfort but are harmless.
>105°F (>40.6°C)	Higher risk of bacterial infections with a very high fever.
>108°F (>42.2°C)	The fever itself can be harmful.

MYTH: Fevers cause brain damage, and fevers over 104°F (40°C) are dangerous.
FACT: Fevers with infections don't cause brain damage. Only body temperatures over 108°F (42.2°C) can cause brain damage. The body temperature only goes this high with high environmental temperatures (e.g., confined in a closed car).

MYTH: Anyone can have a febrile seizure.
FACT: Only 4% of children ever have a febrile seizure.

MYTH: Febrile seizures are harmful.
FACT: Febrile seizures are scary to watch, but they usually stop within 5 minutes. They cause no permanent harm. Children with febrile seizures have no higher incidence for developmental delays, learning disabilities, or seizures without fever.

MYTH: All fevers need to be treated with fever medicine.
FACT: Fevers only need to be treated if they cause discomfort—usually fevers over 102° or 103°F (38.9° or 39.5°C).

MYTH: Without treatment, fevers will keep going higher.
FACT: Fevers from infection top out at 105° or 106°F (40.6° or 41.1°C) or lower, because of the brain's thermostat.

MYTH: With treatment, fevers should come down to normal.
FACT: With treatment, fevers usually come down 2° or 3°F (1°–1.5°C).

MYTH: If the fever doesn't come down (if you can't "break the fever"), the cause is serious.
FACT: Fevers that don't respond to fever medicine can be caused by viruses or bacteria. It doesn't relate to the seriousness of the infection.

MYTH: If the fever is high, the cause is serious.
FACT: If your child looks very sick, the cause is serious.

MYTH: The exact number of the temperature is very important.
FACT: How your child looks is what's important.

MYTH: Temperatures between 98.6° and 100°F (37.0° and 37.8°C) are low-grade fevers.
FACT: The normal temperature changes throughout the day and peaks in the late afternoon and evening.

- A reading of 99.4°F (37.5°C) is just the average rectal temperature. It normally can change from 98.4°F (36.9°C) in the morning to a high of 100.3°F (38.0°C) in the late afternoon.
- A reading of 98.6°F (37°C) is just the average oral temperature. It normally can change from a low of 97.6°F (36.5°C) in the morning to a high of 99.5°F (37.5°C) in the late afternoon.

Instructions for Pediatric Patients, 2nd Edition, ©1999 by WB Saunders Company.
Written by Barton D. Schmitt, MD, pediatrician and author of *Your Child's Health,* Bantam Books, a book for parents.

Nonsmoking children who live in homes with smokers are involuntarily exposed to cigarette smoke. The smoke comes from two sources—secondhand smoke and side-stream smoke. Secondhand smoke is exhaled by the smoker. Side-stream smoke rises off the end of a burning cigarette and accounts for most of the smoke in a room. Side-stream smoke contains two or three times more harmful chemicals than secondhand smoke because it does not pass through the cigarette filter. At worst, a child in a very smoky room for 1 hour with several smokers inhales as many bad chemicals as he or she would by smoking 10 or more cigarettes. In general, children of smoking mothers absorb more smoke into their bodies than children of smoking fathers because they spend more time with their mothers. Children who are breast-fed by a smoking mother are at the greatest risk because chemicals are found in the breast milk as well as the surrounding air.

HARMFUL EFFECTS OF PASSIVE SMOKING ON CHILDREN

Children who live in a house where someone smokes have an increased rate of all respiratory infections. Their symptoms are also more severe and last longer than those of children who live in a smoke-free home. The impact of passive smoke is worse during the first 5 years of life when children spend most of their time with their parents. The more smokers there are in a household and the more they smoke, the more severe a child's symptoms. Passive smoking is especially hazardous to children who have asthma. Exposure to smoke causes more severe asthma attacks, more emergency room visits, and increased admissions to the hospital. These children are also less likely to outgrow their asthma. The following conditions are worsened by passive smoking:

- Pneumonia
- Coughs or bronchitis
- Croup or laryngitis
- Wheezing or bronchiolitis
- Asthma attacks
- Influenza
- Ear infections
- Middle ear fluid and blockage
- Colds or upper respiratory infections
- Sinus infections
- Sore throats
- Eye irritation
- Crib deaths (SIDS)
- Elevated blood cholesterol level
- School absenteeism for all of the above

HOW TO PROTECT YOUR CHILD FROM PASSIVE SMOKING

1. **Give up active smoking.** Sign up for a stop-smoking class or program. Giving up smoking is even more urgent if you are pregnant because your unborn baby has twice the risk for prematurity and newborn complications if you smoke during pregnancy. It is also important to avoid smoking if you are breast-feeding because smoke-related, harmful chemicals get into your breast milk. You can stop smoking if you get help. If you need some self-help reading materials, call your local American Lung Association or American Cancer Society office. The Surgeon General would like us to become a smoke-free society by the year 2000. For more information call the National Cancer Institute on their toll-free line: 1-800-4-CANCER. If you want your child not to smoke, set a good example.

2. **Never smoke inside your home.** Some parents find it difficult to give up smoking, but all parents can change their smoking habits. Restrict your smoking to times you are away from home. If you have to smoke when you are home, smoke only in your garage or on the porch. If these options are not available to you, designate a smoking room within your home. Keep the door to this room closed, and periodically open the window to let fresh air into the room. Wear a special overshirt in this room to protect your underlying clothing from collecting the smoke. Never allow your child inside this room, and don't smoke in other parts of the house. Apply the same rule to visitors.

3. **Never smoke while holding your child.** If your smoking habit cannot be controlled to the degree mentioned above, at a minimum protect your child from smoking when you are close to him or her. This precaution will reduce the child's exposure to smoke and protect him or her from cigarette burns. Never smoke in a car when your child is a passenger. Never smoke when you are feeding or bathing him or her. Never smoke in your child's bedroom. Even doing this much will help your child to some degree.

4. **Avoid leaving your child with a caretaker who smokes.** Inquire about smoking when you are looking for day care centers or babysitters. If your child has asthma, this safeguard is crucial.

Instructions for Pediatric Patients, 2nd Edition, ©1999 by WB Saunders Company.
Written by Barton D. Schmitt, MD, pediatrician and author of *Your Child's Health,* Bantam Books, a book for parents.

PREVENTION OF INFECTIONS

Public health methods have had the greatest impact in preventing the spread of infectious diseases. Proper sewage disposal and safe water supplies have largely eliminated epidemics such as typhoid fever and cholera. Immunizations and vaccinations constitute the other aspect of modern medicine that has controlled infectious diseases such as smallpox and polio.

Precautions within the home can limit the spread of gastrointestinal illnesses. Unfortunately, controlling the spread of colds, coughs, and sore throats within a family unit is impractical.

HOW INFECTIOUS DISEASES ARE SPREAD

- Nose, mouth, and eye secretions are the most common sources of respiratory infections. These secretions are usually spread by contaminated hands or occasionally by kissing. Toddlers are especially prone to spreading these infections because of their habits of touching or mouthing everything.
- Droplet spread from coughing or sneezing is a less common means of transmission of respiratory infections. Droplets can travel up to 6 feet.
- Fecal contamination of hands or other objects accounts for the spread of most diarrhea, as well as infectious hepatitis. Unlike urine, which is usually sterile, bowel movements are composed of up to 50% bacteria.
- The discharge from sores such as chickenpox and fever blisters can be contagious. However, most red rashes without a discharge are not contagious by skin contact.
- Contaminated food or water accounted for many epidemics in earlier times. Even today some foods frequently contain bacteria that cause diarrhea. (For example, 50% of raw turkey or chicken contains *Campylobacter* or *Salmonella* organisms. By contrast, only 1% of raw eggs are contaminated with *Salmonella* organisms.)
- Contaminated objects such as combs, brushes, and hats can lead to the spread of lice or ringworm.

PREVENTION OR REDUCTION OF SPREAD OF INFECTIOUS DISEASES

The following preventive actions can help reduce the spread of disease within your household.

Encourage Hand Washing. Hand washing helps to prevent the spread of gastrointestinal infections more than all other approaches combined. Rinsing your hands vigorously with plain water is probably as effective as using soap and water. Hand washing is especially important after using the toilet, changing diapers, and coming in contact with turtles or aquarium water. Choose a day care center where the staff practices good hand washing after changing diapers. Young children must be supervised in their use of toilets and sinks. Recent studies have found that hand washing is also the mainstay in preventing the spread of respiratory disease. (Wash the hands after blowing or touching the nose.)

Discourage Habits of Touching the Mouth and Nose. Again, this advice is helpful in preventing the spread of respiratory infections to others. Also, touching the eyes after touching the nose is a common cause of eye infections.

Don't Smoke Around Your Children. Passive smoking increases the frequency and severity of colds, coughs, croup, ear infections, and asthma.

Discourage Your Child from Kissing Pets. Pets (especially puppies) can transmit bloody diarrhea, worms, and other things. Pets are for petting.

Cook All Poultry Thoroughly. Undercooked poultry is a common cause of diarrhea. If the poultry is frozen, thaw it in the refrigerator rather than at room temperature to prevent multiplication of the bacteria. After preparation, carefully wash your hands and any object that comes in contact with raw poultry (such as the knife and cutting board) before using them with other foods. Never serve chicken that is still pink inside (a common problem with outdoor grilling). Don't place the cooked meat on the same platter that the uncooked meat was removed from.

Use a Plastic Cutting Board. Germs can't be completely removed from wooden cutting boards.

Avoid Eating Raw Eggs. Don't undercook your eggs. If you make your own eggnog or ice cream, use pasteurized eggs.

Choose a Small Day Care Home over a Day Care Center. Day care provided in private homes has a lower rate of infectious disease. Children who are cared for in their own homes by babysitters have the lowest rate of infection. Since colds have more complications during the first year of life, try to arrange for home-based day care if you child is in this age group.

Clean Contaminated Areas with Disinfectants. These products kill most bacteria, including *Staphylococcus* organisms. Disinfecting the diaper-changing area, cribs, strollers, play equipment, and food service items limits intestinal diseases at home and in day care centers.

Contact Our Office If Your Child Is Exposed to Meningitis or Hepatitis. Antibiotics can prevent some types of bacterial meningitis in exposed children under 4 years of age. An injection of gamma globulin helps to prevent hepatitis in children who have had intimate contact (longer than 4 hours) with someone with this disease.

Keep Your Child's Immunizations Up-to-Date. Check with our office if you don't have a record of your child's immunization schedule.

Don't Attempt to Isolate Your Child. Isolation to stop an infection is mentioned last because its value within a family unit is questionable. By the time a child shows symptoms, he or she has already shared the germs with the family. Also, isolation at home is impossible to enforce.

Instructions for Pediatric Patients, 2nd Edition, ©1999 by WB Saunders Company.
Written by Barton D. Schmitt, MD, pediatrician and author of *Your Child's Health,* Bantam Books, a book for parents.

If you are thinking about having sex for the first time or you already are sexually active, you probably want to know about preventing an unplanned pregnancy. We'll discuss birth control methods most commonly used by teenagers. Although most methods depend on the woman to do or take something, it is important for the man to understand what is involved so that he can support his girlfriend. Also, don't forget that it is only the male method of birth control, condoms, that can also prevent sexually transmitted diseases (STDs).

DECIDING TO HAVE SEX

There are no methods of birth control that are 100% effective. Unless you decide not to have sexual intercourse (abstinence), you are always taking some risk of pregnancy. However, if you are correctly using one of the birth control methods described, the risk can be quite small. Many sexual activities are almost always safe without having to take any special precautions. These include holding hands, hugging, touching, and kissing. Still, some teens decide to have sexual intercourse also.

Having sex can be a very loving and special experience between two people. However, there are several important issues you should think about before you make the decision. Not only does sex have the potential for giving you a sexually transmitted disease or making you pregnant, but you also can get hurt emotionally since it involves such strong feelings between two people. Decide ahead of time what is right for you. Find an adult whom you trust and can discuss your feelings and opinions with, and ask questions. Some teens know that they can discuss sexual issues with their parents, even though it is sometimes awkward to start the conversation. Other adults who may be able to give you valuable information include ministers or rabbis at your church or synagogue, school counselors or teachers, or adult relatives. Also, trained professionals in your doctor's office can help you. You can usually ask questions confidentially.

COMMON BIRTH CONTROL METHODS

In addition to using a condom each time, often a young woman and her male partner want additional protection from pregnancy. If used correctly, condoms prevent pregnancy 85% of the time. The condom is very effective at preventing STDs but there are better methods for preventing pregnancy. The three hormonal birth control methods are birth control pills, "Depo" shots, and Norplant surgical implants. These methods use female hormones to stop ovulation (the female egg does not leave the ovary, so fertilization with the male sperm can't occur), or they also make the mucus that is at the opening of a women's cervix thick, so that male sperm can't travel through the cervix and get to the female egg. They prevent pregnancy 99% of the time.

Birth control pills must be taken once every day. Many women like them because they know exactly when they are going to get their period, and usually the period is lighter, shorter, and has less cramping than before they started "the pill." All medicines have side effects, so you would need to talk with your health care provider about these. Most girls on "the pill" have no problems at all. If you have a problem, usually your birth control pill can be switched to a slightly different one by your doctor and that takes care of it.

"Depo" (Depo-Provera is the brand name for medroxyprogesterone acetate) shots are injections of female hormones given in the arm or buttocks of a young woman every 3 months. You don't have to think about taking a pill every day and you are protected from pregnancy for 3 months until you get the next shot. Usually the shot area is not sore. Most women using "Depo" have irregular periods while they are receiving this hormone.

Norplant surgical implants contain a female hormones (levonorgestrel) in small capsules that are placed just underneath your skin on the inside of your upper arm. This must be done in the doctor's office. Norplant protects a woman from getting pregnant for 5 years. When 5 years have elapsed, the Norplant is removed from the arm (also in the doctor's office) and the woman then decides whether to have new capsules implanted or to change to a different method. If you have any problems with the capsules or you plan to get pregnant, then you can have them taken out before 5 years. As with the "Depo" shots, you probably will have irregular periods. Because the capsules are thin and underneath the skin, they usually can't be seen.

THE "MORNING AFTER" PILL

You may have heard about *emergency contraception*, also known as the "morning after" pill. This type of birth control is sometimes used in an emergency, that is, when a couple who always use condoms finds out *after* the man ejaculates that the condom has broken. Another emergency can happen when a woman who isn't taking birth control pills unexpectedly has sex and her partner doesn't use a condom. Emergency contraception can't prevent all pregnancies, but it can help a lot. The thing is, you have to call the doctor's office less than 72 hours (less than 3 days) from the time it happens, and the sooner the better. If you have sex without any birth control protection on a Friday and can't reach your doctor over the weekend, call first thing on Monday morning. It might be helpful to tell a trusted adult that you are worried about being pregnant and what happened. With emergency contraception, the doctor gives you a few special hormone pills to take right away, and some others to take 12 hours later. In most cases, a pregnancy can be prevented. After that you can decide what birth control method will work best for you in the future.

USING CONDOMS

1. Hold the condom at the tip to squeeze out the air.
2. Roll the condom all the way down the erect (hard) penis. (Don't try to put a condom on a soft penis.)
3. After sex, hold onto the condom while the penis is being pulled out.

Besides knowing the correct way to use a condom, other things to know about condoms follow:

- If the woman also puts spermicidal jelly or foam (available in the drug store without a prescription) inside her vagina right before sex, it helps make the condom method even better at preventing pregnancy. The jelly can kill sperm, but it doesn't work if used without a condom.
- Never reuse the same condom. It is a good idea to have two available in case one breaks.
- If a condom breaks, as soon as you realize it, take it off and put another one on or stop having sex until you can get another condom.
- The man should pull out of his sexual partner while he is still hard. If his penis gets soft first, the sperm can leak around the condom.
- Condoms are sold in drug stores. Buy latex rubber or plastic condoms. Never use condoms made from animal skins, which can leak.
- If you use a lubricant with condoms, make sure it is water-based (like K-Y jelly). Do not use petroleum jelly or Crisco; these can cause the condom to break.
- Some condoms are lubricated with a chemical, nonoxynol-9, which helps kill some of the germs that cause STDs. Others are dry condoms. It doesn't matter which one you use as long as you use a condom every time you have sex.

There is a female condom, one that lines a woman's vagina, but it is more difficult to use and you should talk with a doctor or nurse before you try it.

OTHER INFORMATION ABOUT PREVENTING PREGNANCY

- The "withdrawal" method, in which the man pulls his penis out of the vagina before he ejaculates, is not a good method to prevent a pregnancy. It is very difficult for a man to pull out exactly at the right time, and some sperm leaks out anyway. However, if you are having sex without a condom and the woman has no birth control protection, it is better to withdraw before ejaculating.
- The "rhythm" method, where by a couple only has sex during certain times of the woman's menstrual cycle when she is not as likely to get pregnant, is also not a very reliable method. This method is mostly used by married couples. It is difficult to learn.

 CALL OUR OFFICE

Within 24 hours if
- You are more than a week late for your period.
- You have questions about sex.
- You know the condom broke or you didn't use one and also the female partner isn't on birth control methods.
- You think you might need emergency contraception (the "morning after" pill).

Contributed by J. Todd Jacobs, M.D.

Instructions for Pediatric Patients, **2nd Edition,** ©1999 **by WB Saunders Company.**
Written by Barton D. Schmitt, MD, pediatrician and author of *Your Child's Health,* Bantam Books, a book for parents.

ABOUT SEXUALLY TRANSMITTED DISEASES (STDs)

STDs are diseases that are spread from one person to another during sexual activity. There are many different types of STDs. Some of the more common ones are herpes, chlamydia infection, gonorrhea, pubic lice, syphilis, condylomas (sexual warts), trichomonas infection, HIV (the human immunodeficiency virus that causes AIDS), and hepatitis B (a liver disease). We have treatments for some of them, but not all. Some can be deadly or make you very sick.

Often a person can have one of these diseases and not know it because he or she doesn't have any signs of it and doesn't feel sick. The person can unknowingly spread the disease to a sexual partner if careful precautions aren't always used (read on). Sometimes a person suspects or knows that he may have an STD, but is too embarrassed to talk about it with his sexual partner. If safe sex isn't practiced every time, then the sexual partner is also at risk for getting the disease.

DECIDING TO HAVE SEX

Having sex can be a very loving and special experience between two people. However, there are several important issues you must think about before you decide to have sex. Sexual intercourse not only has the potential for giving you a sexually transmitted disease but you also can get hurt emotionally, since it involves such strong feelings between two people. Decide ahead of time what is right for you. Find an adult with whom you can discuss your feelings and opinions, and ask questions. Some teens know that they can discuss these things with their parents, even though it is sometimes awkward to start the conversation. Other adults who may be able to give you valuable information include officials at your church, school counselors or teachers, or adult relatives. Also the trained staff in your doctor's office can help you; you can usually ask questions of them confidentially.

SAFER SEX

When talking about sex and sexual diseases, the only absolutely risk-free activity is to not have sex (also known as abstinence). Many teens decide to delay having sex until they are older, married, or feel more comfortable. There are also many sexual activities that are almost always safe without taking any special precautions. These include holding hands, hugging, touching, and kissing.

Other sexual activities, especially having sex, are very risky if precautions aren't taken and if you don't think things through and talk with your sexual partner. If you have vaginal or anal intercourse, you can protect yourself against almost all of the STDs by using condoms each time (see "Using Condoms").

USING CONDOMS

1. Hold the condom at the tip to squeeze out the air.
2. Roll the condom all the way down the erect (hard) penis. (Don't try to put a condom on a soft penis.)
3. After sex, hold onto the condom while the penis is being pulled out.
4. Other information about condoms follows:

- Never reuse the same condom. It is a good idea to have two available in case one breaks.
- If a condom breaks, as soon as you realize it, take it off and put on another one. If you don't have another, stop having sexual intercourse until you can get another condom.
- The man should pull out of his sexual partner while he is still hard. If his penis gets soft first, the sperm can leak around the condom.
- Condoms are sold in drug stores. Buy latex rubber or plastic condoms. Never use condoms made from animal skins, which can leak.
- If you use a lubricant with condoms, make sure it is water-based (like K-Y jelly). Do not use petroleum jelly or Crisco; these can cause the condom to break.
- There is a female condom, one that lines a woman's vagina, but it is more difficult to use and you should talk with a doctor or nurse before you try it.

OTHER INFORMATION ABOUT SEXUALLY TRANSMITTED DISEASES

- Your chance of getting an STD is greater if you have more than one sexual partner.
- Douching the vagina or showering after sex does not prevent STDs.
- Withdrawal (when a man pulls his penis out before he ejaculates) is not a way to prevent STDs or pregnancy. However, if a man is not wearing a condom, it reduces the risk somewhat if he withdraws before he ejaculates.
- You can get the same STD again, even if you have had it once and been treated.
- You can get an STD even if you have sex just once.
- Other birth control methods, such as the birth control pill or "Depo" shots, don't prevent you from getting an STD. You still need to protect yourself with condoms.

 ## CALL OUR OFFICE

Within 24 hours if
- You are having any symptoms that you think might be an STD.
- You think you might have been exposed to someone with an STD.
- You had sex without a condom and might need emergency contraception (the "morning after" pill) to prevent a pregnancy.

Contributed by J. Todd Jacobs, M.D.

SLEEP POSITION FOR YOUNG INFANTS

THE PREFERRED POSITION: ON THE BACK (SUPINE)

In 1992 the American Academy of Pediatrics (AAP) recommended that all healthy infants be positioned for sleep on their backs (supine) or on their sides for the first 6 months of life. In 1996, the AAP recommended the back as being preferred over the side position. In 1992, only 30% of U.S. infants slept on their backs or sides. Now about 75% of U.S. infants sleep supine or on their sides.

RESEARCH LINKING THE PRONE (TUMMY) POSITION AND THE SUDDEN INFANT DEATH SYNDROME

Most infants in the world are put to sleep lying on their backs. In the 1980s, research studies from Europe, Australia, and New Zealand showed that the supine sleep position reduces sudden infant death syndrome (SIDS) 20% to 67%. The prone (or tummy) position has a three to nine times greater risk of SIDS than the supine position. The side position has a two times greater risk of SIDS than the supine position. Although none of these studies was perfect, in 1992 the AAP recommended the supine position because of the 6000 to 7000 SIDS deaths each year in the United States. Although this change in sleeping position won't eliminate all SIDS risk factors, it should reduce the number of SIDS deaths.

REASONS THE PRONE (TUMMY) POSITION MIGHT INCREASE THE RISK FOR THE SUDDEN INFANT DEATH SYNDROME

The tummy (prone) position puts pressure on a child's jaw bone. As a result, the airway in the back of the mouth becomes narrower. Also, if the child sleeps on a soft surface, the nose and mouth may sink in, causing the child to breathe from a small pocket of stale air. In fact, the increased SIDS rate in countries such as New Zealand may be due not to the prone position alone but to placing children prone on sheepskin pads. Everyone now agrees that young infants should never be placed on waterbeds, sheepskin, soft pillows, bean-filled pillows, or other soft, spongy surfaces. Soft surfaces are also potentially dangerous when a child is placed in the crib in the supine (on the back) position because he or she may roll over during the night.

RISKS OF THE SUPINE (BACK) POSITION

The main reason for the earlier recommendation of the prone position was the concern that if a child spits up or vomits while lying on the back, he or she could inhale (aspirate) and choke on the vomited material.

However, the AAP has found no evidence to support the belief that choking occurs more commonly in the supine position. Choking is an extremely rare cause of infant death in healthy, full-term infants. During the last 4 years, the rate of choking in infants has not increased.

THE EXCEPTIONS: WHEN THE PRONE (TUMMY) POSITION IS RECOMMENDED

The AAP recommends the prone, or tummy, position for infants in the following three categories:

1. **Infants with complications of gastroesophageal reflux (spitting up).** These complications include recurrent pneumonia from aspiration, choking episodes, interruption of breathing (apnea) episodes, or acid damage to the lower esophagus (esophagitis). Although spitting up is common, these complications are rare.
2. **Infants with birth defects of the upper airway that interfere with breathing.** Examples are a large tongue, a small mouth, or a floppy larynx.
3. **Premature babies who are having difficulty breathing or require oxygen.** (Research shows that premature babies breathe better in the prone position.) By the time they come home, most premature babies can sleep on their backs.

Any baby who needs to sleep prone must be placed on a firm sleeping surface.

PRONE (TUMMY) POSITION FOR PLAYTIME

The back position is recommended for bedtime and naps. It is not necessary if your infant is awake. Yet many parents keep their infant in the back position throughout the day. This can cause some flattening of the back of the head and also some decreased strength of the shoulder muscles. Avoid these side effects by keeping your infant prone for some of his or her playtime and waking hours. In their cribs, babies tend to turn slightly toward the side where they can see people. Therefore, every week reverse the direction you lay your baby in his or her crib.

SUMMARY

Several years have passed since 1992, when the AAP recommended that infants sleep on their backs. Now over 75% of parents follow this advice. By 1995, national data showed a 30% drop in the SIDS rate. Provide your baby an added margin of safety by placing him on his back for sleep. If you use a child care center, be sure the staff are aware of your preference.

Other ways to reduce the risk of SIDS are to use a firm mattress (avoid soft bedding), breast-feed if possible, and protect your infant from exposure to cigarette, cigar, or pipe smoke.

Instructions for Pediatric Patients, 2nd Edition, ©1999 by WB Saunders Company.
Written by Barton D. Schmitt, MD, pediatrician and author of *Your Child's Health,* Bantam Books, a book for parents.

DEFINITION

Most infant suffocations occur when babies are placed face down on a soft surface that the mouth and nose sink into. Infants who are 0 to 4 months old have the greatest risk of suffocating. These young infants don't have enough strength to lift their heads and turn their faces so that they can breathe. Many of these deaths occur when a baby naps at the home of a friend who doesn't have a crib.

Another cause of suffocation in young infants should be mentioned. Small babies have been smothered by mothers who inadvertently fell asleep on top of them. If you nurse your baby in your bed at night, be careful. Try to keep your baby in a crib next to your bed.

Suffocation deaths account for some deaths that used to be attributed to crib death. Despite extensive research, the cause of crib deaths or sudden infant death syndrome (SIDS) remains unknown. True SIDS can't be predicted or prevented. There is one exception: smoking in the house greatly increases the risk of SIDS and should be avoided.

PREVENTION OF SUFFOCATION IN INFANTS

To be safe, place your young baby on his or her back in a crib with a firm mattress. As of 1992, this is the sleep position recommended by the American Academy of Pediatrics for healthy infants during the first 6 months of life. Sleeping on the side is an acceptable alternative, but the back is safer.

Soft surfaces are unsafe for babies even if they are placed on their backs because someone (e.g., another child) might turn them over. You can prevent these tragic deaths from suffocation by never putting young infants on the following soft surfaces:

- Waterbeds
- Sheepskin rugs or mattress covers
- Soft pillows, such as bean-bag or bead-filled pillows
- Any weak, spongy surface (soft mattress or comforter)
- Mattresses covered with plastic bags

PREVENTION OF SUFFOCATION IN TODDLERS

Older infants and toddlers can be suffocated by plastic bags or sheets of plastic. These accidents usually occur when they pull the plastic over their heads or crawl into plastic bags. Carefully dispose of any plastic bags, including the following products, or keep them away from children less than 3 years old:

- Plastic dry-cleaning bags
- Plastic shopping bags
- Plastic trash bags

PART 4

COMMON INFECTIONS OF CHILDHOOD

BRONCHIOLITIS (RESPIRATORY SYNCYTIAL VIRUS)

CHICKENPOX (VARICELLA)

COLDS

COUGH (VIRAL BRONCHITIS)

CROUP

EAR INFECTION (OTITIS MEDIA)

DIARRHEA (VIRAL GASTROENTERITIS)

EYE INFECTION WITHOUT PUS (VIRAL)

EYE INFECTION WITH PUS (BACTERIAL)

FEVER—See Part 3, Preventive Pediatrics

THE TEMPERATURE: HOW TO MEASURE IT—See Part 3, Preventive Pediatrics

EMERGENCY SYMPTOMS: HOW TO RECOGNIZE—See Part 3, Preventive Pediatrics

FREQUENT INFECTIONS

FIFTH DISEASE (ERYTHEMA INFECTIOSUM)

GASTROENTERITIS—See DIARRHEA; VOMITING

INFLUENZA

LYME DISEASE

LYMPH NODE INFECTION IN THE NECK (CERVICAL ADENITIS)

LYMPH NODES OR GLANDS, SWOLLEN

MEASLES (RUBEOLA)

MONONUCLEOSIS

MUMPS

PIERCED-EAR INFECTION

PNEUMONIA

PREVENTION OF INFECTIONS—See Part 3, Preventive Pediatrics

ROSEOLA

RUBELLA (GERMAN MEASLES)

SCARLET FEVER

SINUS INFECTION (SINUSITIS)

SORE THROAT (PHARYNGITIS)

STREP THROAT INFECTION

SWIMMER'S EAR (OTITIS EXTERNA)

URINARY TRACT INFECTION

PAIN WITH URINATION (CHEMICAL URETHRITIS)

VAGINAL IRRITATION AND ITCHING (CHEMICAL VULVITIS)

VOMITING (VIRAL GASTRITIS)

WOUND INFECTION (SKIN INFECTION)

BRONCHIOLITIS (RESPIRATORY SYNCYTIAL VIRUS)

DEFINITION

- Wheezing: a high-pitched whistling sound produced during breathing out
- Rapid breathing with a rate of over 40 breaths/minute
- Tight breathing (your child has to push the air out)
- Coughing, often with very sticky mucus
- Onset of lung symptoms often preceded by fever and a runny nose
- Lots of sticky nasal mucus is a problem
- An average age of 6 months, always less than 2 years
- Symptoms similar to asthma
- This diagnosis must be confirmed by a physician

Cause

The wheezing is caused by a narrowing of the smallest airways in the lung (bronchioles). This narrowing results from inflammation (swelling) caused by any of a number of viruses, usually the respiratory syncytial virus (RSV). RSV occurs in epidemics almost every winter. Whereas infants with RSV develop bronchiolitis, children over 2 years of age and adults just develop cold symptoms. This virus is found in nasal secretions of infected individuals. It is spread by sneezing or coughing at a range of less than 6 feet or by hand-to-nose or hand-to-eye contact. People do not develop permanent immunity to the virus.

Expected Course

Wheezing and tight breathing (difficulty breathing out) become worse for 2 or 3 days and then begin to improve. Overall, the wheezing lasts approximately 7 days and the cough about 14 days. The most common complication of bronchiolitis is an ear infection, occurring in some 20% of infants. Bacterial pneumonia is an uncommon complication. Only 1% or 2% of children with bronchiolitis are hospitalized because they need oxygen or intravenous fluids. In the long run, approximately 30% of the children who develop bronchiolitis go on to develop asthma. Recurrences of wheezing (asthma) occur mainly in children who come from families where close relatives have asthma. Asthma is very treatable with current medications.

HOME TREATMENT FOR BRONCHIOLITIS

Medicines. Some children with bronchiolitis respond to asthma medicines; others do not.

Your child's medicine is _____.

Give _____

every _____ hours.

Continue the medicine until your child's wheezing is gone for 24 hours. In addition, your child can be given acetaminophen every 4 to 6 hours if the fever is over 102°F (39°C).

Warm Fluids for Coughing Spasms. Coughing spasms are often caused by sticky secretions in the back of the throat. Warm liquids usually relax the airway and loosen the secretions. Offer warm lemonade, warm apple juice or warm herbal tea if your child is over 4 months old. In addition, breathing warm moist air helps to loosen the sticky mucus that may be choking your child. You can provide warm mist by placing a warm wet washcloth loosely over your child's nose and mouth, or you can fill a humidifier with warm water and have your child breathe in the warm mist it produces. Avoid steam vaporizers because they can cause burns.

Humidity. Dry air tends to make coughs worse. Use a humidifier in your child's bedroom. The new ultrasonic humidifiers not only have the advantage of quietness, but also kill molds and most bacteria that might be in the water.

Nasal Washes for a Blocked Nose. If the nose is blocked up, your child will not be able to drink from a bottle or nurse. Most stuffy noses are blocked by dry or sticky mucus. Suction alone cannot remove dry secretions. Warm tap water or saline nose drops (nasal washes) are better than any medicine you can buy for loosening up mucus. Place three drops of warm water or saline in each nostril. After about 1 minute, use a soft rubber suction bulb to suck it out. You can repeat this procedure several times until your child's breathing through the nose becomes quiet and easy.

Feedings. Encourage your child to drink adequate fluids. Eating is often tiring, so offer your child formula or breast milk in smaller amounts at more frequent intervals. If your child vomits during a coughing spasm, feed the child again.

No Smoking. Tobacco smoke aggravates coughing. The incidence of wheezing increases greatly in children who have an RSV infection *and* are exposed to passive smoking. Don't let anyone smoke around your child. In fact, try not to let anybody smoke inside your home.

 ## CALL OUR OFFICE

IMMEDIATELY if
- Breathing becomes labored or difficult.
- Breathing becomes faster than 60 breaths/minute (when your child is not crying).
- Your child starts acting very sick.

Within 24 hours if
- There is any suggestion of an earache.
- A fever lasts more than 3 days.
- You have other questions or concerns.

CHICKENPOX (VARICELLA)

DEFINITION

- Multiple small, red bumps that progress to thin-walled water blisters; then cloudy blisters or open sores, which are usually less than ¼ inch across; and finally dry, brown crusts (all within 24 hours)
- Repeated crops of these sores for 4 to 5 days
- Rash on all body surfaces but usually starts on head and back
- Some ulcers (sores) in the mouth, eyelids, and genital area
- Fever (unless the rash is mild)
- Exposure to a child with chickenpox 14 to 16 days earlier

Cause

Chickenpox is caused by exposure to a highly contagious virus 14 to 16 days earlier. A chickenpox vaccine is available for preventing chickenpox.

Expected Course

New eruptions continue to crop up daily for 4 to 5 days. The fever is usually the highest on the third or fourth day. Your child will start to feel better and stop having a fever once he or she stops getting new bumps. The average child gets a total of 500 sores.

Chickenpox rarely leaves any permanent scars unless the sores become badly infected with impetigo or your child repeatedly picks off the scabs. However, normal chickenpox can leave temporary marks on the skin that take 6 to 12 months to fade. One attack gives lifelong immunity. Very rarely, a child may develop a second mild attack.

HOME CARE

Itching and Cool Baths. The best treatment for skin discomfort and itching is a cool bath every 3 to 4 hours for the first few days. Baths don't spread the chickenpox. Calamine lotion can be placed on the most itchy spots after the bath. Itchy spots can also be massaged with an ice cube for 10 minutes. If the itching becomes severe or interferes with sleep, give your child a nonprescription antihistamine such as diphenhydramine (Benadryl).

Fever. Acetaminophen or ibuprofen may be given in the dose appropriate for your child's age for a few days if your child develops a fever over 102°F (39°C). Aspirin should be avoided in children and adolescents with chickenpox because of the link with Reye's syndrome.

Sore Mouth. Since chickenpox sores also occur in the mouth and throat, your child may be picky about eating. Encourage cold fluids. Offer a soft, bland diet and avoid salty foods and citrus fruits. For infants, give fluids by cup rather than a bottle because the nipple can cause pain. If the mouth ulcers become troublesome and your child is over age 4, have him gargle or swallow 1 teaspoon of an antacid solution 4 times per day after meals.

Sore Genital Area. Sores also normally occur in the genital area. If urination becomes very painful, apply some 2½% lidocaine (Xylocaine) or 1% dibucaine (Nupercainal) ointment (no prescription needed) to the genital ulcers every 2 to 3 hours to relieve pain.

Prevention of Impetigo (Infected Sores). To prevent the sores from becoming infected with bacteria, trim your child's fingernails short. Also, wash his hands with an antibacterial soap (such as Dial or Safeguard) frequently during the day. For young babies who are scratching badly, you may want to cover their hands with cotton socks.

Contagiousness and Isolation. Children with chickenpox are contagious until all the sores have crusted over, usually about 6 to 7 days after the rash begins. To avoid exposing other children, try not to take your child to the physician's office. If you must, leave your child in the car with a sitter while you check in. Your child does not have to stay home until all the scabs fall off (this may take 2 weeks).

Most adults who think they didn't have chickenpox as a child had a mild case. Only 4% of adults are not protected. If you lived in the same household with siblings who had chickenpox, consider yourself protected. Siblings will come down with chickenpox in 14 to 16 days. The second case in a family always has many more chickenpox than the first case.

 CALL OUR OFFICE

IMMEDIATELY if
- The chickenpox look infected (yellow pus, spreading redness, red streaks).
- Your child develops a speckled red rash.
- Bleeding occurs into the chickenpox.
- Your child starts acting very sick.

Within 24 hours if
- The fever lasts over 4 days.
- The itching is severe and doesn't respond to treatment.
- You have other concerns or questions.

Instructions for Pediatric Patients, 2nd Edition, ©1999 by WB Saunders Company.
Written by Barton D. Schmitt, MD, pediatrician and author of *Your Child's Health,* Bantam Books, a book for parents.

DEFINITION

- Runny or stuffy nose
- Usually associated with fever and sore throat
- Sometimes associated with a cough, hoarseness, red eyes, and swollen lymph nodes in the neck
- Also called an upper respiratory infection (URI)

Similar Conditions

1. *Vasomotor rhinitis.* Many children and adults have a profusely runny nose in the winter when they are breathing cold air. This usually clears within 15 minutes of coming indoors. It requires no treatment beyond a handkerchief and has nothing to do with infection.
2. *Chemical rhinitis.* Chemical rhinitis is a dry stuffy nose from excessive and prolonged use of vasoconstrictor nose drops (more than 1 week). It will be better within a day or two of stopping the nose drops.

Cause

A cold or URI is a viral infection of the nose and throat. The cold viruses are spread from one person to another by hand contact, coughing, and sneezing—not by cold air or drafts. Since there are up to 200 cold viruses, most healthy children get at least six colds each year.

Expected Course

Usually the fever lasts less than 3 days, and all nose and throat symptoms are gone by 1 week. A cough may last 2 to 3 weeks. The main things to watch for are secondary bacterial infections such as ear infections, yellow drainage from the eyes, sinus pressure or pain (often indicating a sinus infection), or difficulty breathing (often caused by pneumonia). In young infants, a blocked nose can interfere so much with the ability to suck that dehydration can occur.

HOME CARE

Not much can be done to affect how long a cold lasts. However, we can relieve many of the symptoms. Keep in mind that the treatment for a runny nose is quite different from the treatment for a stuffy nose.

Treatment for a Runny Nose with Profuse Discharge: Suctioning or Blowing. The best treatment is clearing the nose for a day or two. Sniffing and swallowing the secretions are probably better than blowing because blowing the nose can force the infection into the ears or sinuses. For younger babies, use a soft rubber suction bulb to remove the secretions gently.

Nasal discharge is the nose's way of eliminating viruses. Medicine is not helpful unless your child has a nasal allergy.

Treatment for a Stuffy or Blocked Nose with Dried Yellow-Green Mucus
Warm-Water or Saline Nose Drops and Suctioning (Nasal Washes). Most stuffy noses are blocked by dry mucus. Blowing the nose or suction alone cannot remove most dry secretions. Nose drops of warm tap water are better than any medicine you can buy for loosening mucus. If you prefer normal saline nose drops, mix ½ level teaspoon of table salt in 8 ounces of water. Make up a fresh solution every day and keep it in a clean bottle. Use a clean dropper to insert drops. Water can also be dripped or splashed in using a wet cotton ball.

- For the younger child who cannot blow her nose: Place three drops of warm water or saline in each nostril. After 1 minute use a soft rubber suction bulb to suck out the loosened mucus gently. To remove secretions from the back of the nose, you will need to seal off both nasal openings completely with the tip of the suction bulb and your fingers. You can get a suction bulb at your drug store for about $2.
- For the older child who can blow her nose: Use three drops as necessary in each nostril while your child is lying on her back on a bed with the head hanging over the side. Wait 1 minute for the water or saline to soften and loosen the dried mucus. Then have your child blow her nose. This can be repeated several times in a row for complete clearing of the nasal passages.
- Errors in using nose drops: The main errors are not putting in enough water or saline, not waiting long enough for secretions to loosen up, and not repeating the procedure until the breathing is easy. The front of the nose can look open while the back of the nose is all gummed up with dried mucus. Obviously, putting in nose drops without suctioning or blowing the nose afterward is of little value.
- Use nasal washes at least 4 times per day or whenever your child can't breathe through the nose.

The Importance of Clearing the Nose in Young Infants. A child can't breathe through the mouth and suck on something at the same time. If your child is breast- or bottle-feeding, you must clear the nose so she can breathe while sucking. Clearing the nasal passages is also important before putting your child down to sleep.

Treatment for Associated Symptoms of Colds
- Fever: Use acetaminophen or ibuprofen for aches or mild fever (over 102°F [38.9°C]).
- Sore throat: Use hard candies for children over 4 years old and warm chicken broth for children over 1 year old.
- Cough: Use cough drops for children over 4 years old and corn syrup for younger children. Run a humidifier.
- Red eyes: Rinse frequently with wet cotton balls.
- Poor appetite: Encourage fluids of the child's choice.

Prevention of Colds. A cold is caused by direct contact with someone who already has one. Over the years, we all become exposed to many colds and develop some immunity to them. Since complications are more common in children during the first year of life, try to avoid undue exposure of young babies to other children or adults with colds, to day care nurseries, and to church nurseries. A humidifier prevents dry mucous membranes, which may be more susceptible to infections. Vitamin C, unfortunately, has not been shown to prevent or shorten colds. Large doses of vitamin C (e.g., 2 grams) cause diarrhea.

Common Mistakes in Treating Colds. Most over-the-counter cold remedies or tablets are worthless. Nothing can shorten the duration of a cold. If the nose is really running, consider a pure antihistamine (such as chlorpheniramine products). Especially avoid drugs that have several ingredients because they increase the risk of side effects. Avoid oral decongestants if they make your child jittery or keep her from sleeping at night. Use acetaminophen or ibuprofen for a cold only if your child also has fever, sore throat, or muscle aches. Leftover antibiotics should not be given for uncomplicated colds because they have no effect on viruses and may be harmful.

 CALL OUR OFFICE

IMMEDIATELY if
- Breathing becomes difficult *and* no better after you clear the nose.
- Your child starts acting very sick.

Within 24 hours if
- The fever lasts more than 3 days.
- The nasal discharge lasts more than 10 days.
- The eyes develop a yellow discharge.
- There is any suggestion of an earache or sinus pain.
- You have other questions or concerns.

Instructions for Pediatric Patients, 2nd Edition, ©1999 by WB Saunders Company.
Written by Barton D. Schmitt, MD, pediatrician and author of *Your Child's Health,* Bantam Books, a book for parents.

DEFINITION

- The cough reflex expels air from the lungs with a sudden explosive noise.
- A coughing spasm is more than 5 minutes of continuous coughing.

Cause

Most coughs are due to a viral infection of the trachea (windpipe) and bronchi (larger air passages). These infections are called tracheitis and bronchitis, respectively. Most children get this infection a couple of times every year as part of a cold. Keep in mind that coughing clears the lungs and protects them from pneumonia. Bronchitis isn't serious. The role of milk in thickening the secretions is doubtful.

Expected Course

Usually bronchitis gives a dry tickly cough that lasts for 2 to 3 weeks. Sometimes it becomes loose (wet) for a few days and your child coughs up a lot of phlegm (mucus). This is usually a sign that the end of the illness is near.

HOME CARE

Medicines to Loosen the Cough and Thin the Secretions

- Cough drops: Most coughs in children over 4 years of age can be controlled by sucking on cough drops freely. Any brand will do.
- Homemade cough syrup: For children under age 4 years, use ½ to 1 teaspoon of corn syrup instead of cough drops. Corn syrup can thin the secretions and loosen the cough.
- Warm liquids for coughing spasms: Warm liquids usually relax the airway and loosen the mucus. Start with warm lemonade, warm apple juice, or warm herbal tea if your child is over 4 months old. Avoid adding any alcohol because inhaling the alcohol fumes stimulates additional coughing and also because there is a risk of intoxication from unintentional overdosage. Children over 4 years old can suck on butterscotch hard candy or cough drops. (Reason: to coat the irritated throat.)

Cough Suppressants. Cough suppressants reduce the cough reflex, which protects the lungs. They are only indicated for dry coughs that interfere with sleep, school attendance, or work. They also help children who have chest pain from coughing spasms. They should not be given to infants under 12 months of age or for wet coughs.

A nonprescription cough suppressant is dextromethorphan (DM). Ask your pharmacist for help in choosing a brand that contains DM without any other active ingredients. Dosage is 0.25 mg/lb every 4 to 6 hours as needed. It usually comes as a liquid in the strength of 15 mg per teaspoon. The following table shows the dosages of DM that you can give a child according to weight or age.

Weight or Age of Child	Dosage of DM (in mg)
20 lb	4
30 lb	6
4–6 yr	7.5
7–12 yr	15
Adults	30

Often corn syrup or cough drops can be given during the day and DM given at bedtime and during the night. DM is also available as a cough lozenge for easy carrying and as a long-acting (12-hour) liquid.

Humidifiers in the Treatment of Cough. Dry air tends to make coughs worse. Dry coughs can be loosened by encouraging a good fluid intake and using a humidifier in your child's bedroom.

The new ultrasonic humidifiers are very quiet, and they kill molds and most bacteria found in the water. Don't add medication to the water in the humidifier because it irritates the cough in some children.

Active and Passive Smoking. Teenagers will find that physical education classes and exercise trigger coughing spasms when they have bronchitis. If so, such physical activity should be avoided temporarily. Don't let anyone smoke around your coughing child. Remind the teenager who smokes that his cough may last weeks longer than it normally would without smoking.

Common Mistakes in Treating Cough. Antihistamines, decongestants, and antipyretics are found in many cough syrups. These ingredients are of unproven value, and the antihistamines carry the risk of sedation. Expectorants are of unproven value but harmless. Stay with the simple remedies mentioned above or use dextromethorphan. Milk does not need to be eliminated from the diet, since restricting it only improves the cough if your child is allergic to milk. Also, never stop breast-feeding because of a cough.

 ## CALL OUR OFFICE

IMMEDIATELY if
- Breathing becomes difficult *and* is not better after you clear the nose.
- Your child starts acting very sick.

During regular hours if
- A fever lasts more than 3 days.
- The cough lasts more than 3 weeks.
- You have other concerns or questions.

DEFINITION

Description of Croupy Cough

- There is a distinctive cough that occurs with infections of the voice box (larynx).
- The cough is tight, low-pitched, and barky (like a barking seal).
- The voice is usually hoarse.

Description of Stridor

- A harsh, raspy, vibrating sound (stridor) is heard when your child breathes in.
- Breathing in becomes very difficult.
- Stridor only occurs with severe croup.
- Stridor is usually only present with crying or coughing.
- As the disease becomes worse, stridor also occurs when a child is sleeping or relaxed.

Cause

Croup is a viral infection of the vocal cords, voice box (larynx), and windpipe (trachea). It is usually part of a cold. The hoarseness is due to swelling of the vocal cords.

Stridor occurs as the opening between the cords becomes more narrow.

Expected Course

Croup usually lasts for 5 to 6 days and generally gets worse at night. During this time, it can change from mild to severe many times. The worst symptoms are seen in children under 3 years of age.

FIRST AID FOR ATTACKS OF STRIDOR WITH CROUP

If your child suddenly develops stridor or tight breathing, do the following:

Inhalation of Warm Mist. Warm, moist air seems to work best to relax the vocal cords and break the stridor. The simplest way to provide this is to have your child breathe through a warm, wet washcloth placed loosely over her nose and mouth. Another good way, if you have a humidifier (not a hot vaporizer), is to fill it with warm water and have your child breathe deeply from the stream of humidity.

The Foggy Bathroom. In the meantime, have the warm shower running with the bathroom door closed. Once the room is all fogged up, take your child into the humidified bathroom for at least 10 minutes. Allay fears by cuddling her.

Results of First Aid. Most children settle down after the above treatments and then sleep peacefully through the night.

Note: If the stridor continues in your child, call our office **immediately.** If your child turns blue, passes out, or stops breathing, call the rescue squad (911).

HOME CARE FOR A CROUPY COUGH

Humidifier. Dry air usually makes coughs worse. Keep the child's bedroom humidified. Use a cool mist humidifier if you have one. Run it 24 hours daily. Otherwise, hang wet sheets or towels in your child's room.

Warm, Clear Fluids for Coughing Spasms. Coughing spasms are often due to sticky mucus caught on the vocal cords. Warm apple juice, lemonade, or herbal tea may help relax the vocal cords and loosen the sticky mucus.

Cough Medicines. Medicines are less helpful than either mist or swallowing warm fluids. Older children (over age 4) can be given cough drops for the cough, and younger children can be given ½ to 1 teaspoon of corn syrup. If your child has a fever (over 102°F [38.9°C]), you may give her acetaminophen or ibuprofen.

Avoid Smoke Exposure. By all means, don't let anyone smoke around your child. Smoke can make croup worse.

Close Observation. While your child is croupy, sleep in the same room with her. Croup can be a dangerous disease.

Contagiousness. The viruses that cause croup are quite contagious until the fever is gone or at least until 3 days into the illness. Since spread of this infection can't be prevented, your child can return to school or child care once she feels better.

 CALL OUR OFFICE

IMMEDIATELY and begin first aid for stridor if
- Breathing becomes difficult (when your child is not coughing).
- Your child develops drooling, spitting, or great difficulty in swallowing.
- Your child develops retractions (tugging in) between the ribs.
- The warm mist fails to clear up the stridor in 20 minutes.
- Your child starts acting very sick.

During regular hours if
- A fever lasts more than 3 days.
- Croup lasts more than 10 days.
- You have other concerns or questions.

Instructions for Pediatric Patients, 2nd Edition, ©1999 by WB Saunders Company.
Written by Barton D. Schmitt, MD, pediatrician and author of *Your Child's Health,* Bantam Books, a book for parents.

DEFINITION

An ear infection is a bacterial infection of the middle ear (the space behind the eardrum). It usually is a complication of a cold, occurring after the cold blocks off the eustachian tube (the passage connecting the middle ear to the back of the throat). The main symptoms are an earache and muffled hearing. Younger children will just cry and fuss. A fever is present with almost half of ear infections. The pain is due to pressure and bulging of the eardrum from trapped, infected fluid. This diagnosis must be confirmed by a physician.

Most children (75%) will have one or more ear infections, and over 25% of these will have repeated ear infections. In 5% to 10% of children, the pressure in the middle ear causes the eardrum to rupture and drain a yellow or cloudy fluid. This small tear usually heals over the next week. The peak age range for ear infections is 6 months to 2 years, but they continue to be a common childhood illness until 8 years of age.

If the following treatment is carried out, your child should do fine. Permanent damage to the ear or to the hearing is very rare.

HOME TREATMENT

Antibiotics. Your child's antibiotic is _____. Your child's dose is _____ given _____ times each day during waking hours for _____ days.

This medicine will kill the bacteria that are causing the ear infection.

Try to remember all doses. If your child goes to school or a babysitter, arrange for someone to give the afternoon dose. If the medicine is a liquid, store it in the refrigerator and use a measuring spoon to be sure that you give the right amount. Give the medicine until all the pills are gone or the bottle is empty. (An antibiotic should not be saved from one illness to the next because it loses its strength.) Even though your child will feel better in a few days, give the antibiotic until it is completely gone to keep the ear infection from flaring up again.

Pain Relief. Acetaminophen or ibuprofen can be given for a few days for the earache or for fever over 102°F (39°C). These medications usually control the pain within 1 to 2 hours.

To help ease the pain, you can put an ice bag or ice wrapped in a wet washcloth over the ear. This may decrease the swelling and pressure inside. Some physicians recommend a heating pad instead. Remove the cold or heat in 20 minutes to prevent unintended frostbite or a burn.

Restrictions. Your child can go outside and does not need to cover the ears. Swimming is permitted as long as there is no perforation (tear) in the eardrum or drainage from the ear. Air travel or a trip to the mountains is safe; just have your child swallow fluids, suck on a pacifier, or chew gum during descent. Your child can return to school or day care when he or she

is feeling better and the fever is gone. Ear infections are not contagious.

Follow-up Visits. Your child has been given a return appointment in 2 to 3 weeks. At that visit we will look at the eardrum to be certain that the infection is cleared up and more treatment isn't needed. We may also want to test your child's hearing. Follow-up exams are important, particularly if the eardrum is perforated.

PREVENTION OF EAR INFECTIONS

If your child has recurrent ear infections, it's time to look closely at how we might prevent some of them. Some of the following factors may apply to your child. If they do, try to change them:

- Protect your child from secondhand tobacco smoke because passive smoking increases the frequency and severity of ear infections. Be sure no one smokes in your home or your child's day care center.
- Reduce your child's exposure to colds during the first year of his life. Most ear infections start with a cold. Try to delay the use of large day care centers during the first year by using a sitter in your home or a small home-based day care center.
- Breast-feed your baby during the first 6 to 12 months of life. Antibodies in breast milk reduce the rate of ear infections. If you're breast-feeding, continue. If you're not, consider it with your next child.
- Avoid bottle propping. If you formula-feed, hold your baby at an angle of 45 degrees. Feeding in the horizontal position can cause a backflow of formula and other secretions into the eustachian tube. Allowing an infant to hold his own bottle also puts milk into the middle ear. This is another reason for weaning your baby from a bottle between 9 and 12 months of age.
- If your infant has continuous nasal secretions, consider an allergy as a contributing factor to the ear infections. This becomes especially likely if your child has other allergies such as eczema. A milk protein allergy is the most likely offender.
- If your toddler has constant snoring and mouth breathing, talk with us about this. Large adenoids may be a cause.

 CALL OUR OFFICE

IMMEDIATELY if
- Your child develops a stiff neck or severe headache.
- Your child starts acting very sick.

Within 24 hours if
- The fever or pain is not gone after your child has taken the antibiotic for 48 hours.
- You feel your child is getting worse.

DIARRHEA (VIRAL GASTROENTERITIS)

DEFINITION

Diarrhea is the sudden increase in the frequency and looseness of bowel movements. Mild diarrhea is the passage of a few loose or mushy stools. Moderate diarrhea gives many watery stools. The best indicator of the severity of the diarrhea is its frequency. A green stool also points to very rapid passage and moderate to severe diarrhea.

The main complication of diarrhea is dehydration from excessive loss of body fluids. Symptoms are a dry mouth, the absence of tears, a reduction in urine production (e.g., none in 8 hours), and a darker, concentrated urine. It's dehydration you need to worry about, not the presence of diarrhea.

Cause

Diarrhea is usually caused by a viral infection of the intestines (gastroenteritis). Occasionally it is caused by bacteria or parasites. Diarrhea can be due to excessive fruit juice or to a food allergy. If only one or two loose stools are passed, the cause was probably something unusual your child ate.

Expected Course

Diarrhea usually lasts from several days to a week, regardless of the treatment. The main goal of therapy is to prevent dehydration by giving enough oral fluids to keep up with the fluids lost in the diarrhea. Don't expect a quick return to solid stools. Since one loose stool can mean nothing, don't start dietary changes until there have been at least two.

HOME CARE: DIET

Dietary changes are the mainstay of home treatment for diarrhea. The optimal diet depends on your child's age and the severity of the diarrhea. Go directly to the part that pertains to your child.

Special Diets for Diarrhea

Mild Diarrhea *and* Child of Any Age
- Continue a regular diet with a few simple changes.
- Continue full-strength formula or milk. Encourage an increased intake of these fluids and extra water.
- Reduce the intake of fruit juices. If given, make them half strength with water.
- Avoid raw fruits and vegetables, beans, spicy foods, and any foods that cause loose stools.

Bottle-Fed Infants *and* Frequent, Watery Diarrhea
Oral Rehydration Solutions (ORS) for 6 to 24 Hours. Children with severe diarrhea need ORS to prevent dehydration. Examples are Infalyte, Kao-Lectrolyte, or Pedialyte. These over-the-counter products are available in all pharmacies or supermarkets. (ORS is not needed for diarrhea unless it's severe.) If your child doesn't like the flavor, add a bit of Kool-Aid powder. Give as much ORS as your baby wants. Diarrhea makes children thirsty, and your job is to satisfy that thirst and prevent dehydration. Never restrict fluids when your child has diarrhea.

Until you get one of these special solutions, continue giving your baby full-strength formula in unlimited amounts. (Avoid giving your baby Jell-O water mixtures or sports drinks. Reason: inadequate sodium content.)

If you can't get an ORS, ask your doctor about making a homemade ORS as follows: Mix ½ cup of dry infant rice cereal with 2 cups (16 ounces) of water and ¼ level teaspoon of salt. Be careful not to add too much salt. (Reason: risk of salt poisoning.)

Continue giving your baby ORS for at least 6 hours. Between 6 and 24 hours, switch back to formula when your baby becomes hungry, the diarrhea becomes less watery, and the child is making lots of urine.

Returning to Formula. After being given ORS for 6 to 24 hours, your baby will be hungry, so begin her regular formula. If the diarrhea continues to be severe, begin with a soy formula. If you give cow's milk formula and the diarrhea doesn't improve after 3 days, change to a lactose-free formula (milk-based lactose-free or a soy formula). Often there is less diarrhea with soy formulas than with cow's milk formulas because the soy formulas don't contain milk sugar (lactose). If you start giving soy formula, plan to keep your baby on the soy formula until the diarrhea is gone for 3 days.

If your baby's bowel movements are very watery, mix the formula with 1 or 2 ounces of extra water per bottle for 24 hours. Then after 24 hours go back to full-strength formula.

Adding Solids. Foods that contain a lot of starch are more easily digested than other foods during diarrhea. If your baby is over 4 months old, has had diarrhea for over 24 hours, and wants to eat solid food, give her the following starchy foods until the diarrhea is gone: any cereal, mashed potatoes, applesauce, strained bananas, strained carrots, and other high-fiber foods.

Breast-Fed Infants and Frequent, Watery Diarrhea
Definition of Diarrhea. No matter how it looks, the stool of the breast-fed infant must be considered normal unless it contains mucus or blood or develops a bad odor. In fact, breast-fed babies can normally pass some green stools or stools with a water ring around them. Frequency of movements is also not much help. As previously stated, during the first 2 or 3 months of life, the breast-fed baby may normally have as many stools as one after each feeding. The presence of something in the mother's diet that causes rapid passage should always be considered in these babies (e.g., coffee, cola, or herbal teas). Diarrhea can be diagnosed if your baby's stools abruptly increase in number. Additional clues are if your baby feeds poorly, acts sick, or develops a fever.

Instructions for Pediatric Patients, 2nd Edition, ©1999 by WB Saunders Company.
Written by Barton D. Schmitt, MD, pediatrician and author of *Your Child's Health*, Bantam Books, a book for parents.

Treatment

- Continue breast-feeding, but at more frequent intervals. Breast-feeding should never be discontinued because of diarrhea.
- If urine production is decreased, offer ORS between breast-feedings for 6 to 24 hours.

Older Children (over 1 Year Old) and Frequent, Watery Diarrhea

- The choice of solids is the key factor—starchy foods are absorbed best. Give cereals (especially rice cereal), oatmeal, bread, noodles, mashed potatoes, carrots, applesauce, strained bananas, etc. Pretzels or salty crackers can help meet your child's sodium needs.
- For fluids, use water (if solids are being consumed) or half-strength Kool-Aid. If solids are not being consumed, offer ORS. Encourage a high fluid intake.
- Avoid all fruit juice or other drinks containing fructose because they usually make diarrhea worse.
- Avoid milk for 2 or 3 days. (Reason: lactose is not as easily absorbed as complex carbohydrates.) Active culture yogurt is fine.
- ORS is rarely needed, unless diarrhea is very watery and urine production is decreased.

HOME CARE: OTHER ASPECTS

Common Mistakes. Using boiled skim milk or any concentrated solution can cause serious complications for babies with diarrhea because they contain too much salt. Kool-Aid and soda pop should not be used as the only foods because they contain little or no salt. Use only the fluids mentioned. Clear fluids alone should only be used for 6 to 24 hours because the body needs more calories than they can provide. Likewise, a diluted formula should not be used for more than 24 hours. The most dangerous myth is that the intestine should be "put to rest"; restricting fluids can cause dehydration. Keep in mind that there is no effective, safe drug for diarrhea and that extra water and diet therapy work best.

Prevention. Diarrhea is very contagious. Hand washing after diaper changing or using the toilet is crucial for keeping everyone in the family from getting diarrhea.

Diaper Rash from Diarrhea. The skin near your baby's anus can become "burned" from the diarrhea stools. Wash it off after each bowel movement and then protect it with a thick layer of petroleum jelly or other ointment. This protection is especially needed during the night and during naps. Changing the diaper quickly after bowel movements also helps.

Overflow Diarrhea in a Child Not Toilet Trained. For children in diapers, diarrhea can be a mess. Place a cotton washcloth inside the diaper to trap some of the more watery stool. Use disposable superabsorbent diapers temporarily to cut down on cleanup time. Use the ones with snug leg bands or cover the others with a pair of plastic pants. Wash your child under running water in the bathtub. Someday she will be toilet trained.

 CALL OUR OFFICE

IMMEDIATELY if

- Any blood appears in the diarrhea.
- Signs of dehydration occur (no urine in more than 8 hours, very dry mouth, no tears).
- Your child has severe diarrhea (more than eight bowel movements in the last 8 hours).
- The diarrhea is watery *and* your child also vomits the clear fluids three or more times.
- Your child starts acting very sick.

Note: If your child has vomited more than once, treatment of the vomiting has priority over the treatment of diarrhea until your child has gone 8 hours without vomiting.

During regular hours if

- A fever lasts more than 3 days.
- Mild diarrhea lasts more than 2 weeks.
- You have other concerns or questions.

DEFINITION

- Redness of the sclera (white part of the eye)
- Redness of the inner eyelids
- A watery discharge
- No yellow discharge or matting of eyelids
- Not caused by crying or allergy

Also called "bloodshot eyes" or "conjunctivitis."

Causes

Red eyes are usually caused by a viral infection, and they commonly accompany colds. If a bacterial superinfection occurs, the discharge becomes yellow and the eyelids are commonly matted together after sleeping. These children need antibiotic eye drops even if the eyes are not red.

The second most common cause is an irritant in the eye. The irritant can be shampoo, smog, smoke, or chlorine from a swimming pool. More commonly in young children it comes from touching the eyes with hands carrying dirt, food, soap, or animal saliva.

Expected Course

Viral conjunctivitis usually lasts as long as the cold (4 to 7 days). Red eyes from irritants usually are cured within 4 hours after washing out the irritating substance.

HOME CARE

Washing with Soap. Wash the face, and then wash the eyelids once with soap and water. Rinse them carefully with water. This will remove any irritants.

Irrigating with Water. For viral infections, rinse the eyes with warm water as often as possible, at least every 1 to 2 hours while your child is awake. Use a fresh, wet cotton ball each time. This usually will keep a bacterial infection from occurring. For mild chemical irritants, irrigate the eye with warm water for 5 minutes.

Vasoconstrictor Eye Drops. Viral conjunctivitis is not helped by eye drops.

Red eyes from irritants usually feel much better after the irritant has been washed out. If the eyes remain uncomfortable and bloodshot, instill some long-acting vasoconstrictor eye drops (a nonprescription item).

Your child's eye drops are _____.

Use 2 drops every _____ hours as necessary.

Contagiousness. Viral conjunctivitis is harmless and mildly contagious. Children with viral conjunctivitis can attend day care or school.

CALL OUR OFFICE

IMMEDIATELY if
- The outer eyelids become very red or swollen.
- Eye pain occurs.
- The vision becomes blurred.

Within 24 hours if
- A yellow discharge develops.
- The redness lasts for more than 7 days.
- You have other concerns or questions.

Instructions for Pediatric Patients, 2nd Edition, ©1999 by WB Saunders Company.
Written by Barton D. Schmitt, MD, pediatrician and author of *Your Child's Health,* Bantam Books, a book for parents.

DEFINITION

- Yellow discharge in the eye
- Eyelids stuck together with pus, especially after naps
- Dried eye discharge on the upper cheek
- The sclera may or may not have some redness or pinkness.
- Eyelids are usually puffy due to irritation from the infection.

Also called "bacterial conjunctivitis," "runny eyes," or "mattery eyes."

Note: A small amount of cream-colored mucus in the inner corner of the eyes after sleeping is normal.

Cause

Eye infections with pus are caused by various bacteria and can be a complication of a cold. Red eyes without a yellow discharge, however, are more common and are due to a virus.

Expected Course

With proper treatment, the yellow discharge should clear up in 3 days. The red eyes (which are due to the cold) may persist for several more days.

HOME TREATMENT

Cleaning the Eye. Before putting in any medicines, remove all the pus from the eye with warm water and wet cotton balls. Unless this is done, the medicine will not have a chance to work.

Antibiotic Eye Drops or Ointments. Bacterial conjunctivitis must be treated with an antibiotic eye medicine.

Your child's eye medicine is _____.

Put in _____, _____ times each day.

Putting eye drops or ointment in the eyes of younger children can be a real battle. It is most easily done with two people. One person can hold the child still while the other person opens the eyelids with one hand and puts in the medicine with the other. One person can do it alone if he sits on the floor holding the child's head (face up) between the knees to free both hands to put in the medication.

If we have prescribed antibiotic eye drops, put 2 drops in each eye every 2 hours while your child is awake. Do this by gently pulling down on the lower lid and placing the drops there. As soon as the eye drops have been put in the eyes, have your child close them for 2 minutes so the eye drops will stay inside. If it is difficult to separate your child's eyelids, put the eye drops over the inner corner of the eye while he is lying down. As your child opens the eye and blinks, the eye drops will flow in. Continue the eye drops until your child has awakened two mornings in a row without any pus in the eyes.

If we have prescribed antibiotic eye ointment, the ointment needs to be used just 4 times daily because it can remain in the eyes longer than eye drops. Separate the eyelids and put in a ribbon of ointment from one corner to the other. If it is very difficult to separate your child's eyelids, put the ointment on the lid margins. As it melts from body heat, it will flow onto the eyeball and give equally good results. Continue until two mornings have passed without any pus in the eye.

Contact Lenses. Children with contact lenses need to switch to glasses temporarily. (Reason: to prevent damage to the cornea.)

Contagiousness. The pus from the eyes can cause eye infections in other people if they get some of it on their eyes. Therefore it is very important for the sick child to have his own washcloth and towel. Your child should be encouraged not to touch or rub the eyes, because it can make the infection last longer and it puts many germs on his fingers. Your child's hands should also be washed often to prevent spreading the infection. After using eye drops for 24 hours and if the pus is minimal, children can return to day care or school.

 ## CALL OUR OFFICE

IMMEDIATELY if
- The outer eyelids become very red or swollen.
- The vision becomes blurred.
- Your child starts acting very sick.

Within 24 hours if
- The infection isn't cleared up after 3 days on treatment.
- Your child develops an earache.
- You have other concerns or questions.

FREQUENT INFECTIONS

DEFINITION
Average Frequencies of Infections

Some children seem to have the constant sniffles. They get one cold after another. Many a parent wonders, "Isn't my child having too many colds?" Children start to get colds after about 6 months of age. During infancy and the preschool years they average seven or eight colds each year. During the school-age years they average five or six colds each year. During adolescence they finally reach an adult level of approximately four colds per year. Colds account for more than 50% of all acute illnesses with fever. In addition, children can have diarrheal illnesses (with or without vomiting) two or three times per year.

Similar Condition: Allergies

If your child is over 3 years of age, sneezes a lot, has a clear nasal discharge that lasts over 1 month, doesn't have a fever, and especially if these symptoms occur during pollen season, your child probably has a nasal allergy. Allergies are much easier to treat than frequent colds because medicines are effective at controlling symptoms.

Causes

The main reason your child is getting all these infections is that she is being exposed to new viruses. There are at least 200 cold viruses. The younger the child, the less the previous exposure and subsequent protection. Your child is exposed more if she attends day care, play group, a church nursery, or a preschool. Your child has more indirect exposures if she has older siblings in school. Therefore colds are more common in large families. The rate of colds triples in the winter when people spend more time crowded together indoors breathing recirculated air. In addition, smoking in the home increases your child's susceptibility to colds, coughs, ear infections, sinus infections, croup, wheezing, and asthma.

WHAT DOESN'T CAUSE FREQUENT INFECTIONS

Most parents are worried that their repeatedly ill child has some serious underlying disease. A child with immune system disease (inadequate antibody or white blood cell production) doesn't experience any more colds than the average child. Instead, the child has two or more bouts per year of pneumonia, sinus infection, draining lymph nodes, or boils and heals slowly from these infections. In addition, a child with serious disease does not gain weight adequately nor appear well between bouts of infection.

DEALING WITH FREQUENT INFECTIONS

Look at Your Child's General Health. If your child is vigorous and gaining weight, you don't have to worry about her basic health. Your child is no sicker than the average child of her age. Children get over colds by themselves. Although you can reduce the symptoms, you can't shorten the course of each cold. Your child will muddle through like every other child. The long-term outlook is good. The number of colds will decrease over the years as your child's body builds up a good antibody supply to the various viruses. For perspective, note the findings of a recent survey: on any given day 10% of children have colds, 8% have fevers, 5% have diarrhea, and 3% have ear infections.

Send Your Child Back to School as Soon as Possible. The main requirement for returning your child to day care or school is that the fever is gone and the symptoms are not excessively noisy or distracting to classmates. It doesn't make sense to keep a child home until we can guarantee that she is no longer shedding any viruses because this could take 2 or 3 weeks. If isolation for respiratory infections were taken seriously, insufficient days would remain to educate children. Also the "germ warfare" that normally occurs in schools is fairly uncontrollable. Most children shed germs during the first days of their illness before they even look sick or have symptoms. In other words, contact with respiratory infections is unavoidable in group settings such as schools or day care.

Also, as long as your child's fever has cleared, there is no reason she cannot attend parties, play with friends after school, and go on scheduled trips. Gym and team sports may need to be postponed for a few days.

Try Not to Miss Work. When both parents work, these repeated colds are extremely inconvenient and costly. Since the complication rate is low and the improvement rate is slow, don't hesitate to leave your child with someone else at these times. Perhaps you have a babysitter who is willing to care for a child with a fever.

If your child goes to day care or preschool, she can go back once the fever is gone. There is no reason to prolong the recovery at home if you need to return to work. Early return of a child with a respiratory illness won't increase the complication rate for your child or the exposure rate for other children. Consider switching to a small home-based day care if your child is less than 2 years old. Also, find another day care if someone on the day care staff smokes on-site.

SUMMARY

There are no instant cures for recurrent colds and other viral illnesses. Antibiotics are not helpful unless your child develops complications such as an ear infection, sinus infection, or pneumonia. Having your child's tonsils removed is not helpful because colds are not caused by bad tonsils. Colds are not caused by poor diet or lack of vitamins. Again, the best time to have these infections and develop immunity is during childhood. Colds are the one infection we can't prevent yet. From a medical standpoint, colds are an unavoidable educational experience for your child's immune system.

Instructions for Pediatric Patients, 2nd Edition, ©1999 by WB Saunders Company.
Written by Barton D. Schmitt, MD, pediatrician and author of *Your Child's Health,* Bantam Books, a book for parents.

DEFINITION

- Bright red or rosy rash on both cheeks for 1 to 3 days ("slapped cheek" appearance)
- Rash on cheeks is followed by pink "lacelike" (or "netlike") rash on extremities
- "Lacy" rash mainly on thighs and upper arms; comes and goes several times over 1 to 3 weeks
- No fever or low-grade fever (less than 101°F [38.4°C])

Similar Conditions

Fifth disease was so named because it was the fifth pink-red infectious rash to be described by physicians. The other four are

1. Scarlet fever
2. Measles
3. Rubella
4. Roseola (controversial)

Cause

Fifth disease is caused by the human parvovirus B19.

Expected Course

This is a very mild disease with either no symptoms or a slight runny nose and sore throat. The lacelike rash may come and go for 5 weeks, especially after warm baths, exercise, and sun exposure.

HOME CARE

Treatment. No treatment is necessary. This distinctive rash is harmless and causes no symptoms that need treatment.

Contagiousness. Over 50% of exposed children will come down with the rash in 10 to 14 days. The disease is mainly contagious during the week before the rash begins. Therefore exposed children should try to avoid contact with pregnant women, but that can be difficult. Once the child has "slapped cheeks" or the lacy rash, he is no longer considered contagious and does not need to stay home from school.

Adults with Fifth Disease. Most adults who get fifth disease develop just a mild pinkness of the cheeks or no rash at all. Adults develop joint pains, especially in the knees, more often than a rash. These pains may last 1 to 3 months. Taking a nonprescription ibuprofen product usually relieves these symptoms. An arthritis workup is not necessary for joint pains that occur after exposure to fifth disease.

Refer Pregnant Women Exposed to Fifth Disease to Their Obstetrician. The risk of fifth disease is to the unborn babies of pregnant women. If a pregnant woman is exposed to a child with fifth disease, she should see her obstetrician. The doctor will obtain an antibody test to see if the mother already had the disease and is therefore protected. If not, the pregnancy will need to be monitored closely. Some fetuses infected with fifth disease before birth develop complications. Ten percent develop severe anemia and 2% may die. Birth defects, however, are never a result of this virus.

 CALL OUR OFFICE

During regular hours if
- The rash becomes itchy.
- Your child develops a fever over 102°F (38.9°C).
- You have other concerns or questions.

INFLUENZA

DEFINITION

Influenza (flu) is a viral infection of the nose, throat, trachea, and bronchi that occurs in epidemics every 3 or 4 years (e.g., Asian influenza). The main symptoms are a stuffy nose, sore throat, and nagging cough. There may be more muscle pain, headache, fever, and chills than with usual colds. For most people, influenza is just a "bad cold" and bed rest is not necessary. The dangers of influenza for healthy people are overrated.

HOME CARE

The treatment of influenza depends on the child's main symptoms and is no different from the treatment for other viral respiratory infections. Bed rest is unnecessary.

Fever or Aches. Use acetaminophen every 6 hours or ibuprofen every 8 hours. Aspirin should be avoided in children and adolescents with suspected influenza because of the possible link with Reye's syndrome.

Cough or Hoarseness. Give your child cough drops if over 4 years old. If your child is younger than 4 years old, give corn syrup ½ to 1 teaspoon as needed.

Sore Throat. A soft diet will help. For children over age 1, offer sips of warm chicken broth. Children over age 4 can suck on hard candy.

Stuffy Nose. Warm-water or saline nose drops followed by suction (or nose blowing) will open most blocked noses. Use nasal washes at least 4 times per day or whenever your child can't breathe through the nose. Saline nose drops are made by adding ½ teaspoon of salt to 1 cup of warm water.

Contagiousness. Spread is rapid because the incubation period is only 24 to 36 hours and the virus is very contagious. Therefore, your child may return to day care or school after the fever is gone and she feels up to it.

 CALL OUR OFFICE

IMMEDIATELY if
- Your child is having difficulty with breathing.
- Your child starts to act very sick.

During regular hours if
- An earache or sinus pain occurs.
- A fever lasts over 3 days.
- You have other questions or concerns.

INFLUENZA VACCINE AND PREVENTION

Influenza vaccine gives protection for only 1 or 2 years. In addition, the vaccine itself can cause fever in 20% of all people and a sore injection site in 10%. Therefore the vaccine is not recommended for healthy children (unless an especially severe form of influenza comes along). Only children with chronic diseases (e.g., asthma) need to have yearly influenza boosters. Talk about this with your physician if you think your child should have flu shots.

Instructions for Pediatric Patients, 2nd Edition, ©1999 by WB Saunders Company.
Written by Barton D. Schmitt, MD, pediatrician and author of *Your Child's Health,* Bantam Books, a book for parents.

DEFINITION

Lyme disease is the most common disease spread by a tick bite. About 7000 cases are reported each year in the United States. Complications, however, are rare. Giving up picnics, hikes, and camping because of this pest is an overreaction to the small risk. Lyme disease has been divided into three stages. If treated with antibiotics, it does not progress from one stage to the next.

Stage 1 occurs 3 to 30 days after the tick bite. A unique rash develops in 70% to 80% of people. The rash (called erythema migrans) consists of a red ring or bull's-eye that starts where the person was bitten and expands in size. The rash at the bite becomes larger than 2 inches across. A rash the size of a dime or quarter is not Lyme disease. The rash is neither painful nor itchy. It lasts 2 weeks to 2 months. About 50% of children also develop smaller spots at several locations. Some also develop a flulike illness, including fever, chills, sore throat, and headache, for several days.

Stage 2 occurs 2 to 12 weeks after the tick bite. It only affects 15% of untreated patients. The main symptoms are neurologic ones such as stiff neck (aseptic meningitis), weak facial muscles (seventh nerve paralysis), and weakness or numbness of the extremities (polyneuritis). A few children develop some abnormalities of heart rhythm (myocarditis).

Stage 3 occurs 6 weeks to 2 years after the tick bite. It affects about 50% of untreated patients, often without any stage 2 symptoms. The main symptom is recurrent attacks of painful, swollen joints (arthritis), usually of the knees. The arthritis becomes chronic in 10% of children.

Cause

Lyme disease is caused by a corkscrew-shaped bacterium called a spirochete. It is transmitted by little deer ticks that are the size of a pinhead, dark brown, and hard to see. Lyme disease is not carried by the more common wood tick, which is ¼ to ½ inch in size. In most states only 2% of deer ticks carry Lyme disease. In Wisconsin, Minnesota, and the New England states, however, up to 50% of ticks are infected. If left undisturbed, a tick will remain attached and feed for 3 to 6 days. How long a tick is attached determines the likelihood of passing on the infection. For Lyme disease to be transmitted, the tick needs to be attached for 18 to 24 hours.

Prevention of Tick Bites

Ticks like to hide in underbrush and shrubbery. Children and adults who are hiking in tick-infested areas should wear long clothing and tuck the ends of the pants into the socks. Apply an insect repellent to shoes and socks. During the hike perform tick checks using a buddy system every 2 to 3 hours to remove ticks on the clothing or exposed skin. Immediately after the hike or at least once each day, do a bare skin check. A brisk shower at the end of a hike will also remove any tick that isn't firmly attached. Because the bite is painless and doesn't itch, the child will usually be unaware of its presence. Favorite hiding places for ticks are in the hair, so carefully check the scalp, neck, armpit, and groin. Removing ticks promptly may prevent infection because transmission of Lyme disease requires 18 to 24 hours of feeding. Also, the tick is easier to remove before it becomes firmly attached. Perform tick checks on the dog if he accompanies you on a hike. Pull off any that are found.

Tick Removal

The simplest and quickest way to remove a tick is to pull it off. Use a tweezers to grasp the tick as close to the skin as possible. (Try to get a grip on its head.) Apply a steady upward traction until it releases its grip. Do not twist the tick or jerk it suddenly, thus breaking off its head or mouth parts. Do not squeeze the tweezers to the point of crushing the tick, because the secretions released may spread disease. If you don't have a tweezers, pull the tick off in the same way using your fingers, a loop of thread around the tick's jaws, or a needle between the tick's jaws for traction. Some tiny ticks need to be scraped off with a knife blade or the edge of a credit card.

If the body is removed but the head is left in the skin, it should be removed. Use a sterile needle (as you would to remove a sliver). Wash the wound and your hands with soap and water after removal.

A recent study showed that embedded ticks do not back out when covered with petroleum jelly, fingernail polish, or rubbing alcohol. We used to think that this would block the tick's breathing pores and take its mind off eating. Unfortunately, ticks breathe only a few times per hour. The study also found that the application of a hot match to the tick failed to cause it to detach and also carried the risk of inducing the tick to vomit infected secretions into the wound.

 ## CALL OUR OFFICE

IMMEDIATELY if
- You can't remove the tick.
- Fever or widespread rash occurs within the 2 weeks following a tick bite.
- Your child starts acting very sick.

During regular hours if
- You think your child might have Lyme disease.
- You have other questions or concerns.

Instructions for Pediatric Patients, 2nd Edition, ©1999 by WB Saunders Company.
Written by Barton D. Schmitt, MD, pediatrician and author of *Your Child's Health,* Bantam Books, a book for parents.

LYMPH NODE INFECTION IN THE NECK (CERVICAL ADENITIS)

DEFINITION

- A bacterial infection of a lymph node in the neck
- Abrupt onset of a tender, firm mass on one side of the neck
- Usually located below the angle of the jaw (the tonsillar node)
- Large node, usually over 1 inch across (can be size of walnut or egg)
- Sometimes the overlying skin is pink
- Fever is usually present

Cause

Lymph nodes are part of our immune system, which helps fight infections. Although viral infections or even a "strep throat" infection usually cause several nodes on both sides of the neck to become swollen, when bacteria actually invade a lymph node, usually only one lymph node is involved. Bacteria present in the nose, tonsils, or adenoids can spread to a lymph node and cause an infection. Also, cavities in the teeth can become infected and the bacteria may then spread to a lymph node under the jaw. The infected lymph node then becomes enlarged, warm, and tender.

Expected Course

Most lymph node infections heal well with oral antibiotics, but sometimes a lymph node needs to be opened and drained. Lymph nodes that need to be drained become soft in the middle or come to a head (form a large pimple).

HOME CARE

Oral Antibiotics. Antibiotics are used to treat the bacterial infection.

Your child's antibiotic is _____. Your child's

dose is _____. Give it _____ times a day for a

total of _____ days.

Local Heat. Apply a heating pad or warm, moist washcloth to the lymph node for 20 minutes, three times a day. This will help deliver the antibiotic to the infection and bring the infection to a head.

Fever and Pain Relief. Give your child acetaminophen or ibuprofen if she develops a fever over 102°F (39°C) or has pain from the neck swelling.

Fluids. Make sure your child is drinking plenty of fluids.

Observation of Lymph Nodes. Your child's lymph node may have been outlined with a pen during your visit. If so, watch to see that the node is not enlarging rapidly outside of the markings after the antibiotic is begun.

Follow-up Visit. All children with lymph node infections should see their doctor at the end of the antibiotic treatment to make sure the lymph node is no longer infected. It may take 1 or 2 months for the node to return to normal size. However, the node won't ever completely disappear.

 ## CALL OUR OFFICE

IMMEDIATELY if
- Your child has any difficulty swallowing liquids or breathing.
- The lymph node is rapidly enlarging even though your child is taking oral antibiotics.
- The fever is not gone 48 hours after starting an antibiotic.
- Your child starts acting very sick.

During regular hours if
- The lymph node becomes soft in the middle.
- The swelling is enlarging after 48 hours of antibiotics and your child is not getting better.
- You have other questions or concerns.

Instructions for Pediatric Patients, 2nd Edition, ©1999 by WB Saunders Company.
Written by Barton D. Schmitt, MD, pediatrician and author of *Your Child's Health,* Bantam Books, a book for parents.

DEFINITION

- Normal noninfected nodes are less than ½ inch across (often the size of a pea or baked bean).
- Nodes infected by a virus are usually ½ to 1 inch across. Slight enlargement and mild tenderness mean the lymph node is fighting infection and succeeding.
- Nodes severely infected with bacteria are usually more than 1 inch across and tender to the touch. If they are over 2 inches across or the overlying skin is pink, the nodes are not controlling the infection and may contain pus.

Cause

Lymph glands stop the spread of infection and protect the bloodstream from invasion (blood poisoning). They enlarge with cuts, scrapes, scratches, splinters, burns, insect bites, rashes, impetigo, or any break in the skin. Try to locate and identify the cause of the swollen gland by remembering that the groin nodes drain lymph from the legs and lower abdomen, the armpit nodes drain the arms and upper chest, the back-of-the-neck nodes drain the scalp, and the front-of-the-neck nodes drain the lower face, nose, and throat. Most enlarged nodes in the neck are due to colds or throat infections. A disease such as chickenpox can cause all the nodes to swell.

Expected Course

With the usual viral infections or skin infections, nodes can quickly double in size over 2 or 3 days and then slowly return to normal size over 2 to 4 weeks. However, you can still see and feel nodes in most normal children, especially in the neck and groin. Don't check for lymph nodes because you can always find some normal ones.

HOME CARE

Facts About Nodes. The body contains more than 500 lymph nodes. They can always be felt in the neck and groin. Normal nodes are largest at age 10 to 12. At this age they can be twice the normal adult size. Minor skin infections and irritations can cause lymph nodes to double in size. It may take 1 month for them to return to normal size. However, they won't completely disappear.

Treat the Cause of the Swelling. In general, no treatment is necessary for swollen nodes associated with viral infections (e.g., upper respiratory infections). For bacterial infections, the underlying disease that's causing the node to react needs to be treated. For example, remove the splinter, treat the ingrown toenail, or have a dentist treat the tooth abscess. Many children with swollen lymph nodes due to a skin infection also require an oral antibiotic.

For pain or fever above 102°F (38.9°C), give acetaminophen or ibuprofen in the appropriate amount.

Don't Squeeze the Nodes. Poking and squeezing lymph nodes may keep them from shrinking back to normal size. Remember that it may take a month for the nodes to return to normal, and they won't completely disappear. There's no need to check them more than once a month. If your child fidgets with them, discourage it if he is old enough to cooperate.

 ## CALL OUR OFFICE

IMMEDIATELY if
- The node swells to more than 2 inches across.
- The overlying skin becomes red.
- Your child starts acting very sick.

During regular hours if
- The node swells to 1 to 2 inches across.
- Your child also develops a sore throat.
- A fever persists more than 3 days.
- You have other concerns or questions.

MEASLES (RUBEOLA)

DEFINITION

- Three or 4 days of red eyes, cough, runny nose, and fever before the rash begins
- Pronounced blotchy red rash starting on the face and spreading downward over the entire body in 3 days
- White specks on the lining of the mouth (Koplik's spots)
- Exposure to a child with measles 10 to 12 days earlier
- This diagnosis must be confirmed by a physician

Cause

The measles virus.

Expected Course

Measles can be a miserable illness. The rash usually lasts 7 days. Your child will usually begin to feel a lot better by the fourth day of the rash. Ear and eye infections are common complications.

HOME CARE

Treatment
- Fever: Use acetaminophen or ibuprofen in the usual dosage for your child's age.
- Cough: Use ½ to 1 teaspoon of corn syrup for children less than 4 years old, or cough drops for children over 4 years old. If the cough interferes with sleep, give a cough suppressant such as dextromethorphan. Also, use a humidifier.

- Red eyes: Wipe your child's eyes frequently with a clean, wet cotton ball. The eyes are usually sensitive to bright light, so your child probably won't want to go outside for several days unless she wears sunglasses.
- Rash: The rash requires no treatment.

Contagiousness. The disease is no longer contagious after the rash is gone. This usually takes 7 days.

Measles Exposure. Any child or adult who has been exposed to your child and who has not had measles or the measles vaccine should call her physician. If given early, a measles vaccine is often protective.

 CALL OUR OFFICE

IMMEDIATELY if
- Breathing becomes labored *and* no better after you clear the nose.
- Your child develops a severe headache.
- Your child starts acting very sick.

Within 24 hours if
- Your child develops an earache.
- The eyes develop a yellow discharge.
- Your child develops sinus pain or pressure.
- The fever lasts more than 3 days (after the start of the rash).
- You have other concerns or questions.

Instructions for Pediatric Patients, 2nd Edition, ©1999 by WB Saunders Company.
Written by Barton D. Schmitt, MD, pediatrician and author of *Your Child's Health,* Bantam Books, a book for parents.

DEFINITION

- Severe sore throat
- Large red tonsils covered with pus
- Swollen lymph nodes in the neck, armpits, and groin
- Fever for 7 to 14 days
- Enlarged spleen (in 50% of children)
- Blood smear showing many atypical (unusual) lymphocytes
- Positive blood test for mononucleosis
- This diagnosis must be confirmed by a physician

Cause

Mononucleosis (mono) is caused by the Epstein-Barr virus. This virus is transmitted in infected saliva through coughing, sneezing, and kissing. Although mononucleosis can occur at any age, it occurs more often in 15- to 25-year-olds, possibly because of more intimate contacts with others. Contrary to popular belief, mono is not very contagious. Household contacts of your child rarely come down with it.

Expected Course

Most children have only mild symptoms for about 1 week. Even those with severe symptoms usually feel completely well in 2 to 4 weeks. Complications are rare and require hospitalization when they occur. The most common complication is dehydration from not drinking enough fluids. Breathing may be obstructed by enlarged tonsils, adenoids, and other lymph tissue in the back of the throat. On rare occasions, the enlarged spleen will rupture if the abdomen is hit or strained. Because over 90% of youngsters with mononucleosis will develop a severe rash if they receive ampicillin or amoxicillin, these medications should be avoided in this condition. In general, mononucleosis is neither lingering nor progressive. All symptoms are gone by 4 weeks after they first appeared.

HOME TREATMENT FOR MONONUCLEOSIS

Fever and Pain Medicines.   No specific medicine will cure mononucleosis. However, symptoms can usually be reduced by medicines. The pain of swollen lymph nodes, sore throats, and fever over 102°F (39°C) can usually be relieved by appropriate doses of acetaminophen or ibuprofen.

Sore Throat Treatment.   Older children over age 6 can gargle with warm salt water (½ teaspoon of salt per glass). Sucking on hard candies for children over age 4 also relieves symptoms (butterscotch seems to be a soothing flavor). Over age 1, children can sip warm chicken broth.

Provide a Soft Diet.   Since swollen tonsils can make some foods hard to swallow, provide a soft diet as long as necessary. To prevent dehydration, be sure that your youngster drinks enough fluids. Milk shakes and cold drinks are especially good. Avoid citrus fruits. Give a daily multiple vitamin pill until the appetite returns to normal.

Activity.   Your child does not need to stay in bed. Bed rest will not shorten the course of the illness or reduce symptoms. Your child can select how much rest he needs. Usually children voluntarily slow down until the fever has resolved. Children can return to school when the fever is gone and they can swallow normally. Most children will want to be back to full activity by 2 to 4 weeks.

Precautions for an Enlarged Spleen.   A blow to the abdomen can cause rupture of an enlarged spleen and bleeding. This is a surgical emergency. Therefore all children with mononucleosis should avoid contact sports for at least 4 weeks. Athletes especially must restrict their activity until the spleen returns to normal size by physical exam. We will check your child weekly until the spleen size returns to normal. Constipation and heavy lifting should also be avoided because of the sudden pressures they can put on the spleen.

Contagiousness.   Infectious mononucleosis is most contagious while your child has a fever. After the fever is gone, the virus is still carried in the saliva for up to 6 months, but in small amounts. Overall, mononucleosis is only slightly contagious from contacts. Boyfriends, girlfriends, roommates, and relatives rarely get it. (The incubation period is 4 to 7 weeks after contact.) The person with mononucleosis does not need to be isolated. However, he should definitely use separate glasses and utensils and avoid kissing until the fever has been gone for several days.

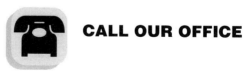 **CALL OUR OFFICE**

IMMEDIATELY if
- Your child develops difficulty breathing.
- Your child becomes dehydrated.
- Abdominal pain occurs (especially high on the left side).
- Left shoulder pain occurs.
- Your child starts acting very sick.

Within 24 hours if
- Your child develops noisy breathing.
- Your child can't drink enough fluids.
- Sinus or ear pain occurs.
- The fever isn't gone within 10 days.
- Your child isn't back to school in 2 weeks.
- You have other questions or concerns.

DEFINITION

- Swollen parotid gland in front of the ear and crossing the corner of the jaw
- Both parotid glands swollen in 70% of children
- Tenderness of the swollen gland
- Pain increased with chewing
- Fever is present
- No prior mumps vaccine
- Exposure to another child with mumps 16 to 18 days earlier (adds weight to the diagnosis)
- This diagnosis must be confirmed by a physician

Cause

Mumps is an acute viral infection of the parotid, a gland that produces saliva and is located in front of and below each ear.

Expected Course

The fever is usually gone in 3 to 4 days. The swelling and pain are cleared in 7 days.

HOME CARE

Pain and Fever Relief. Give acetaminophen or ibuprofen. Cold compresses applied to the swollen area may also relieve pain.

Diet
- Avoid sour foods or citrus fruits that increase saliva production and parotid swelling.
- Avoid foods that require much chewing.
- Consider a liquid diet if chewing is very painful.

Contagiousness. The disease is contagious until the swelling is gone (usually 6 or 7 days). Your child should be kept out of school and away from other children who have not had mumps or mumps vaccine.

Mumps Exposure. Mumps exposure is important if a person has never received the mumps vaccine or had mumps, but only 10% of adults who have no record of mumps are really susceptible. Adults who as children lived in the same household with siblings who had mumps can be considered protected. Those who are not protected should call our office during office hours to see if the mumps vaccine would be helpful and should use the following guidelines:

- Children: All should receive the mumps vaccine.
- Adolescent or adult males: The mumps vaccine is optional. (The risk of testicular infection [orchitis] is 2.5%.)
- Adult females: The mumps vaccine is unnecessary. No serious complications occur.

 CALL OUR OFFICE

IMMEDIATELY if
- Your child develops a stiff neck or severe headache.
- Your child vomits repeatedly.
- Your child starts acting very sick.

During regular hours if
- The swelling lasts for more than 7 days.
- The fever lasts for more than 4 days.
- The skin over the mumps gland becomes reddened.
- In adolescent males, the testicle becomes painful.
- You have other concerns or questions.

Instructions for Pediatric Patients, 2nd Edition, ©1999 by WB Saunders Company.
Written by Barton D. Schmitt, MD, pediatrician and author of *Your Child's Health,* Bantam Books, a book for parents.

DEFINITION

Symptoms of an infection of a pierced ear are tenderness, a yellow discharge, redness, and some swelling.

Causes

The most common causes of infection are piercing the ears with unsterile equipment, inserting unsterile posts, or frequently touching the earlobes with dirty hands.

Another frequent cause is earrings that are too tight either because the post is too short (the thickness of earlobes varies) or the clasp is closed too tightly. Tight earrings don't allow air to enter the channel through the earlobe. Also, the pressure from tight earrings reduces blood flow to the earlobe and makes it more vulnerable to infection.

Some inexpensive earrings have rough areas on the posts that scratch the channel and can result in infection. Inserting the post at the wrong angle also can scratch the channel, so a mirror should be used until insertion becomes second nature. Posts containing nickel can also cause an itchy, allergic reaction.

Expected Course

With proper care, most mild earlobe infections will clear up in 1 to 2 weeks. Recurrences are common if the youngster is not conscientious in ear and earring care.

HOME CARE FOR MILD PIERCED-EAR INFECTIONS

Remove the earring and post three times a day. Cleanse them with rubbing alcohol. Clean both sides of the earlobe with rubbing alcohol. Apply bacitracin ointment (a nonprescription item) to the post and reinsert it. Continue the antibiotic ointment for 2 days beyond the time the infection seems cleared. Carefully review and follow all the recommendations on preventing infections given below.

PREVENTION OF INFECTIONS

Recommended Age for Pierced Ears. Pierced earrings should not be worn until a child is old enough (usually older than 4 years) to know not to fidget with them (which can lead to infections) or take them out and put them in her mouth (which can lead to swallowing or choking on them). Ideally, the ears should not be pierced until a child can play an active part in the decision (usually past age 8).

Prevention of Infections When Ears Are First Pierced
- Do not pierce your child's ears if she has a tendency to bleed easily, form thick scars (keloids), or get staphylococcal skin infections.
- Have your child's earlobes pierced by someone who is experienced and understands sterile technique. Piercing by someone inexperienced can result in infections or a cosmetically poor result.
- The initial posts should be 14-karat gold or stainless steel.
- Do not remove the posts for 6 weeks.
- Apply the earring clasp loosely to allow for swelling.
- After washing the hands and cleaning both sides of the earlobes with rubbing alcohol, turn the posts approximately three rotations. Do this twice a day.
- By the end of 6 weeks, the lining of the channels should be healed and earrings may be changed as often as desired.

Prevention of Later Infections
- Remind your child not to touch the earrings except when inserting or removing them. Fingers are often dirty and can contaminate the area.
- Clean earrings, posts, and earlobes with rubbing alcohol before each insertion.
- Apply the clasps loosely to prevent any pressure on the earlobes and to provide an air space on both sides of each earlobe.
- Polish or discard any posts with rough spots.
- At bedtime, remove the earrings so that the channel is exposed to the air during the night.

Prevention of Injury to the Earlobe. Remind your youngster that dangling earrings can lead to a torn earlobe requiring plastic surgery. Such earrings should not be worn during sports. Your child should also take precautions while dancing, hair washing, or handling young children who might yank the earrings.

 CALL OUR OFFICE

IMMEDIATELY if
- The earring clasp becomes embedded in the earlobe and can't be removed.
- Your child develops a fever.

During regular hours if
- Swelling or redness spreads beyond the pierced area.
- Your child develops a fever (over 100°F, or 37.8°C).
- The infection is not improving after 48 hours of treatment.
- You have other concerns or questions.

PNEUMONIA

DEFINITION

- Labored breathing (respiratory distress)
- Rapid breathing
- Occasionally painful breathing
- Coughing
- Fever, sometimes with chills
- Abnormal patch ("infiltrate") on chest x-ray film
- This diagnosis must be confirmed by a physician
  Note: Most rattly breathing is not pneumonia.

Causes

Pneumonia is an infection of the lung that causes fluid to collect in the air sacs (alveoli). Approximately 80% of pneumonia cases are caused by viruses and 20% by bacteria. Viral pneumonia is usually milder than bacterial pneumonia. Bacterial pneumonia tends to have a more abrupt onset, higher fevers (often over 104°F [40°C]) and a larger infiltrate (greater lung involvement) visible on the chest x-ray film. Only bacterial pneumonia is helped by antibiotics. Because it's difficult to distinguish bacterial from viral pneumonia in all cases, antibiotics are prescribed for some children with viral pneumonia. Because pneumonia is usually a complication of a cold, it is not considered contagious.

Expected Course

Before antibiotics were available, bacterial pneumonia was dangerous. With antibiotics, it improves within 24 to 48 hours. On the other hand, viral pneumonia can continue for 2 to 4 weeks. Most children with pneumonia can be cared for at home. Admission to the hospital for oxygen or intravenous fluids is required in less than 10% of cases. Most children admitted to the hospital are young infants or children who have extensive involvement of the lungs. Recovery from viral pneumonia is gradual but complete. Recurrences of pneumonia are rare.

HOME TREATMENT

Antibiotics. Children with bacterial pneumonia need an antibiotic.

Your child's antibiotic is _____.

Give _____ every _____ hours. Continue the antibiotic for a full _____ days.

Medicines for Fever. Use acetaminophen or ibuprofen for moderate fever (over 102°F [38.9°C]). These medicines can also help chest pain.

Warm Fluids for Coughing Spasms. Coughing spasms are often caused by sticky secretions in the back of the throat. Warm liquids usually relax the airway and loosen the secretions. Offer your child warm lemonade, warm apple juice, or herbal tea. In addition, breathing warm moist air helps to loosen the sticky mucus that may be choking your child. You can provide warm mist by placing a warm, wet washcloth loosely over your child's nose and mouth; or you can fill a humidifier with warm water and have your child breathe in the warm mist it produces. Avoid steam vaporizers because they can cause burns. Don't give cough suppressant medicines (such as those containing dextromethorphan) to children with pneumonia. The infectious secretions need to be coughed up.

Humidity. Dry air tends to make coughs worse. Use a humidifier in your child's bedroom. The new ultrasonic humidifiers not only have the advantage of quietness, but also kill molds and most bacteria that might be in the water.

No Smoking. Tobacco smoke aggravates coughing and makes coughs last longer. Don't let anyone smoke around your child. In fact, try not to let anybody smoke inside your home. Remind a teenager with pneumonia, if he smokes, that the cough will last weeks longer than it normally would without smoking.

 ## CALL OUR OFFICE

IMMEDIATELY if
- Breathing becomes more labored or difficult.
- Your child starts acting very sick.

Within 24 hours if
- The fever lasts over 48 hours on an antibiotic.
- The cough lasts over 3 weeks.
- You have other questions or concerns.

Instructions for Pediatric Patients, 2nd Edition, ©1999 by WB Saunders Company.
Written by Barton D. Schmitt, MD, pediatrician and author of *Your Child's Health,* Bantam Books, a book for parents.

DEFINITION

- Age 6 months to 3 years
- Presence of a fine pink rash, mainly on the trunk
- High fever during the preceding 2 to 4 days that cleared within 24 hours before the rash appeared
- Child only mildly ill during the time with fever
- Child acting fine now

Cause

Roseola is caused by the human herpesvirus-6.

Expected Course

The rash lasts 1 or 2 days, followed by complete recovery. Some children have 3 days of fever without a rash.

HOME CARE

No particular treatment is necessary. Roseola is contagious until the rash is gone. Other children of this age who have been with your child may come down with roseola in about 12 days.

 CALL OUR OFFICE

IMMEDIATELY if
- The spots become purple or blood-colored.

During regular hours if
- The rash lasts more than 3 days.
- The fever lasts more than 4 days.
- You have other questions or concerns.

RUBELLA (GERMAN MEASLES)

DEFINITION

- Widespread pink-red spots
- Rash beginning on the face and moving rapidly downward, covering the body in 24 hours
- Lasts 3 to 4 days ("3-day measles")
- Rubella rash is not distinctive. Many other viral rashes look like it
- Enlarged lymph nodes at back of neck
- Mild fever
- Child never given the rubella vaccine
- This diagnosis must be confirmed by a physician

Cause

Rubella is caused by a virus. The incubation period is 14 to 21 days.

Expected Course

The disease is mild. Your child should be completely recovered in 3 or 4 days. Complications in general are very rare. However, complications to the unborn child of a pregnant woman with rubella are disastrous and include deafness, cataracts, heart defects, growth retardation, and encephalitis. Pregnant women should avoid anyone with suspected rubella.

HOME CARE

If we have determined that your child probably has rubella, the following may be helpful.

Treatment. No treatment is probably necessary. Give acetaminophen or ibuprofen for fever over 102°F (38.9°C), sore throat, or other pains.

Avoid Pregnant Women. If your child might have rubella, keep her away from any pregnant women. Your child is contagious for 5 days after the start of the rash.

Exposure of Adult Women to Rubella. The nonpregnant woman exposed to rubella should avoid pregnancy during the following 3 months.

A pregnant woman exposed to rubella should see her obstetrician. If she has already received the rubella vaccine, she (and her unborn child) are probably protected. Even if she thinks she had the German measles disease as a child and the present exposure was minor or brief, she should have a blood test to determine her immunity against rubella.

Rubella Vaccine. Get your children immunized against rubella at 12 to 15 months of age so we won't have to worry about pregnant women getting exposed to rubella when a child gets a pink or red rash. It's quite safe to immunize the child who has a pregnant mother.

 CALL OUR OFFICE

IMMEDIATELY if
- The rash becomes purple or blood-colored.
- Your child starts acting very sick.

During regular hours if
- The fever lasts more than 3 days.
- You have other concerns or questions.

Instructions for Pediatric Patients, 2nd Edition, ©1999 by WB Saunders Company.
Written by Barton D. Schmitt, MD, pediatrician and author of *Your Child's Health*, Bantam Books, a book for parents.

DEFINITION

- Reddened, sunburned-looking skin (especially of the chest and abdomen). On close inspection, the redness is speckled (tiny pink dots)
- Increased redness in skinfolds (especially the groin, armpits, and elbow creases)
- Full-blown rash within 24 hours
- Rough feeling of reddened skin, somewhat like sandpaper
- Flushed face with paleness around the mouth
- Sore throat and fever (usually preceding the rash by 18 to 24 hours)
- This diagnosis must be confirmed by a physician

Cause

Scarlet fever is a strep throat infection with a rash. The complication rate is no different than the complication rate for strep throat alone. The rash is caused by a special rash-producing toxin that is produced by some strep bacteria.

Expected Course

The red rash usually clears in 4 or 5 days. Sometimes the skin peels in 1 to 2 weeks where the rash was most prominent (e.g., the groin). The skin on the fingertips also commonly peels. Your child will stop having a sore throat and fever after 1 or 2 days of taking penicillin or other antibiotic.

HOME TREATMENT

Antibiotics

Your child's antibiotic is _____. Your child's dose is _____ 3 times daily during waking hours (i.e., before breakfast, midafternoon, and at bedtime) for 10 days.

Try not to forget any doses. If your child goes to school or a babysitter, arrange for someone to give the midafternoon dose. Give the medicine until all the pills are gone or the bottle is empty. Even though your child will feel better in a few days, give the antibiotic for 10 days to keep the strep throat from flaring up again.

If the medicine is a liquid, store it in the refrigerator. Use a measuring spoon to be sure that you give the right amount.

A long-acting penicillin (Bicillin) injection can be given if your child will not take oral medicines or if it will be impossible for you to give the medicine regularly.

(*Note:* If given correctly, the oral antibiotic works just as rapidly and effectively as a shot.)

For Relief of Sore Throat. Acetaminophen or ibuprofen are very helpful. Children over age 1 can sip warm chicken broth or warm apple juice. Children over age 4 can suck on hard candy or lollipops.

The Rash. The rash itself needs no treatment. It generally clears in 4 to 5 days.

Contagiousness. Your child is no longer contagious after he has been on an antibiotic for 24 hours. Therefore your child can return to school after 1 day if he is feeling better. The rash itself is not contagious.

Throat Cultures for the Family. Scarlet fever and strep throat can spread to others in the family. Any child or adult who lives in your home and has a fever, sore throat, runny nose, headache, vomiting, or sores; or who doesn't want to eat; or who develops these symptoms in the next 5 days should be brought in for a throat culture. In most homes we need to culture only those who are sick. We will call you if any of the cultures are positive for a strep infection.

(*Exception:* In families where relatives have had rheumatic fever or frequent strep infections, everyone should have a throat culture.)

Follow-up Visit. Repeat throat cultures are not necessary if your child takes all of the antibiotic.

 ## CALL OUR OFFICE

IMMEDIATELY if
- Your child develops drooling or great difficulty in swallowing.
- Your child starts acting very sick.

Within 24 hours if
- The fever lasts over 48 hours after your child starts taking an antibiotic.
- You have other concerns or questions.

SINUS INFECTION (SINUSITIS)

DEFINITION

A sinus infection is a bacterial infection of one of the seven sinuses that normally drain into the nose. Sinus congestion can occur without an infection if one of the sinus openings becomes blocked from a cold or hay fever. As bacteria multiply within the sinuses, pain and pressure occur above the eyebrow, behind the eye, or over the cheekbone. Other symptoms can include a profuse yellow nasal discharge, postnasal drip, a blocked nose, fever, and bad breath. Until recent years, we didn't recognize that a chronic cough can be caused by a sinus infection. Swallowing sinus secretions is normal and harmless but may lead to some nausea. Most sinus infections can be diagnosed without sinus x-ray studies. The following treatment should reduce pain and fever within 48 hours or less.

HOME TREATMENT

Antibiotics

Your child's antibiotic is _____. Your child's dose is _____ given _____ times per day by mouth during waking hours for _____ days.

This medicine will kill bacteria that are causing the sinus infection. Try not to forget any of the doses. If your child goes to school or to a babysitter, arrange for someone to give the afternoon dose. If the medicine is a liquid, use a measuring spoon so you give the right amount. Also, an antibiotic should not be saved from one illness to the next because it loses its strength. Even though your child will feel better in a few days, give all the medicine to prevent the infection from flaring up.

Nasal Washes. Use warm water or saline nose drops followed by suction or nose blowing to wash dried mucus or pus out of the nose. Do nasal washes at least four times a day or whenever your child can't breathe through the nose. If the air in your home is dry, run a humidifier.

Decongestant Nose Drops or Spray. To drain the sinuses, use a generic, long-acting vasoconstrictor nose drop or spray (such as oxymetazoline), which is nonprescription. The usual dose for adolescents is 2 drops or sprays per nostril twice daily. For younger children use 1 drop or spray each day. Use the medicine routinely for the first 2 or 3 days of treatment. Thereafter don't use the spray or nose drops unless the sinus congestion or pain recurs. Stop the drops or spray after 5 days to prevent rebound swelling.

Pain Relief Medicines. Acetaminophen or ibuprofen can be given for a few days for sinus pain or any fever over 102°F (39°C).

Oral Antihistamines. If your child also has hay fever, give her allergy medicine. Otherwise, avoid antihistamines because they can slow down the movement of secretions out of the sinuses.

Contagiousness. Sinus infections are not contagious. Your child can return to school or day care when she is feeling better and the fever is gone.

 ## CALL OUR OFFICE

IMMEDIATELY if
- Redness or swelling occurs on the cheek, eyelid, or forehead.
- Your child starts acting very sick.

Within 24 hours if
- The fever or pain is not gone after your child has taken the antibiotic for 48 hours.
- You have other questions or concerns.

Instructions for Pediatric Patients, 2nd Edition, ©1999 by WB Saunders Company.
Written by Barton D. Schmitt, MD, pediatrician and author of *Your Child's Health,* Bantam Books, a book for parents.

DEFINITION

- The child complains of a sore throat.
- In children too young to talk, a sore throat may be suspected if they refuse to eat or begin to cry during feedings.
- When examined with a light, the throat is bright red.

Cause

Most sore throats are caused by viruses and are part of a cold. About 10% of sore throats are due to the strep bacteria. A throat culture or rapid strep test is the only way to distinguish strep pharyngitis from viral pharyngitis. Without treatment, a strep throat can have some rare but serious complications. Tonsillitis (temporary swelling and redness of the tonsils) is usually present with any throat infection, viral or bacterial. The presence of tonsillitis does not have any special meaning.

Children who sleep with their mouths open often wake in the morning with a dry mouth and sore throat. It clears within an hour of having something to drink. Use a humidifier to help prevent this problem. Children with a postnasal drip from draining sinuses often have a sore throat from frequent throat clearing.

Expected Course

Sore throats with viral illnesses usually last 3 or 4 days. Strep throat responds well to penicillin. After taking the medication for 24 hours, your child is no longer contagious and can return to day care or school if the fever is gone and he is feeling better.

HOME CARE

Local Pain Relief. Children over 8 years of age can gargle with warm salt water (¼ teaspoon of salt per glass). Children over 4 years of age can suck on hard candy (butterscotch seems to be a soothing flavor) or lollipops as often as necessary. Children over age 1 can sip warm chicken broth or warm apple juice.

Soft Diet. Swollen tonsils can make some foods hard to swallow. Provide your child with a soft diet for a few days if he prefers it.

Fever. Acetaminophen or ibuprofen may be given for a few days if your child has a fever over 102°F (39°C) or a great deal of throat discomfort.

Common Mistakes in Treating Sore Throat

- Avoid expensive throat sprays or throat lozenges. Not only are they no more effective than hard candy, but they also may contain an ingredient (benzocaine) that may cause a drug reaction.
- Avoid using leftover antibiotics from siblings or friends. These should be thrown out because they deteriorate faster than other drugs. Unfortunately, antibiotics only help strep throats. They have no effect on viruses, and they can cause harm. They also make it difficult to find out what is wrong if your child becomes sicker.

Rapid Strep Tests. Rapid strep tests are helpful only when their results are positive. If they are negative, a throat culture should be performed to pick up the 20% of strep infections that the rapid tests miss. Avoid rapid strep tests performed in shopping malls or at home because they tend to be inaccurate.

 CALL OUR OFFICE

IMMEDIATELY if
- Your child is drooling, spitting, or having great difficulty in swallowing.
- Breathing becomes difficult.
- Your child is acting very sick.

During regular hours
- To make an appointment for a throat culture for any other child with a sore throat present for more than 24 hours.

(Exception: If the sore throat is very mild *and* the main symptom is croup, hoarseness, or a cough, a throat culture is probably not needed. Throat cultures are recommended for all other sore throats because a resurgence of acute rheumatic fever began in 1987. Rheumatic fever is a complication of strep infections that can lead to permanent damage to the valves of the heart.)

- If a fever lasts more than 3 days.
- If you have other questions or concerns.

STREP THROAT INFECTION

DEFINITION

Your child has a strep throat infection if diagnosis is confirmed by a throat culture or rapid strep test. The treatment of strep throats can prevent some rare but serious complications, namely, rheumatic fever (heart disease) or glomerulonephritis (kidney disease). In addition, treatment usually eliminates the fever and much of the sore throat within 24 hours.

HOME TREATMENT

Antibiotics

Your child's antibiotic is _____. Your child's dose is _____ given _____ times each day during waking hours for _____ days.

Try not to forget any doses. If your child goes to school or a babysitter, arrange for someone to give the midafternoon dose. If the medicine is a liquid, store the antibiotic in the refrigerator and use a measuring spoon to be sure that you give the right amount. Give the medicine until all the pills are gone or the bottle is empty. Even though your child will feel better in a few days, give the antibiotic for 10 days to keep the strep throat from flaring up.

A long-acting penicillin (Bicillin) injection can be given if your child refuses oral medicines or if it will be impossible for you to give the oral medicine regularly. (*Note:* If given correctly, the oral antibiotic works just as rapidly and effectively as a shot.)

Local Pain Relief. Children over age 1 can sip warm chicken broth or warm apple juice. Children over age 4 can suck on hard candy or lollipops. Children over age 8 can gargle with warm salt water (¼ teaspoon of salt per glass).

Soft Diet. Since swollen tonsils can make some foods hard to swallow, provide your child with a soft diet for a few days.

Fever. Acetaminophen or ibuprofen may be given if your child has a fever over 102°F (39°C) or a great deal of throat discomfort.

Contagiousness. Your child is no longer contagious after he or she has taken the antibiotic for 24 hours. Therefore your child can return to school after 1 day if the fever is gone.

Throat Cultures for the Family. Strep throat can spread to others in the family. Any child or adult who lives in your home and has a fever, sore throat, runny nose, headache, vomiting, or sores; doesn't want to eat; or develops these symptoms in the next 5 days should be brought in for a throat culture. In most homes we need to culture only those who are sick. We will call you if any of these cultures are positive for strep infection.

(*Exception:* In families where relatives have had rheumatic fever or frequent strep infections, everyone should come in for a throat culture.)

Follow-up Visit. Repeat cultures are unnecessary if your child receives all of the antibiotic.

 CALL OUR OFFICE

IMMEDIATELY if
- Your child develops drooling.
- Your child develops great difficulty with swallowing.
- Your child is acting very sick.

Within 24 hours if
- The fever lasts over 48 hours after starting an antibiotic.
- You have other questions or concerns.

Instructions for Pediatric Patients, 2nd Edition, ©1999 by WB Saunders Company.
Written by Barton D. Schmitt, MD, pediatrician and author of *Your Child's Health*, Bantam Books, a book for parents.

DEFINITION

- Itchy and painful ear canals
- Currently engaged in swimming
- Pain when the outer ear is moved up and down
- Pain when the tab of the outer ear overlying the ear canal is pushed in
- A feeling that the ear is plugged up
- Slight, clear discharge initially; without treatment, it becomes yellowish

Cause

Swimmer's ear is an infection of the skin lining the ear canal. The cause is prolonged contact with water (any type of water). When water gets trapped in the ear canal the lining becomes damp, swollen, and prone to infection. Ear canals were meant to be dry. Children are more likely to get swimmer's ear from swimming in lake water, compared with swimming pools or the sea. During the hottest weeks of summer, some lakes have high levels of bacteria. Narrow ear canals also increase the risk of swimmer's ear.

Expected Course

With treatment, symptoms should be better in 3 days.

HOME TREATMENT

Antibiotic-Steroid Ear Drops

Your child's ear drops are _____. Put in _____ drops _____ times each day.

Run the ear drops down the side of the ear canal's opening so that air isn't trapped under them. Move the earlobe back and forth to help the ear drops pass downward. Continue the ear drops for 48 hours until all the symptoms are cleared up.

Generally, your child should not swim until the symptoms are gone. If she is on a swim team, continue the sport, but make sure she uses the ear drops as a rinse after each session. Continued swimming may cause a slower recovery but won't cause any serious complications.

White Vinegar Ear Drops. For mild swimmer's ear, use ½ strength white vinegar ear drops instead of antibiotic-steroid ear drops. Fill the ear canal with white vinegar diluted with equal parts of water. After 5 minutes, remove the solution by turning the head to the side. Do this twice a day.

Pain Relief. Use acetaminophen or ibuprofen as needed for pain relief.

Prevention. First, limit how many hours a day your child spends in the water. The key to prevention is keeping the ear canals dry when your child is not swimming. After swimming, get all water out of the ear canals by turning the head to the side and pulling the earlobe in different directions to help the water run out. Dry the opening to the ear canal carefully. If recurrences are a big problem, rinse your child's ear canals with rubbing alcohol for 1 minute each time she finishes swimming or bathing to help it dry the ear canals and to kill germs. Another helpful home remedy is a solution of 50% rubbing alcohol and 50% white vinegar. The vinegar restores the normal acid balance to the ear canal.

Common Mistakes. Don't use earplugs of any kind for prevention or treatment. They tend to jam ear-wax back into the ear canal. Also, they don't keep all water out of the ear canals. Cotton swabs also shouldn't be inserted in ear canals. Wax buildup traps water behind it and increases the risk of swimmer's ear. A rubbing alcohol mixture is helpful for preventing swimmer's ear but not for treating it because it would sting too much.

CALL OUR OFFICE

IMMEDIATELY if
- Your child starts acting very sick.
- The ear pain becomes severe.

During regular hours if
- The symptoms are not cleared up in 3 days.
- A fever (over 100°F [37.8°C]) occurs.
- You have other concerns or questions.

URINARY TRACT INFECTION

DEFINITION

A urinary tract infection (UTI) is an infection of the bladder (cystitis) and sometimes the kidneys (pyelonephritis). It is important to treat UTIs so that the kidneys are not damaged.

Various symptoms are possible:

- Painful urination
- Bladder frequency or urgency
- Daytime and night-time wetting
- Dribbling
- Foul-smelling urine
- Fever
- Stomachaches (especially lower abdomen)
- Vomiting

Cause

Urinary tract infections are caused by bacteria. The bacteria enter the bladder by traveling up the urethra. In general, the urethra is protected, but if the opening of the urethra (or the vulva in girls) is irritated, bacteria can grow there. Common irritants are bubble bath, shampoo, or fecal soiling. A rare cause of UTIs (1% in girls and 5% in boys) is obstruction of the urinary tract that leads to incomplete emptying of the bladder.

Expected Course. With treatment, your child's fever should be gone and symptoms should be better by 48 hours after starting the antibiotic. The chances of getting another UTI are about 50%. Read the advice on preventing UTIs to decrease your child's risk.

HOME TREATMENT

Antibiotics

Your child's antibiotic is _____. Your child's dose is _____ given _____ times per day during waking hours for _____ days. This medicine will kill the bacteria that are causing the UTI.

If the medicine is liquid, store it in the refrigerator and shake the bottle well before measuring each dose. Use a measuring spoon to be sure that you give the right amount.

Try not to forget any of the doses. If your child goes to school or a babysitter, arrange for someone to give the afternoon dose. Give the medicine until all the pills are gone or the bottle is empty. Even though your child will feel better in a few days, give the antibiotic for the full 10 days to keep the UTI from flaring up.

Extra Fluids. Encourage your child to drink extra fluids to help clear the infection.

Fever and Pain Relief. Acetaminophen or ibuprofen may be given if your child develops a fever over 102°F (39°C) or if urination is quite painful.

Medical Follow-up. Two days after your child begins antibiotics, it is important to contact us to find out the results of the urine culture and make sure that your child's symptoms are responding to the antibiotic.

About two weeks after your initial visit we will want to see your child for another urine culture. Because the chances are high that your daughter will develop a second infection (occurs in 50% of cases), we would like to recheck the urine at the following times: 1, 4, and 12 months after the first infection is cleared up.

Instructions for Collecting a Midstream, Clean-Catch Urine Specimen at Home. If you are told to bring in a urine sample, try to collect the first one in the morning. Use a sterile jar.

Wash off the genital area several times with cotton balls and warm water. Have your child then sit on the toilet seat with her legs spread widely so that the labia (skinfolds of the vagina) don't touch. Have her start to urinate into the toilet, and then place the clean container directly in line with the urine stream. Remove it after you have collected a few ounces but before she stops urinating. The first or last drops that come out of the bladder may be contaminated with bacteria.

Keep the urine in the refrigerator until you take it to the office. Bring it in chilled (put the jar in a plastic bag with some ice).

PREVENTION OF UTIs

- Wash the genital area with water, not soap.
- Don't use bubble bath before puberty; it's extremely irritating. Don't put shampoo or other soaps into the bath water. Don't let a bar of soap float around in the tub.
- Keep bath time less than 15 minutes. Have your child urinate after baths.
- Teach your daughter to wipe herself correctly from front to back, especially after a bowel movement.
- Try not to let your child become constipated.
- Encourage her to drink enough fluids each day to keep the urine light-colored.
- Encourage her to urinate at least every 3 to 4 hours during the day and not "hold back."
- Have her wear loose cotton underpants. Discourage wearing underpants at night.

 CALL OUR OFFICE

IMMEDIATELY if
- Back pain occurs.
- Your child can pass only very small amounts of urine.
- Your child starts acting very sick.

Within 24 hours if
- Fever or painful urination is not gone after your child has taken the antibiotic for 48 hours.
- You have other concerns or questions.

Instructions for Pediatric Patients, 2nd Edition, ©1999 by WB Saunders Company.
Written by Barton D. Schmitt, MD, pediatrician and author of *Your Child's Health,* Bantam Books, a book for parents.

DEFINITION

- Discomfort with passing urine (dysuria)
- Burning or stinging with passing urine
- Urgency and frequency are occasionally present
- Uses bubble bath, bathes in soapy water, or washes genitals with soap
- Prepubertal girl
- No evidence for a urinary tract infection

Cause

The most common cause of mild pain or burning with urination in young girls is an irritation of the vulva (vulvitis) and the opening of the urethra (urethritis). The irritation is usually caused by bubble bath, shampoo, or soap that was left on the genital area. Occasionally, it is due to poor cleansing of the genital area after passing a bowel movement. This chemical urethritis occurs almost exclusively before puberty. At that age, the lining of the vulva is very thin and sensitive. However, since 5% of young girls get urinary tract infections (UTIs), one must always consider this diagnosis. A UTI is a bacterial infection of the bladder (cystitis) and sometimes the kidneys.

Expected Course of Bubble Bath (Chemical) Urethritis

With warm soaks, the pain and burning usually clear in 12 hours.

HOME CARE

Warm Baking Soda–Water Soaks. Have your daughter soak her bottom in a basin or bathtub of warm water for 20 minutes. Put 4 tablespoons of baking soda in the water.

(**Note:** Baking soda is much better than vinegar for young girls who have not entered puberty.) Be sure she spreads her legs and allows the water to cleanse the genital area. No soap should be used. Repeat this every 4 hours while she is awake for 1 day. This will remove any soap, concentrated urine, or other irritants from the genital area. It will also promote healing. With soaks the burning will usually clear in 24 hours. Thereafter, cleanse the genital area once daily with warm water.

Prevention of Recurrences of Pain with Urination

- Wash the genital area with water. Don't wash the genitals with soap until after puberty.
- Don't use bubble bath before puberty; it's extremely

irritating. Don't put any soaps or shampoo into the bath water. Don't let a bar of soap float in the bathtub. If you are going to shampoo your child's hair, do this at the end of the bath.
- Keep bath time less than 15 minutes. Have your child urinate immediately after baths.
- Teach your daughter to wipe herself correctly from front to back, especially after a bowel movement.
- Encourage her to drink enough fluids each day to keep the urine light-colored.
- Encourage her to urinate at least every 4 hours during the day.
- Sexually active young women should urinate after sexual intercourse.
- Have her wear cotton underpants. Underpants made of synthetic fibers (polyester or nylon) don't allow the skin to "breathe." Discourage wearing underpants at night.

Instructions for Collecting a Midstream, Clean-Catch Urine Specimen at Home. If you are told to bring in a urine sample, try to collect the first one in the morning. Use a jar and lid that have been sterilized by boiling them for 10 minutes.

Wash off the genital area several times with cotton balls and warm water. Have your child then sit on the toilet seat with her legs spread widely so that the labia (skinfolds of the vagina) don't touch. Have her start to urinate into the toilet, and then place the clean container directly in line with the urine stream. Remove it after you have collected a few ounces but before she stops urinating. The first or last drops that come out of the bladder may be contaminated with bacteria.

Keep the urine in the refrigerator until you take it to the office. Bring it in chilled (put the jar in a plastic bag with some ice).

 CALL OUR OFFICE

IMMEDIATELY if
- The pain with urination becomes severe.
- Any abdominal or back pain occurs.
- Your child starts acting very sick.

Within 24 hours if
- The pain and burning continue for more than 24 hours after warm baking soda–water soaks.
- Your child develops any fever (over 100°F [37.8°C]).
- You have other concerns or questions.

VAGINAL IRRITATION AND ITCHING (CHEMICAL VULVITIS)

DEFINITION

- Pain, soreness, burning, or itching in genital area
- No pain or burning with urination
- Uses bubble bath, bathes in soapy water, or washes genitals with soap
- Prepubertal girl

Causes

Most vaginal itching or discomfort is due to a chemical irritation of the vulva or outer vagina. The usual irritants are bubble bath, shampoo, or soap left on the genital area. Occasionally, it is due to poor hygiene. This chemical vulvitis almost always occurs before puberty. At that age, the lining of the vulva is very thin and sensitive. If the vagina becomes infected, there will be a vaginal discharge.

Expected Course

The discomfort goes away after 1 to 2 days of proper treatment.

HOME CARE

Baking Soda–Warm Water Soaks. Have your daughter soak her bottom in a basin or bathtub of warm water with baking soda for 20 minutes. Add 4 tablespoons of baking soda per tub of warm water. (*Note:* Baking soda is better than vinegar soaks for young girls who have not entered puberty.) Be sure she spreads her legs and allows the water to cleanse the genital area. No soap should be used. Repeat this every 4 hours while your daughter is awake for the next 2 days. This will remove any soap, concentrated urine, or other irritants from the genital area and promote healing. After symptoms resolve, cleanse the genital area once a day with warm water.

Hydrocortisone Cream. Apply 1% hydrocortisone cream (a nonprescription item) to the genital area after soaks.

Prevention of Recurrences

- Don't use bubble bath before puberty because it's extremely irritating. Don't put any other soaps or shampoo into the bath water. Don't let a bar of soap float around in the bathtub. Wash the genital area with plain water, not soap. If necessary, use baby oil to remove secretions from between the labia that don't come off with water. If you are going to shampoo your child's hair, do this at the end of the bath.
- Keep bath time less than 15 minutes. Have your child urinate immediately after baths.
- Wear cotton underpants. Underpants made of synthetic fibers (polyester or nylon) don't allow the skin to "breathe." Discourage wearing underpants during the night so the genital area has a chance to "air out."
- Teach your daughter to wipe herself correctly from front to back, especially after a bowel movement.
- Encourage her to drink enough fluids each day to keep the urine light-colored. Concentrated urine can be an irritant.

 CALL OUR OFFICE

During regular hours if
- The itching is not gone after 48 hours of treatment.
- A vaginal discharge or bleeding occurs.
- Passing urine becomes painful.
- You have other concerns or questions.

Instructions for Pediatric Patients, 2nd Edition, ©1999 by WB Saunders Company.
Written by Barton D. Schmitt, MD, pediatrician and author of *Your Child's Health,* Bantam Books, a book for parents.

DEFINITION

Vomiting is the forceful ejection of a large portion of the stomach's contents through the mouth. The mechanism is strong stomach contractions against a closed stomach outlet. By contrast, regurgitation is the effortless spitting up of one or two mouthfuls of stomach contents that is commonly seen in babies under 1 year of age.

Cause

Most vomiting is caused by a viral infection of the stomach (viral gastritis) or eating something that disagrees with your child. Often, the viral type is associated with diarrhea.

Expected Course

The vomiting usually stops in 6 to 24 hours. Dietary changes usually speed recovery. If diarrhea is present, it usually continues for several days.

HOME CARE FOR VOMITING

Special Diet for Vomiting
For Bottle-Fed Infants (less than 1 year old). Offer oral rehydration solutions (ORS) for 8 hours.

- ORS includes Infalyte, Kao-Lectrolyte, and Pedialyte (over-the-counter products).
- For vomiting once, offer half-strength formula.
- For vomiting two or more times, offer ORS.
- Give small amounts (1 teaspoon) every 10 minutes.
- After 4 hours without vomiting, increase the amount.
- After 8 hours without vomiting, return to formula.
- For infants more than 4 months old, also return to cereal, strained bananas, etc.
- A normal diet is okay in 24 to 48 hours.

For Breast-Fed Infants. Reduce the amount per feeding.

- Provide breast milk in smaller amounts. Your goal is to avoid filling the stomach.
- If your baby vomits twice, nurse on only one side every 1 to 2 hours.
- If he vomits more than two times, nurse for 4 to 5 minutes every 30 to 60 minutes.
- After 8 hours without vomiting, return to regular breast-feeding.

For Older Children (more than 1 year old). Offer clear fluids in small amounts for 8 hours.

- Water or ice chips are best for vomiting without diarrhea because water is directly absorbed across the stomach wall (ORS is unnecessary).

- Other options: Half-strength flat lemon-lime soda or popsicles. Stir soda until the fizz is gone because the bubbles can inflate the stomach.
- Give small amounts (1 tablespoon) every 10 minutes.
- After 4 hours without vomiting, increase the amount.
- For severe vomiting, rest the stomach completely for 1 hour, then start over with smaller amounts.
- For older children (more than 1 year old), add bland foods after 8 hours without vomiting.
- Stay on bland, starchy foods (any complex carbohydrates) for 24 hours.
- Start with saltine crackers, white bread, rice, mashed potatoes, etc.
- A normal diet is okay in 24 to 48 hours.

Sleep. Help your child go to sleep. Sleep often empties the stomach and relieves the need to vomit. Your child doesn't have to drink anything if he feels nauseated.

Medicines. Discontinue all medicines for 8 hours. Oral medicines can irritate the stomach and make vomiting worse. If your child has a fever over 102°F (38.9°C), use acetaminophen suppositories. Call our office if your child needs to be taking a prescription medicine.

Common Mistakes in Treatment of Vomiting. A common error is to give as much clear fluid as your child wants rather than gradually increasing the amount. This almost always leads to continued vomiting. Keep in mind that there is no effective drug or suppository for vomiting and that diet therapy is the answer. Vomiting alone rarely causes dehydration unless you give drugs by mouth, milk, or too much clear fluid.

 ## CALL OUR OFFICE

IMMEDIATELY if
- Any signs of dehydration occur (no urine in over 8 hours, very dry mouth, etc.).
- Any blood appears in the vomited material.
- Abdominal pain develops and lasts more than 4 hours.
- Your child starts acting very sick.

Within 24 hours if
- The vomiting continues for more than 24 hours in children under age 2 or for more than 48 hours if over age 2.
- You have other concerns or questions.

WOUND INFECTION (SKIN INFECTION)

DEFINITION

A break in the skin shows signs of infection, such as:

- Pus or cloudy fluid is draining from the wound.
- A pimple or yellow crust has formed on the wound (impetigo).
- The scab has increased in size.
- Increasing redness occurs around the wound (cellulitis).
- A red streak is spreading from the wound toward the heart (lymphangitis).
- The wound has become extremely tender.
- Pain or swelling has increased 48 hours after the wound occurred.
- The lymph node draining that area of skin may become large and tender.
- Your child may develop a fever over 100°F (37.8°C).
- The wound hasn't healed within 10 days.
- Most of these diagnoses must be confirmed by a physician.

Causes

Most skin infections follow breaks in the skin (e.g., from cuts, puncture wounds, animal bites, splinters, thorns, or burns). Bacteria (especially staphylococcus or streptococcus) then invade the wound through the "portal of entry" and cause the infection. Some infections start with a closed rash (that is, the skin is *not* broken). Examples are insect bites, chickenpox, scabies, or acne. If a child picks at these rashes, the skin can become broken and then infected.

Deeper wounds (e.g., puncture wounds) are more likely to become infected than superficial wounds (such as scrapes). The hands are at increased risk for infection from puncture wounds. The penetrating teeth or claws of cats pose a major risk for infection.

Expected Course

With appropriate antibiotics and warm soaks, the wound infection should improve within 24 to 48 hours. By that time, your child should stop having any fever caused by the infection. Any red streaking (lymphangitis) or red patches (cellulitis) should stop spreading. The area of the wound should also be much less tender within 48 hours. Within 1 week after your child starts taking antibiotics, all signs of active infection should be completely gone.

TREATMENT

Antibiotics

Your child's antibiotic is _____. Your child's dose is _____. Give it _____ times a day during waking hours for _____ days.

This medicine will kill the germs that are causing the wound infection. Try not to forget any of the doses. If your child goes to school or stays with a babysitter, arrange for someone to give the afternoon dose. Even though your child will feel better in a few days, give the antibiotic until it is completely gone to keep the infection from flaring up again.

Warm Soaks or Local Heat. Proper cleansing of an open wound is important for healing. Soak the wounded area in warm water or put a warm, wet cloth on the wound for 20 minutes three times a day. Use a warm salt water solution containing 2 teaspoons of table salt per quart of water. Use this solution to remove all the pus and loose scabs. (Don't use hydrogen peroxide because it is a feeble germ killer.) Your physician may give you a syringe to help irrigate the wound. Continue soaking the wound three times a day until it looks clear of infection. Then continue to cleanse it and change the dressing once a day until the wound has healed.

If the wound is closed (e.g., cellulitis), apply a heating pad or warm, moist washcloth to the reddened area for 20 minutes three times a day. This will help deliver the antibiotic to the infection.

Fever and Pain Relief. Give your child acetaminophen or ibuprofen if he develops a fever over 102°F (39°C) or the wound is painful.

Contagiousness. The pus from wound infections is somewhat contagious. It can cause skin infections in other people if the pus gets on other people's skin or on an open cut. Be certain that other people in the family do not use your child's towel or washcloth. Encourage your child not to touch the wound because it puts germs on his fingers. Also, ask your child to wash the hands more often than usual, or wash your child's hands for him. Cut the fingernails short. Keep your child out of school until he has been treated with antibiotics for 24 hours and is free of fever.

Prevention of Wound Infections. Wash all new wounds vigorously with soap and water for 5 to 10 minutes to remove dirt and bacteria. Soak puncture wounds in warm, soapy water for 15 minutes. Do this as soon as possible after the injury occurs. Applying an antibiotic ointment after cleaning may be helpful. Encourage your child not to pick at insect bites, scabs, or other areas of irritated skin. Teach your children not to kiss an open wound because it will become contaminated by the many germs in the mouth.

 ## CALL OUR OFFICE

IMMEDIATELY if
- The redness keeps spreading.
- The wound becomes extremely painful.
- Your child starts acting very sick.

During regular hours if
- The fever is not gone 48 hours after your child starts taking an antibiotic.
- The wound infection doesn't look better in 3 days.
- The wound isn't completely healed within 10 days.
- You have other questions or concerns.

Instructions for Pediatric Patients, 2nd Edition, ©1999 by WB Saunders Company.
Written by Barton D. Schmitt, MD, pediatrician and author of *Your Child's Health,* Bantam Books, a book for parents.

PART 5

PEDIATRIC DERMATOLOGY

DEFINITION

- Blackheads, whiteheads (pimples), or red bumps
- Face, neck, and shoulders involved
- Adolescent and young adult years
- Larger red lumps quite painful

Cause

Acne is due to plugging of the oil glands. More than 90% of teenagers have some acne. The main cause of acne is increased levels of hormones during adolescence. It is not caused by diet, and it is unnecessary to restrict fried foods, chocolate, or any other food. Acne is not caused by sexual activity of any kind, nor by dirt or not washing the face often enough. The tops of blackheads are black because of the chemical reaction of the oil plug with the air.

Expected Course

Acne usually lasts until 20 or 25 years of age. It is rare for acne to leave any scars, and people worry needlessly about this.

HOME CARE

There is no magic medicine at this time that will cure acne. However, good skin care can keep acne under control and at a mild level.

Basic Treatment for All Acne
- Soap: The skin should be washed twice each day and after exercise. The most important time is before bedtime. A mild soap such as Dove should be used.
- Hair: The hair should be shampooed daily. Hair can make acne worse by friction if it is too long.
- Avoid picking. Picking keeps acne from healing.

Treatment for Pimples.
Pimples are infected oil glands. They should be treated with the following:

- Benzoyl peroxide 5% lotion or gel. This lotion helps to open pimples and unplug blackheads, and it also kills bacteria. It is available without a prescription. Ask your pharmacist to recommend a brand. The lotion should be applied daily at bedtime. In redheads and blonds it should be applied every other day initially. An amount the size of a pea should cover most of the face. If the skin becomes red or peels, you are using too much of the medicine or applying it too often, so slow down. This lotion may be needed for several years.
- Pimple opening: In general, it is better not to "pop" pimples, but teenagers do it anyway. Therefore do it safely. Never open a pimple before it has come to a head. Wash your face and hands first. Use a sterile needle (sterilized by alcohol or a flame). Nick the surface of the yellow pimple with the tip of the needle. The pus should run out without squeezing. Wipe away the pus and wash the area with soap and water. Scarring will not result from opening small pimples, but it can result from squeezing boils or other large, red, tender lumps.

Treatment for Blackheads (Comedones).
Blackheads are the plugs found in blocked-off oil glands. They should be treated with the following:

- Benzoyl peroxide: This agent is also excellent for removing thickened skin that blocks the openings to oil glands. It should be used as described above for treating pimples.
- Blackhead extractor: Blackheads that are a cosmetic problem can sometimes be removed with a blackhead extractor. This instrument costs about $1 and is available at any drugstore. By placing the hole in the end of the small metal spoon directly over the blackhead, uniform pressure can be applied that does not hurt the normal skin. This method is much more efficient than anything you can accomplish with your fingers. Soak your face with a warm washcloth before you try to remove blackheads. If the blackhead does not come out the first time, leave it alone.

Treatment for Red Bumps.
Large red bumps mean the infection has spread beyond the oil gland. If you have several red bumps, you probably also need an antibiotic. Antibiotics come as solutions for the skin or pills.

Your antibiotic is _____. Use it _____ a day.

Common Mistakes in Treating Acne
- Avoid scrubbing the skin. Hard scrubbing of the skin is harmful because it irritates the openings of the oil glands and can cause them to be more tightly closed.
- Avoid applying any oily or greasy substances to the face. They make acne worse by blocking off oil glands. If you must use cover-up cosmetics, use water-based ones and wash them off at bedtime.
- Avoid hair tonics or hair creams (especially greasy ones). With sweating, these will spread to the face and aggravate the acne.
- Don't stop your acne medicine too soon. It takes 8 weeks to see a good response.

 CALL OUR OFFICE

During regular hours if
- It looks infected (large, red, tender lump).
- Acne is not improved after treating it with benzoyl peroxide for 2 months.
- Benzoyl peroxide makes the face itchy or swollen.
- You have other concerns or questions.

ATHLETE'S FOOT (TINEA PEDIS)

DEFINITION

- A red, scaly, cracked rash between the toes
- Itchy, burning rash
- Rash raw and weepy with scratching
- Often spreads to instep
- Unpleasant foot odor
- Mainly occurs in adolescents

Cause

Athlete's foot is caused by a fungus infection that grows best on warm, damp skin.

Expected Course

With proper treatment, it usually clears in 2 to 3 weeks.

HOME CARE

Antifungal Cream. Buy Tinactin, Micatin, or Lotrimin cream at your drugstore. You won't need a prescription. First rinse the feet in plain water or water with a little white vinegar added. Dry the feet carefully, especially between the toes. Then apply the cream to the rash area and well beyond its borders twice a day. Continue the cream for several weeks or for at least 7 days after the rash seems to have cleared. Successful treatment often takes 3 to 4 weeks.

Dryness. Athlete's foot improves dramatically if the feet are kept dry. It helps to go barefoot or wear sandals or thongs as much as possible. Wear shoes that allow the feet to breathe. Cotton socks should be worn because they absorb sweat and keep the feet dry. Change the socks twice daily. Dry the feet thoroughly after baths and showers.

Foot Odor. Foot odor will often clear as the athlete's foot improves. Rinsing the feet and changing the socks twice daily are essential. If that doesn't work, rinse the feet in a basin of warm water containing 1 ounce of vinegar. If you can still smell your child coming, take off his tennis shoes and wash them in your washing machine with some soap and bleach.

Discourage Scratching. Scratching infected feet will delay a cure.

Contagiousness. The condition is not very contagious. The fungus won't grow on dry, normal skin. Your child may take physical education and continue with sports.

 CALL OUR OFFICE

IMMEDIATELY if
- It looks infected (yellow pus, spreading redness, red streaks).

During regular hours if
- The athlete's foot is not improved in 1 week.
- It is not completely cured after using this treatment for 4 weeks.
- You have other concerns or questions.

Instructions for Pediatric Patients, 2nd Edition, ©1999 by WB Saunders Company.
Written by Barton D. Schmitt, MD, pediatrician and author of *Your Child's Health,* Bantam Books, a book for parents.

DEFINITION

- Tender, red lump in skin
- Causes pain even when not being touched
- Usually ½ to 1 inch across

Cause

A bacterial infection of a hair root or skin pore caused by *Staphylococcus* organisms.

Expected Course

Without treatment, the body will wall off the infection. After about 1 week, the center of the boil becomes soft and mushy (filled with pus). The overlying skin then develops a pimple or becomes thin and pale. The boil is now ready for draining. Without lancing, it will drain by itself in 3 or 4 days. Until it drains, a boil is extremely painful.

HOME TREATMENT

Antibiotics. Boils heal faster and are less likely to recur if your child receives an antibiotic that kills *Staphyloccocus* bacteria.

Your child's antibiotic is _____. Your child's dosage is _____ given _____ times each day for _____ days.

Lancing or Draining the Boil. In general, it's better not to open a boil on your own child because it's a very painful procedure. Until the abscess comes to a head or becomes soft, apply warm compresses three times daily for 20 minutes. When the boil is ready, contact our office. If you must open it yourself, use a sterile needle (sterilized with alcohol or a flame), make a large opening, and squeeze very gently or not at all. Once opened, it will drain pus for 2 or 3 days and then heal. Since the pus is contagious, the boil must be covered by a large 4-inch × 4-inch piece of gauze and microporous tape. This bandage should be changed and the area washed with an antiseptic soap (e.g., Dial or Safeguard) three times daily.

Prevention of More Boils. Boils can easily become a recurrent problem. The *Staphylococcus* bacteria on the skin can be decreased by showering and washing the hair daily with an antibacterial soap. Showers are preferred because during a bath, bacteria are just relocated to other parts of the skin.

Contagiousness. Boils are contagious. Be certain that other people in your family do not use your child's towel or washcloth. Any clothes, towels, or sheets that are contaminated with drainage from the boils should be washed with Lysol. Any bandages with pus on them should be carefully thrown away.

Common Mistakes in Treatment of Boils. Sometimes friends or relatives may advise you to squeeze a boil until you get the core out. The pus in a boil will come out easily if the opening is large enough. Vigorous squeezing is not only very painful but also entails the risk of forcing bacteria into the bloodstream or causing other boils in the same area. Again, squeezing should be done very gently or not at all (as on the face).

 ## CALL OUR OFFICE

IMMEDIATELY if
- The boil is not better within 48 hours after starting the antibiotic.
- Your child starts acting very sick.

During regular hours if
- The boil has come to a head and needs to be opened.
- You have other concerns or questions.

Instructions for Pediatric Patients, 2nd Edition, ©1999 by WB Saunders Company.
Written by Barton D. Schmitt, MD, pediatrician and author of *Your Child's Health,* Bantam Books, a book for parents.

DEFINITION

Dry skin is mainly caused by removing the skin's natural oils through too much bathing and soap. Dry climates make it worse, as does winter weather ("winter itch"). The problem is less common in teenagers because their oil glands are more active. Dry, rough, bumpy skin on the back of the upper arms is called keratosis pilaris. Dry, pale spots on the face are called pityriasis alba. Both are complications of scrubbing dry skin with soap. The dry areas are often itchy, and this is the main symptom.

Cracked skin most commonly occurs on the soles of the feet, especially the heels and big toes (called juvenile plantar dermatosis). Deep cracks are painful and periodically bleed. The main cause is wearing wet shoes and socks or swimming a lot. Cracks can also develop on the hands in children who frequently wash dishes or suck their thumbs. The lips can become cracked (chapped) in children with a habit of licking their lips or from excessive exposure to sun or wind.

HOME CARE

Soap and Bathing. For children with dry skin, avoid all soaps. They take the natural oils out of the skin. Have your child bathe or shower with plain water—perhaps twice weekly. Avoid soaps, detergents, and bubble baths.

Teenagers can get by with applying soap only to the armpits, genitals, and feet. Buy a special soap for dry skin (such as Dove). Rinse well. Don't let a bar of soap float in the tub. Use no soap on itchy areas. Don't lather up (the outer arms are often affected for this reason).

Lubricating Cream for Dry Skin. Buy a large bottle of lubricating cream (special hand lotion). Apply the cream to any dry or itchy areas several times daily, especially after bathing. You will probably have to continue this throughout the winter. If the itch persists after 4 days, use 1% hydrocortisone cream (nonprescription) temporarily.

Humidifier. If your winters are dry, run a room humidifier. The presence of static electricity means your home is much too dry. During cold weather, have your child wear gloves outside to protect against the rapid evaporation of moisture from the hands.

Bath Oils. It does not make much sense to pour bath oils into the bath water; most of the oil goes down the drain. It also makes the bathtub slippery and dangerous. If you prefer a bath oil over hand lotion, apply it immediately after baths. Baby oil (mineral oil) is inexpensive and keeps the skin moisture from evaporating.

Ointments for Cracked Skin. Even deep cracks of many years' duration can be healed in about 2 weeks if they are constantly covered with an ointment (such as petroleum jelly). If the crack seems mildly infected, use an antibiotic ointment (no prescription needed). Covering the ointment with a Band-Aid, socks, or gloves speeds recovery even more. For chapped lips, a lip balm can be applied frequently. Apply ointments 4 times a day.

 CALL OUR OFFICE

During regular hours if
- No improvement occurs within 2 weeks.
- The cracks develop a yellow discharge (pus).
- You have other concerns or questions.

Instructions for Pediatric Patients, 2nd Edition, ©1999 by WB Saunders Company.
Written by Barton D. Schmitt, MD, pediatrician and author of *Your Child's Health*, Bantam Books, a book for parents.

DEFINITION

- Red, extremely itchy rash
- Often starts on the cheeks at 2 to 6 months of age
- Most common on flexor surfaces (creases) of elbows, wrists, and knees
- Occasionally, neck, ankles, and feet involved
- Rash raw and weepy if scratched
- Constant dry skin
- This diagnosis must be confirmed by a physician

Cause

Eczema is an inherited type of sensitive skin. A personal history of asthma or hay fever or a family history of eczema makes it more likely that your child has eczema. Flare-ups occur when there is contact with irritating substances (e.g., soap or chlorine).

In 30% of infants with eczema, certain foods cause the eczema to flare up. If you suspect a particular food item (e.g., cow's milk, eggs, or peanut butter) is causing your child's flare-ups, feed that food to your child one time (a "challenge") after avoiding it for 2 weeks. If it does cause flare-ups, the eczema should become itchy or develop hives within 2 hours of ingestion. If this occurs, avoid ever giving this food to your child and talk to us about food substitutes.

Expected Course

This is a chronic condition and will usually not go away before adolescence. Therefore early treatment of any itching is the key to preventing a severe rash.

HOME TREATMENT

Steroid Creams. Steroid cream is the main treatment for itchy eczema.

Your child's cream is _____.

Apply this cream _____ times daily when the eczema flares up.

When the rash quiets down, use it at least once daily for an additional 2 weeks. After that, use it immediately on any spot that itches. When you travel with your child, always take the steroid cream with you. If your supply starts to run out, get the prescription renewed.

Bathing and Hydrating the Skin. Hydration of the skin followed by lubricating cream is the main way to prevent flare-ups of eczema. Your child should have one bath each day for 10 minutes. Water-soaked skin is far less itchy. Eczema is very sensitive to soaps. Young children can usually be cleaned without any soap. Teenagers need a soap to wash under the arms, the genital area, and the feet. They can use a nondrying soap such as Dove for these areas. Keep shampoo off the eczema.

Lubricating Cream. Children with eczema always have dry skin. After a 10-minute bath, the skin is hydrated and feels good. Help trap the moisture in the skin by applying an outer layer of lubricating cream to the entire skin surface while it is damp. Apply it after steroid cream has been applied to any itchy areas. Apply the lubricating cream once daily (twice daily during the winter). Some lubricating creams are Keri, Lubriderm, Nivea, and Nutraderm. Avoid applying any ointments, petroleum jelly, or vegetable shortening because they can block the sweat glands, increase itching, and worsen the rash (especially in warm weather). Also, soap is needed to wash them off. For severe eczema, ointments may be needed temporarily to heal the skin.

Itching. At the first sign of any itching, apply the steroid cream to the area that itches. Keep your child's fingernails cut short. Also, wash your child's hands with water frequently to avoid infecting the eczema.

Prevention. Wool fibers and clothes made of other scratchy, rough materials make eczema worse. Cotton clothes should be worn as much as possible. Avoid triggers that cause eczema to flare up, such as excessive heat, sweating, excessive cold, dry air (use a humidifier), chlorine, harsh chemicals, and soaps. Never use bubble bath. Also, keep your child off the grass during grass pollen season (May and June). Keep your child away from anyone with fever blisters since the herpesvirus can cause a serious skin infection in children with eczema. Try to breast-feed all high-risk infants. Otherwise, use a soy formula. Also try to avoid cow's milk products, eggs, peanut butter, wheat, and fish during the first year of life.

 ## CALL OUR OFFICE

IMMEDIATELY if
- The rash looks infected (yellow pus or scabs, spreading redness, red streaks).
- The rash flares up after contact with someone who has fever blisters (herpes).
- Your child starts acting very sick.

During regular hours if
- The rash becomes raw and open in several places.
- The rash hasn't greatly improved after 7 days of using this treatment.
- You have other concerns or questions.

DEFINITION

- A large pimple at the junction of the cuticle and the fingernail
- Redness and tenderness of this area
- Occasionally, pus draining from this area

Cause

Those with a large pimple or draining pus are usually infected with the *Staphylococcus* bacteria. The original cause is usually a break in the skin resulting from pulling on or chewing on the cuticle. Those limited to redness and swelling of the cuticle are due to *Candida* (yeast). The *Candida* superinfections usually occur in thumb suckers or finger suckers, swimmers, or other children who have waterlogged cuticles.

Expected Course

With proper treatment, this infection should clear up in 7 days. If not, your physician will probably prescribe an oral antibiotic.

HOME TREATMENT

Antiseptic Soaks. For bacterial infections, soak the infected finger 3 times daily for 10 minutes in warm water and a liquid antibacterial soap. Do this for 4 days or longer if the infection has not healed.

Antibiotic Ointments. For bacterial infections, apply an antibiotic ointment 6 times daily.

Your child's ointment is _____.

Cover the area with an adhesive bandage. Continue to apply the ointment until no signs of infection remain.

Open Any Large Pimple. Open and drain any visible pus pocket using a needle sterilized with rubbing alcohol or a flame. Make a large opening where the pus pocket joins with the nail. If the pus doesn't run out, gently squeeze the pus pocket.

Yeast (Candida) Infections.

For yeast infections, apply _____ 3 times daily.

Also, try to keep the area dry. Do not cover it with a Band-Aid.

Prevention. Discourage any picking or chewing of hangnails (loose pieces of cuticle). Instead, cut these off with nail clippers.

 CALL OUR OFFICE

IMMEDIATELY if
- Fever develops.
- A red streak spreads beyond the cuticle.

During regular hours if
- The infection is not improved by 48 hours on home treatment.
- The infection is not totally cleared up by 7 days.
- You have other concerns or questions.

Instructions for Pediatric Patients, 2nd Edition, ©1999 by WB Saunders Company.
Written by Barton D. Schmitt, MD, pediatrician and author of *Your Child's Health*, Bantam Books, a book for parents.

DEFINITION

- Small ulcers in the mouth
- A mildly painful mouth
- Small water blisters or red spots located on the palms and soles and on the webs between the fingers and toes
- Five or fewer blisters per limb
- Sometimes, small blisters or red spots on the buttocks
- Low-grade fever between 100° and 102°F (37.8° and 38.9°C)
- Mainly occurs in children 6 months to 4 years of age

Cause

Hand, foot, and mouth disease is always caused by a Coxsackie A-16 virus. It has no relationship to hoof and mouth disease of cattle.

Expected Course

The fever and discomfort are usually gone by day 3 or 4. The mouth ulcers resolve in 7 days, but the rash on the hands and feet can last 10 days. The only complication seen with any frequency is dehydration from refusing fluids.

HOME CARE

Antacid Solution. Use an antacid solution for pain relief. For younger children, put ½ teaspoon antacid solution in the front of their mouth 4 times a day after meals. Children over age 4 can use 1 teaspoon of an antacid solution as a mouthwash after meals.

Diet. Change to a soft diet for a few days and encourage plenty of clear fluids. Cold drinks, Popsicles, and sherbert are often well received. For a younger child, give fluids by cup rather than from a bottle. Avoid giving your child citrus, salty, or spicy foods. Also avoid foods that need much chewing.

Fever. Acetaminophen or ibuprofen may be given for a few days for severe mouth pain or a fever above 102°F (38.9°C).

Contagiousness. Hand, foot, and mouth disease is quite contagious and usually some of your child's playmates will develop it at about the same time. The incubation period after contact is 3 to 6 days. Because the spread of infection is extremely difficult to prevent and the condition is harmless, these children do not need to be isolated. They can return to day care or school when the fever returns to normal range. Although most children are contagious from 2 days before to 2 days after the rash, avoidance of other children is unnecessary.

 ## CALL OUR OFFICE

IMMEDIATELY if
- Your child has not urinated for more than 8 hours.
- Your child starts acting very sick.

During regular hours if
- The fever lasts more than 3 days.
- The mouth pain becomes severe.
- You have other concerns or questions.

HEAT RASH (MILIARIA)

DEFINITION
- Tiny, pink bumps
- Occasionally, some are pinpoint-size water blisters
- Mainly neck and upper back/chest
- Occurs during hot, humid weather
- Heat rash can be itchy
- Older children report a "prickly" pins-and-needles sensation
- No fever or sickness
- Also called "prickly heat"

Cause
Heat rash is caused by blocked-off sweat glands. Lots of children get it during hot, humid weather when sweat glands are overworked. Infants can also get it in the wintertime with fever, overdressing, or ointments applied to the chest for coughs. (Reason: ointments block off the sweat glands.) Older children can get it with exercise.

Expected Course
With treatment, heat rash usually clears up completely in 2 to 3 days.

HOME CARE
Cooling. Use techniques that cool off the skin:
- Give cool baths every 2 to 3 hours, without soap. Let the skin air-dry.
- For localized rashes, apply a cool, wet washcloth to the area for 5 to 10 minutes.
- Dress in as few layers of clothing as possible.
- Lower the temperature in your home or use a fan when your child is asleep.
- Have the child lie on a cotton towel to absorb perspiration.

Hydrocortisone Cream. Apply 1% hydrocortisone cream (no prescription necessary) 3 times a day to itchy spots. Avoid hydrocortisone ointments. Calamine lotion is another option.

Avoid Ointments. Avoid all ointments or oils, because they can block off sweat glands. Be sure the rash isn't caused by a mentholated ointment being used for a cough.

 CALL OUR OFFICE

During regular hours if:
- The rash lasts more than 3 days on this treatment.
- You have other concerns or questions.

Instructions for Pediatric Patients, **2nd Edition,** ©1999 by WB Saunders Company.
Written by Barton D. Schmitt, MD, pediatrician and author of *Your Child's Health,* Bantam Books, a book for parents.

DEFINITION

- Very itchy rash
- Raised pink spots with pale centers (hives look like mosquito bites.)
- Size range of ½ inch to several inches across
- Shapes quite variable
- Rapid and repeated changes of location, size, and shape

Cause

Widespread hives are an allergic reaction to a food, drug, viral infection, insect bite, or a host of other substances. Often the cause is not found. Localized hives are usually due to skin contact with plants, pollen, food or pet saliva. Localized hives are not caused by drugs, infections or swallowed foods. Hives are not contagious.

Expected Course

More than 10% of children get hives. Most children who develop hives have it only once. The hives come and go for 3 or 4 days and then mysteriously disappear. Large swellings are common around the eyes, lips, and genitals if hives occur there. Some young children become sensitized to mosquito or flea bites. They develop big hives (called papular urticaria) at the sites of old and new bites that can last for months.

HOME TREATMENT

Antihistamine Medicine. The best drug for hives is an antihistamine. An antihistamine won't cure the hives, but it will reduce their number and relieve itching. Benadryl, one of the most commonly used drugs for hives, has recently become available without prescription. The main side effect of this drug is drowsiness. If you have another antihistamine (e.g., any drug for hay fever) at home, you can use it if you know the dosage until you can get some Benadryl. Give Benadryl four times daily in the following dosages:

BENADRYL DOSAGE

Child's weight more than (lb)	22	33	44	55	110
Total amount (mg)	10	15	20	25	50
Liquid 12.5 mg/5 mL (tsp)	¾	1	1½	2	—
Chewable 12.5 mg	—	1	1½	2	4
Capsules 25 mg	—	—	—	1	2

Your child's drug is _____.

Give _____ every _____ hours. Continue the medicine until the hives are completely gone for 24 hours.

Itching. Give a cool bath to relieve itching. Rub very itchy areas with an ice cube for 10 minutes.

Avoidance. Avoid anything you think might have caused the hives. For hives triggered by pollen or animal contact, take a cool shower or bath. For localized hives, wash the allergic substance off the skin with soap and water. If itchy, massage the area with a cold washcloth or ice for 10 minutes. Localized hives usually disappear in a few hours and don't need Benadryl.

Common Mistakes in Treatment of Hives. Many parents wait to give the antihistamine until new hives have appeared. This means your child will become itchy again. The purpose of the medicine is to keep your child comfortable until the hives go away. Therefore give the medicine regularly until you are sure the hives are completely gone. Since hives are not contagious, your child can be with other children.

 ## CALL OUR OFFICE

IMMEDIATELY if
- Breathing or swallowing becomes difficult.
- Your child starts acting very sick.

During regular hours if
- The itch is not controlled after your child has been taking continuous antihistamines for 24 hours.
- The hives last more than 1 week.
- You have other concerns or questions.

Instructions for Pediatric Patients, 2nd Edition, ©1999 by WB Saunders Company.
Written by Barton D. Schmitt, MD, pediatrician and author of *Your Child's Health,* Bantam Books, a book for parents.

A bite involves biting with the insect's mouth parts and removing a drop of blood from the human. A sting involves injecting a poison into the human from the insect's stinger. The following three types of bites or stings are covered:

- Bee and yellow jacket stings
- Itchy or painful bites
- Tick bites

1. BEE AND YELLOW JACKET STINGS

DEFINITION

Your child was stung by a honeybee, bumblebee, hornet, wasp, or yellow jacket. Over 95% are from yellow jackets. These stings cause immediate painful red bumps. Although the pain is usually better in 2 hours, the swelling may increase for up to 24 hours. Multiple stings (more than 10) can cause vomiting, diarrhea, a headache, and fever. This is a toxic reaction related to the amount of venom received (i.e., not an allergic reaction). A sting on the tongue can cause swelling that interferes with breathing.

HOME CARE

Treatment. If you see a little black dot in the bite, the stinger is still present (this occurs only with honeybee stings). Remove it by scraping it off. If only a small fragment remains, don't worry about it. Then rub each sting for 20 minutes with a cotton ball soaked in a meat tenderizer solution. This will neutralize the venom and relieve the pain. If meat tenderizer is not available, apply aluminum-based deodorant or a baking soda solution for 20 minutes. For persistent pain, massage with an ice cube for 10 minutes. Give acetaminophen or ibuprofen immediately for relief of pain and burning.

PREVENTION

Some bee stings can also be prevented by avoiding gardens and orchards and by not going barefoot. Insect repellents are not effective against these stinging insects.

 ## CALL OUR OFFICE

IMMEDIATELY if
- Breathing or swallowing is difficult (call 911).
- Hives are present.
- There are 10 or more stings.
- Your child starts acting very sick.

During regular hours if
- Swelling of the hand (or foot) spreads past the wrist (or ankle).
- You have other questions or concerns.

2. ITCHY OR PAINFUL INSECT BITES

DEFINITION

Bites of mosquitoes, chiggers, fleas, and bedbugs usually cause itchy, red bumps. The size of the swelling can vary from a dot to ½ inch. The larger size does not mean that your child is allergic to the insect bite. Mosquito bites near the eye always cause massive swelling. The following are clues that a bite is due to a mosquito: itchiness, a central raised dot in the swelling, bites on surfaces not covered by clothing, summertime, and the age of the child (i.e., she is an infant). In contrast to mosquitoes, fleas and bedbugs don't fly; therefore, they crawl under clothing to nibble. Flea bites often turn into little blisters in young children.

Bites of horseflies, deerflies, gnats, fire ants, harvester ants, blister beetles, and centipedes usually cause a painful, red bump. Within a few hours, fire ant bites change to blisters or pimples.

HOME CARE

Itchy Insect Bites. Apply calamine lotion or a baking soda paste to the area of the bite. If the itch is severe (as with chiggers), apply nonprescription 1% hydrocortisone cream 4 times daily. Another way to reduce the itch is to apply firm, sharp, direct, steady pressure to the bite for 10 seconds. A fingernail, pen cap, or other object can be used. Encourage your child not to pick at the bites or they will leave marks.

Painful Insect Bites. Rub the area of the bite with a cotton ball soaked in meat tenderizer solution for 20 minutes. This will relieve the pain. If you don't have any meat tenderizer, use a baking soda solution. Give acetaminophen or ibuprofen for pain relief.

PREVENTION

Mosquitoes and Chiggers. Many of these bites can be prevented by applying an insect repellent sparingly to the clothing or exposed skin before your child goes outdoors or into the woods. Repellents are essential for infants (especially those less than 1 year old) because they cannot bat the insects away.

Bedbugs. The bed and baseboards can be sprayed with 1% malathion, but young children must be kept away from the area because this substance is somewhat poisonous. You may need to call an exterminator.

Fleas. Usually you will find the fleas on your dog or cat. If the bites started after a move into a different home, fleas from the previous owner's pet are the most common cause. Fleas can often be removed by

Instructions for Pediatric Patients, 2nd Edition, ©1999 by WB Saunders Company.
Written by Barton D. Schmitt, MD, pediatrician and author of *Your Child's Health,* Bantam Books, a book for parents.

bringing a dog or cat inside the house for 2 hours to collect the fleas (they prefer the dog or cat to living in the carpet) and then applying flea powder or soap to the animal outdoors. Careful daily vacuuming will usually capture any remaining fleas.

Precautions with Diethylduamide (DEET) Insect Repellents. Insect repellents containing DEET must be used with caution. DEET can be absorbed across the skin into the bloodstream and products with high concentrations can cause seizures or coma. Young children may also have reactions to DEET from licking it off the skin. To prevent harmful reactions, take the following precautions:

- Use DEET products formulated for children. These contain 10% or less DEET. Even adults don't need more than a 30% DEET concentration.
- Apply repellent mainly to clothing and shoes.
- To prevent contact with the mouth or eyes, don't put any repellent on the hands.
- Don't put any repellent on areas that are sunburned or have rashes because the DEET is more easily absorbed in these areas.
- Warn older children who apply their own repellent that a total of 3 or 4 drops can protect the whole body.
- Because one application of repellent lasts 4 to 8 hours, apply it no more than twice daily.
- If repellent is put on the skin, wash it off after your child comes indoors.

 ## CALL OUR OFFICE

IMMEDIATELY if
- The bite looks infected (yellow pus, spreading redness, red streaks).

During regular hours if
- Itching or pain is severe after treatment.
- You have other questions or concerns.

3. TICK BITES

DEFINITION

A tick is a small brown bug that attaches to the skin and sucks blood for 3 to 6 days. The bite is usually painless and doesn't itch. The wood tick (or dog tick), which transmits Rocky Mountain spotted fever and Colorado tick fever, is up to ½ inch in size. The deer tick, which transmits Lyme disease, is the size of a pinhead.

HOME CARE

Tick Removal. The simplest and quickest way to remove a wood tick is to pull it off. Use a pair of tweezers to grasp the tick as close to the skin as possible (try to get a grip on its head). Apply a steady upward traction until the tick releases its grip. Do not twist the tick or jerk it suddenly because these maneuvers can break off the tick's head or mouth parts. Do not squeeze the tweezers to the point of crushing the tick; the secretions released may contain germs that cause disease.

If tweezers aren't available, use fingers, a loop of thread around the tick's jaws, or a needle between the jaws for traction. Tiny deer ticks need to be scraped off with a knife blade or the edge of a credit card. If the body is removed but the head is left in the skin, use a sterile needle to remove the head (in the same way that you would remove a sliver). Apply antibiotic ointment to the bite once.

Wash the wound and your hands with soap and water after removal. A recent study by Dr. G. R. Needham showed that embedded ticks do not back out with the application of a hot match or when covered with petroleum jelly, fingernail polish, or rubbing alcohol. We formerly thought that petroleum jelly, fingernail polish, or alcohol would block the tick's breathing pores and take its mind off eating. Unfortunately ticks breathe only a few times per hour.

PREVENTION

Children and adults who are hiking in tick-infested areas should wear long clothing and tuck the end of the pants into the socks. Apply an insect repellent to shoes and socks (permethrin products are more effective than DEET products against ticks). During the hike perform tick checks using a buddy system every 2 to 3 hours to remove ticks on the clothing or exposed skin. Immediately after the hike or at least once daily, do a bare skin check. A brisk shower at the end of a hike will also remove any tick that isn't firmly attached. Because the bite is painless and doesn't itch, the child will usually be unaware of its presence. Favorite hiding places for ticks are in the hair, so carefully check the scalp, neck, armpit, and groin. Removing ticks promptly may prevent infection because transmission of Lyme disease requires 18 to 24 hours of feeding. Also the tick is easier to remove before it becomes firmly attached.

 ## CALL OUR OFFICE

IMMEDIATELY if
- You can't remove the tick.
- A fever or rash occurs within the 2 weeks following the bite.
- Your child starts acting very sick.

During regular hours if
- You think your child might have Lyme disease.
- You have other questions or concerns.

IMPETIGO (INFECTED SORES)

DEFINITION

- Sores are less than 1 inch in diameter.
- Sores begin as small red bumps that rapidly change to cloudy blisters, then pimples, and finally sores.
- Sores (any wounds that don't heal) increase in size.
- Sores are often covered by a soft, yellow-brown scab.
- Scabs may be draining pus.
- Impetigo often spreads and increases in number from scratching and picking at the initial sore.
- Any wound that doesn't heal or increases in size usually has become infected.

Cause

Impetigo is a superficial infection of the skin, caused by *Streptococcus* or *Staphylococcus* bacteria. It is more common in the summer when the skin is often broken by cuts, scrapes, and insect bites. When caused by a strep infection of the nose, the impetigo usually first appears near the nose or mouth.

Expected Course

With proper treatment, the skin will be completely healed in 1 week. Some blemishes will remain for 6 to 12 months, but scars are unusual unless your child repeatedly picks her sores.

HOME TREATMENT

Antibiotic (Oral or Injectable). Most children with impetigo need an antibiotic.

Your child's antibiotic is _____. Your child's dosage is _____ given _____ each day for _____ days.

One or two sores following an insect bite or cut may respond to an antibiotic ointment.

Antibiotic Ointment. After the crust has been removed, antibiotic ointment should be applied to the raw surface three times daily. You won't need a prescription. Apply for 7 days or longer if necessary. The area should be washed with an antibacterial soap each time. Any new crust that forms should not be removed since this delays healing. After applying an antibiotic ointment, cover the sore with a Band-Aid to prevent scratching and spread.

Removing the Scabs. The bacteria live underneath the soft scabs, and until these are removed, the antibiotic ointment has difficulty getting through to the bacteria to kill them. Scabs can be soaked off using warm water and an antibacterial soap. Take your time. The area may need to be gently rubbed, but it should not be scrubbed. A little bleeding is common if you remove all the crust.

Preventing Spread of Impetigo to Other Areas of the Body. Every time your child touches the impetigo and then scratches another part of the skin with that finger, she can start a new site of impetigo. To prevent this, discourage your child from touching or picking at the sores. Keep the fingernails cut short, and wash her hands often with one of the antibacterial soaps.

Contagiousness to Other People. Impetigo is quite contagious. Be certain that other people in the family do not use your child's towel or washcloth. Your child should be kept out of school until she has taken oral antibiotics for 24 hours. For mild impetigo treated with an antibiotic ointment, the child can continue to attend day care or school if the sore is covered with a Band-Aid.

 ## CALL OUR OFFICE

IMMEDIATELY if
- Spreading redness or red streaks occur.
- Your child starts to act very sick.

Within 24 hours if
- The impetigo increases in size and number of sores after 48 hours of treatment.
- A fever or a sore throat occurs.
- The impetigo is not completely healed in 1 week.
- You have other concerns or questions.

Instructions for Pediatric Patients, 2nd Edition, ©1999 by WB Saunders Company.
Written by Barton D. Schmitt, MD, pediatrician and author of *Your Child's Health,* Bantam Books, a book for parents.

DEFINITION

- Pink, scaly rash
- Usually extremely itchy
- Inner thighs, groin, and scrotum involved (*Note:* The penis is not involved.)
- Almost exclusively in males
- Also called ringworm of the crotch or tinea cruris

Cause

Jock itch is caused by a fungus, often the same one that causes athlete's foot. Sometimes it's transferred by a towel because a teenager with athlete's foot dries the groin after drying the feet.

Expected Course

With appropriate treatment, the symptoms are better in 2 or 3 days and the rash is cured in 3 to 4 weeks.

HOME CARE

Antifungal Medicine. Buy Tinactin, Micatin, or Lotrimin powder or spray (nonprescription) at your drug store. It needs to be applied twice daily to the rash and at least 1 inch beyond the borders. Make sure you get it in all the creases. Continue it for several weeks or for at least 7 days after the rash seems to have cleared. Successful treatment often takes 3 to 4 weeks.

Dryness. Jock itch will improve dramatically if the groin area is kept dry. Loose-fitting cotton shorts should be worn. Shorts and athletic supporters should be washed frequently. The rash area should be carefully cleansed daily with plain water and carefully dried. Avoid using soap on the rash.

Scratching. Scratching will delay the cure, so have your child avoid scratching the area.

Contagiousness. The condition is not very contagious. The fungus won't grow on dry, normal skin. Your child may continue to take physical education and play sports.

 ## CALL OUR OFFICE

During regular hours if
- There is no improvement in 1 week.
- The rash is not completely cured in 1 month.
- You have other questions or concerns.

Instructions for Pediatric Patients, 2nd Edition, ©1999 by WB Saunders Company.
Written by Barton D. Schmitt, MD, pediatrician and author of *Your Child's Health,* Bantam Books, a book for parents.

LICE (PEDICULOSIS), HEAD

DEFINITION

- Nits (white eggs) are firmly attached to hairs.
- Unlike dandruff, nits can't be shaken off.
- Gray bugs (lice) are 1/16 inch long, move quickly, and are difficult to see.
- The scalp itches and has a rash.
- The back of the neck is the favorite area.
- The nits are easier to see than the lice because they are white and very numerous.

Cause

Head lice only live on human beings and can be spread quickly by using the hat, comb, or brush of an infected person or simply by close contact. Anyone can get lice despite good health habits and frequent hair washing. The nits (eggs) normally hatch into lice within 1 week. Pubic lice ("crabs") are slightly different but are treated the same way. They can be transmitted from bedding or clothing and do not signify sexual contact.

Expected Course

With treatment, all lice and nits will be killed. A recurrence usually means another contact with an infected person or the shampoo wasn't left on for 20 minutes. There are no lasting problems from having lice and they do not carry other diseases.

HOME TREATMENT

Antilice Shampoo or Rinse.

Your child's antilice shampoo or rinse is _____.

Wash the hair with your regular shampoo, rinse it and towel-dry it. Pour about 2 ounces of the shampoo into the damp hair. Scrub the hair and scalp for 10 to 20 minutes. Rinse the hair thoroughly and dry it with a towel. These shampoos kill both the lice and the nits. Most antilice shampoos need to be repeated once in 7 days to prevent reinfection.

(*Note:* A new antilice shampoo called Nix only requires one application.)

Removing Nits. Remove the nits by back combing with a fine-tooth comb or pull them out individually. The nits can be loosened from the hair shafts using a mixture of half vinegar and half water applied for 30 minutes under a towel wrap. Even though the nits are dead, most schools will not allow children to return if nits are present. Obviously, the hair does not need to be shaved to cure lice.

Lice in the Eyelashes. If you see any lice or nits in the eyelashes, apply petroleum jelly to the eyelashes twice a day for 8 days. The lice won't survive.

Cleaning the House. Lice can't live for more than 72 hours (3 days) off the human body. Your child's room should be vacuumed. Combs and brushes should be soaked for 1 hour in a solution made from the antilice shampoo. Wash your child's sheets, blankets, and pillowcases in hot water. Items that can't be washed (hats or coats) can be set aside in plastic bags for 3 weeks (the longest that nits can survive). Antilice sprays or fumigation of the house is unnecessary.

Contagiousness. Check the heads of everyone else living in your home. If any have scalp rashes, sores, or itching, they should be treated with the antilice shampoo even if lice and nits are not seen. Your child can return to school after one treatment with the shampoo. Reemphasize to your child that he or she should not share combs and hats.

 CALL OUR OFFICE

During regular hours if
- The rash and itching are not cleared by 1 week after treatment.
- The sores start to spread or look infected.
- The lice or nits return.
- You have other questions or concerns.

Instructions for Pediatric Patients, 2nd Edition, ©1999 by WB Saunders Company.
Written by Barton D. Schmitt, MD, pediatrician and author of *Your Child's Health,* Bantam Books, a book for parents.

DEFINITION

- The rash begins with a single herald or mother patch that looks like large ringworm.
- The herald patch has a scaly, raised border and a pink center.
- The herald patch is 1 to 3 inches across.
- A widespread rash of smaller matching spots on both sides of the body occurs 7 to 14 days after the herald patch first appears.
- This rash consists of pink, oval-shaped spots that are ¼ to ½ inch across. The spots are covered with fine scales, which give the rash a crinkled appearance.
- The rash appears mainly on the chest, abdomen, and back. Sometimes the rash is worse in the groin and armpits. Usually the rash does not appear on the face.
- The rash can be itchy during the first 1 or 2 weeks.
- This rash primarily affects people between the ages of 6 and 30 years.
- Usually a physician needs to examine the rash to diagnose it.

Cause

The rash is probably caused by a virus.

Expected Course

This condition is harmless. The rash will disappear without treatment. The skin will return to a normal appearance. The difficult part of this rash is that it lasts 6 to 10 weeks. During this time, however, your youngster will feel fine.

HOME CARE

Skin Creams. In general treatment is unnecessary. If the skin is dry, a moisturizing cream may be helpful. For itchiness, use 1% hydrocortisone cream (no prescription necessary) 2 or 3 times a day. For itchiness unresponsive to this, recontact our office for a stronger steroid cream.

Sunlight Exposure. One dose of ultraviolet light may stop itching and shorten the course of pityriasis. Have your youngster sunbathe for 30 minutes (enough to make the skin pink). If this is impossible, use a sun lamp or consider a tanning salon. (*Caution:* Avoid sunburn.)

Contagiousness. Pityriasis is not contagious. Your child can attend school and take gym during the 6 to 10 weeks the rash is present.

 CALL OUR OFFICE

During regular hours if
- The rash becomes very itchy.
- The rash becomes infected with pus or draining scabs.
- The rash lasts longer than 3 months.
- You have other questions or concerns.

POISON IVY

DEFINITION

- Redness and blisters
- Eruption on exposed body surfaces (e.g., hands)
- Shaped like streaks or patches
- Extreme itchiness
- Onset 1 or 2 days after the patient was in a forest or field

Cause

Poison ivy, poison oak, and poison sumac cause the same type of rash and are found throughout the United States. More than 50% of people are sensitive to the oil of these plants.

Expected Course

Poison ivy usually lasts 2 weeks. Treatment reduces the symptoms but doesn't cure the disease. The best approach is prevention.

HOME TREATMENT

Cool Soaks. Soak the involved area in cold water or massage it with an ice cube for 20 minutes as often as necessary. Then let it air-dry. This will reduce itching and oozing.

Steroid Creams

If applied early, a steroid cream can reduce the itching.

Your child's cream is _____.

Apply it _____ times per day for _____ days.

The sores should be dried up and no longer itchy in 10 to 14 days. In the meantime, cut your child's fingernails short and encourage your child not to scratch himself or herself.

Benadryl. If itching persists, give Benadryl orally (no prescription needed) every 6 hours as needed.

Contagiousness. The fluid from the sores themselves is not contagious. However, anything that has poison ivy oil or sap on it is contagious for about 1 week. This includes the shoes and clothes the patient last wore into the woods, as well as any pets that may have oil on their fur. Be sure to wash them off with soap and water. The rash begins 1 to 2 days after skin contact.

PREVENTION

Learn to recognize these plants. Otherwise, avoid all plants with three large shiny, green leaves. Another clue is the presence of shiny black spots on damaged leaves. (The sap of the plant turns black when exposed to air.)

Wear long pants or socks when walking through woods that may contain poison ivy, poison oak, or poison sumac. If you think your child has had contact with one of these plants wash the exposed areas of skin with any available soap for 5 minutes. Strong laundry soap has no added benefits. Do this as soon as possible, because after 1 hour it is of little value in preventing absorption of the oil.

 CALL OUR OFFICE

IMMEDIATELY if
- The rash looks infected (yellow pus, spreading redness, red streaks).

During regular hours if
- The face, eyes, or lips become involved.
- The itching becomes severe even with treatment.
- Poison ivy lasts longer than 2 weeks.
- You have other concerns or questions.

Instructions for Pediatric Patients, 2nd Edition, ©1999 by WB Saunders Company.
Written by Barton D. Schmitt, MD, pediatrician and author of *Your Child's Health,* Bantam Books, a book for parents.

DEFINITION

- Ring-shaped pink patch
- Scaly, raised border
- Ring slowly increases in size
- Clearing of the center as the patch grows
- Usually ½ to 1 inch in size
- Mildly itchy

Cause

Ringworm is caused by a fungus infection of the skin, often transferred from puppies or kittens who have it.

Expected Course

It responds well to appropriate treatment.

HOME CARE

Antifungal Cream. Buy Tinactin, Micatin, or Lotrimin cream at your drug store. You won't need a prescription. Apply the cream twice daily to the rash and 1 inch beyond its borders. Continue this treatment for 1 week after the ringworm patch is smooth and seems to be gone. Successful treatment often takes 3 to 4 weeks. Encourage your child to avoid scratching the area.

Contagiousness. Ringworm of the skin is mildly contagious. It requires direct skin-to-skin contact. The type acquired from pets is not transmitted human-to-human, only animal-to-human. After 48 hours of treatment, it is not contagious at all. Your child doesn't have to miss any school (or day care).

Treatment of Pets. Kittens and puppies with ringworm usually do not itch and may not have any rash. If ringworm patches are seen, call your veterinarian. If no patches are present but ringworm recurs in your child, also contact your veterinarian. Also have your child avoid close contact with the animal until he or she is treated. Natural immunity will develop in animals after 4 months even without treatment.

 CALL OUR OFFICE

During regular hours if
- The ringworm continues to spread after 1 week of treatment.
- The rash has not cleared up in 4 weeks.
- You have other concerns or questions.

RINGWORM OF THE SCALP (TINEA CAPITIS)

DEFINITION

- Round patches of hair loss that slowly increase in size
- A black-dot, stubbled appearance of the scalp from hair shafts that are broken off at the surface
- The scalp may have scaling
- Mild itching of the scalp
- Ringworm of the face may also be present
- Usually occurs in children age 2 to 10 years
- This diagnosis requires a positive microscope test (potassium hydroxide [KOH prep]) or fungus culture.

Cause

A fungus infects the hairs and causes them to break. Ringworm is not caused by a worm. Over 90% of cases are due to *Trichophyton tonsurans*, which is transmitted from other children who are infected. Combs, brushes, hats, barrettes, seat backs, pillows, and bath towels can transmit the fungus. Less than 10% of the cases are caused by infected animals. The animal type causes more scalp irritation, redness, and scaling. If your child has the animal type of fungus, he is not contagious to other children.

Expected Course

Ringworm of the scalp is not dangerous. Without treatment, however, the hair loss and scaling may spread to other parts of the scalp. Some children develop a kerion, which is a boggy, tender swelling of the scalp that can drain pus. Kerions are an allergic reaction to the fungus and may require additional treatment with an oral steroid. Hair regrowth is normal after treatment but will take 6 to 12 months. In the meantime, your child can wear a hat or scarf to hide the bald areas.

TREATMENT

Oral Antifungal Medicine. The main treatment for ringworm of the scalp is griseofulvin taken orally for 8 weeks.

Your child's dosage is _____

taken 2 times a day.

(The product comes in a 125 mg/5 mL suspension and 250-mg capsules.) Griseofulvin is best absorbed if taken with fatty foods such as milk or ice cream. Antifungal creams or ointments are not effective in killing the fungus that causes ringworm of the scalp.

Antifungal Shampoo. The use of an antifungal shampoo makes your child less contagious and allows him to return to day care or school. Purchase a nonprescription shampoo containing selenium sulfide (e.g., Selsun). Lather up and leave it on for 10 minutes before rinsing. Use the antifungal shampoo twice a week for the next 8 weeks. On other days, use a regular shampoo.

Contagiousness. Ringworm is mildly contagious. In the days before antifungal medications, about 5% of school contacts usually became infected. However, 25% of siblings (close contacts) developed ringworm. Once your child has been started on griseofulvin and received one washing with the special shampoo, he can return to school. Caution your child not to share combs or caps with other children. Check the scalps of your child's siblings and close friends. If you see any scaling or patches of hair loss, refer that child to their doctor's office.

Common Mistakes. It is psychologically harmful and unnecessary to shave the hair, give a close haircut, or to force your child to wear a protective skull cap.

Follow-up Appointment. In 4 weeks return for lab tests of your child's hair to be certain we have achieved a cure. If not, the griseofulvin will need to be given for longer than 8 weeks.

 CALL OUR OFFICE

During regular hours if
- The ringworm looks infected with pus or a yellow crust.
- The scalp becomes swollen or boggy.
- The ringworm continues to spread after 2 weeks of treatment.
- You have questions or concerns.

Instructions for Pediatric Patients, 2nd Edition, ©1999 by WB Saunders Company.
Written by Barton D. Schmitt, MD, pediatrician and author of *Your Child's Health*, Bantam Books, a book for parents.

DEFINITION

- Scabies are little bugs (mites) that burrow under the skin and cause severe itching and little red bumps. They are so small that they can only be seen with a microscope.
- They rarely attack the skin above the neck, except in infants.
- Usually more than one person in a family has them.
- This diagnosis must be confirmed by a physician.

HOME CARE

Scabies Cream

Your child's medicine is _____.

(Elimite cream is usually prescribed.)

Apply the cream to every square inch of the body from the neck down. (Infants less than 1 year old also need it carefully applied to the scalp, forehead, temples, and neck. Avoid the lower face.) Don't forget the navel, between the toes, or other creases. Leave some under the fingernails. Areas that don't seem infected should still be covered.

Eight to 12 hours later give your child a bath and remove the cream. One treatment is usually effective. For severe rashes, repeat the treatment once in 1 week.

Kwell Precautions. If Kwell is used, babies under 1 year of age should have it washed off in 4 hours. Leaving Kwell on longer than this can cause side effects. Swallowing Kwell can be quite harmful, so cover the hands with gloves or socks if your child is a thumb sucker.

Pregnant Women. Pregnant women need special medicines for scabies. Pregnant women cannot use Kwell. If you use Elimite cream, wash it off in 8 hours. If you use Eurax, leave the first coat on. Apply a second coat 24 hours later. Wash the Eurax off 48 hours after the second application. The Eurax 2-day treatment needs to be repeated in 1 week.

Itching. The itching and rash may last for 2 to 3 weeks after successful treatment with Kwell or Eurax. This itch can be helped by frequent cool baths without use of soap, followed by 1% hydrocortisone cream, which you can buy without a prescription.

Contagiousness. Children can return to school after one treatment with the scabies medicine.

Family Contacts. Scabies is highly contagious. The symptoms take 30 days to develop after exposure. Therefore everyone living in the house should be treated preventively with one application of the scabies medicine. Close contacts of the infected child (such as a friend who spent the night or a babysitter) should also be treated.

Cleaning the House. Machine wash all your child's sheets, pillowcases, underwear, pajamas, and recently worn clothing. Blankets can be put away for 3 days. Scabies cannot live outside the human body for more than 3 days.

 CALL OUR OFFICE

During regular hours if
- It looks infected (sores that enlarge or drain pus).
- New scabies occur after treatment is completed.
- You have other concerns or questions.

SUNBURN

DEFINITION

Sunburn is due to overexposure of the skin to the ultraviolet rays of the sun or a sunlamp. Most people have been sunburned many times. Vacations can quickly turn into painful experiences when the power of the sun is overlooked. Unfortunately, the symptoms of sunburn do not begin until 2 to 4 hours after the sun's damage has been done. The peak reaction of redness, pain, and swelling is not seen for 24 hours. Minor sunburn is a first-degree burn that turns the skin pink or red. Prolonged sun exposure can cause blistering and a second-degree burn. Sunburn never causes a third-degree burn or scarring.

Increased leisure time can lead to increased sun damage. Repeated sun exposure and suntans cause premature aging of the skin (wrinkling, sagging, and brown sunspots). Repeated sunburns increase the risk of skin cancer in the damaged area. Each blistering sunburn doubles the risk of developing malignant melanoma, which is the most serious type of skin cancer.

HOME CARE

Pain Relief. The sensation of pain and heat will probably last for 48 hours.

- Ibuprofen products started early and continued for 2 days can reduce the discomfort.
- Nonprescription 1% hydrocortisone cream or moisturizing creams applied 3 times each day may also cut down on swelling and pain, but only if used early. (Avoid petroleum jelly or other ointments because they keep heat and sweat from escaping.)
- The symptoms can also be helped by cool baths or wet compresses several times daily.
- Showers are usually too painful.
- Peeling will usually occur in about a week. Apply a moisturizing cream.
- Offer extra water to replace the fluid lost into the swelling of sunburned skin and to prevent dehydration and dizziness.
- For broken blisters, trim off the dead skin with a small scissors and apply an antibiotic ointment. Wash off and reapply the antibiotic ointment twice daily for 3 days.

Common Mistakes in Treatment of Sunburn. Avoid applying ointments or butter to a sunburn; they are painful to remove and not helpful. Don't buy any first aid creams or sprays for burns. They often contain benzocaine that can cause an allergic rash. Don't confuse sunscreens that block the sun's burning rays with suntan lotions or oils that mainly lubricate the skin.

PREVENTION OF SUNBURNS

The best way to prevent skin cancer is to prevent sunburn. Although skin cancer occurs in adults, it is caused by the sun exposure and sunburns that occurred during childhood. Every time you apply sunscreen to your child, you are preventing skin cancer down the line.

- Apply sunscreen anytime your child is going to be outside for more than 30 minutes per day.
- For teenagers who are determined to acquire a suntan, teach them the limits of sun exposure without a sunscreen.
- After 1 hour of sun exposure, always apply a sunscreen.
- Protect high-risk children. About 15% of white people have skin that never tans but only burns. These fair-skinned children need to be extremely careful about the sun throughout their lives. The big risk factors for sunburn are red hair, blond hair, blue eyes, green eyes, freckles, or excessive moles. These children are also at increased risk for skin cancer. They need to be instructed repeatedly to use a sunscreen throughout the summer even for brief exposure and to avoid the sun whenever possible.
- Protect infants. The skin of infants is thinner and more sensitive to the sun. Therefore, babies under 6 months of age should be kept out of direct sunlight. Keep them in the shade whenever possible. If sun exposure must occur, sunscreens, longer clothing, and a hat with a brim are essential. Don't apply sunscreen to areas where the infant may lick it off.
- Try to keep sun exposure to small amounts early in the season until a tan builds up. (*Caution:* Although people with a suntan can tolerate a little more sun, they can still get a serious sunburn.) Start with 15 or 20 minutes per day and increase by 5 minutes per day. Decrease daily exposure time if the skin becomes reddened. Because of the 2- to 4-hour delay before sunburn starts, don't expect symptoms to tell you when it's time to get out of the sun.
- Avoid the hours of 10:00 AM to 3:00 PM, when the sun's rays are most intense. Even if it's not hot outside, avoid the mid-day sun. Find other activities for your children during these hours.
- Don't let overcast days give you a false sense of security. Over 70% of the sun's rays still get through the clouds. Over 30% of the sun's rays can also penetrate loosely woven fabrics (for instance, a T-shirt).
- Sun exposure increases by 4% for each 1000 feet of elevation. A sunburn can occur quickly when hiking above the timberline.
- Water, sand, or snow increases sun exposure. The shade from a hat or umbrella won't protect you from reflected rays.
- Also protect your child's eyes. Years of exposure to ultraviolet (UV) light increase the risk of cataracts. Buy sunglasses with UV protection.
- Set a good example. Did you apply your sunscreen? Are you wearing a baseball cap to protect your face?

Sunscreens. There are good sunscreens on the market that prevent sunburn but still permit gradual tanning to occur. Choose a broad-spectrum sunscreen that screens out both ultraviolet A and B (UVA and

Instructions for Pediatric Patients, 2nd Edition, ©1999 by WB Saunders Company.
Written by Barton D. Schmitt, MD, pediatrician and author of *Your Child's Health,* Bantam Books, a book for parents.

UVB) rays. The sun protection factor (SPF) or filtering power of the product determines what percent of the UV rays gets through to the skin. An SPF of 15 allows only 1/15 (7%) of the sun's rays to get through and thereby extends safe sun exposure from 20 minutes to 5 hours without sunburning. For practical purposes, an SPF higher than 15 is rarely needed because sun exposure beyond 5 hours is unusual. Fair-skinned whites (with red or blond hair) may need a sunscreen with an SPF of 30. The simplest approach is to use an SPF of 15 or greater on all children.

Apply the sunscreen 30 minutes before exposure to the sun to give it time to penetrate the skin. Give special attention to the areas most likely to become sunburned, such as your child's nose, ears, cheeks, and shoulders. Most products need to be reapplied every 3 to 4 hours, as well as immediately after swimming or profuse sweating. A "waterproof" sunscreen stays on for about 30 minutes in water. Do not towel off after swimming. Most people apply too little (the average adult requires 1 ounce of sunscreen per application).

To prevent sunburned lips, apply a lip coating that also contains para-aminobenzoic acid (PABA). If your child's nose or some other area has been repeatedly burned during the summer, protect it completely from all the sun's rays with zinc oxide ointment.

 ## CALL OUR OFFICE

IMMEDIATELY if
- An unexplained fever over 102°F (38.9°C) occurs.
- The sunburn looks infected (yellow pus, spreading redness, red streaks).
- Your child starts acting very sick.

During regular hours if
- You have other questions or concerns.

SHINGLES (ZOSTER)

DEFINITION

- There is a linear rash that follows the path of a nerve.
- The rash occurs on only one side of the body.
- The rash starts with clusters or red bumps, changes to water blisters, and finally becomes dry crusts. (It looks like a small group of chickenpox).
- The back, chest, and abdomen are the most common sites.
- The rash usually doesn't burn or itch in children (in contrast to the adult form).
- Your child does not have a fever or feel sick.
- Your child had chickenpox in the past.

Cause

Zoster is caused by the chickenpox virus. The disease is not caught from other people with active shingles or chickenpox. The chickenpox virus lies dormant in the bodies of some people and is reactivated for unknown reasons as zoster. Children with zoster are usually over 3 years old.

Expected Course

New shingles continue to appear for several days. All the rash dries up by 7 to 10 days. Complications do not occur unless the eye is involved. If zoster involves the nose, the cornea is usually also involved. Most people have shingles just once; a second attack occurs in 5% of children who get zoster.

HOME CARE

Relief of Symptoms. Most children have no symptoms. For pain, give acetaminophen or ibuprofen as necessary. Avoid giving aspirin for zoster because of the possible link with Reye's syndrome. Discourage itching or picking the rash. The rash does not need any cream.

Contagiousness. Children with zoster can transmit chickenpox (but not zoster) to others. Transmission occurs by touching the zoster rash. Although they are far less contagious than children with chickenpox, children with zoster should stay home from school for 7 days unless they can keep the rash covered until it crusts over. Children or adults who have not had chickenpox should avoid visiting the child with zoster (unless the rash is covered).

 CALL OUR OFFICE

IMMEDIATELY if
- Zoster rash involves the eye or nose.

During regular hours if
- The rash becomes very painful or very itchy.
- The rash lasts more than 14 days.
- The rash looks infected with pus or soft yellow scabs.
- You have other questions or concerns.

Instructions for Pediatric Patients, 2nd Edition, ©1999 by WB Saunders Company.
Written by Barton D. Schmitt, MD, pediatrician and author of *Your Child's Health*, Bantam Books, a book for parents.

DEFINITION

- The name means "multicolored ringworm."
- The condition occurs in adolescents and adults.
- Numerous spots and patches appear on the neck, upper back, and shoulders.
- The spots are covered by a fine scale.
- The spots vary in size.
- In summer, the spots are light and don't tan like normal skin.
- In winter as normal skin fades, the spots look darker (often pink or brown) than normal Caucasian skin.

Cause

This superficial infection is caused by a yeastlike fungus call *Malassezia furfur*. It is more common in warm, humid climates.

Expected Course

The problem tends to wax and wane for many years. Since complications do not occur, tinea versicolor is solely a cosmetic problem. Itching is uncommon.

HOME CARE

Selsun Blue Shampoo. Selsun Blue (selenium sulfide) is a nonprescription medicated shampoo that can cure this condition. Apply this shampoo once each day for 14 days. Apply it to the affected skin areas as well as 2 or 3 inches onto the adjacent normal skin. Rub it in and let it dry. Be careful to keep it away from the eyes and genitals, since it is irritating to these tissues. After 30 minutes, take a shower. In 2 weeks the scaling should be stopped, and the rash temporarily cured. Normal skin color will not return for 6 to 12 months.

Prevention of Recurrences. Tinea versicolor tends to recur. Prevent this by applying Selsun Blue shampoo to the formerly involved areas once each month for several years. Leave it on for 1 to 2 hours, then shower. This precaution is especially important in the summer months, because this fungus thrives in warm weather.

Contagiousness. Tinea versicolor is not contagious. This fungus is a normal inhabitant of the hair follicles in many people. Only a few develop the overgrowth of the fungus and a rash.

 CALL OUR OFFICE

During regular hours if
- The rash is not improved with this treatment after 2 weeks.
- You feel your child is getting worse.
- You have other questions or concerns.

DEFINITION

If your child has tenderness, redness, and swelling of skin surrounding the corner of the toenail on one of the big toes, proceed with this guideline. Occasionally, some pus drains from this area. Ingrown toenails are usually due to tight shoes (e.g., cowboy boots) or improper cutting of the toenails. They take several weeks to clear up.

HOME CARE

Soaking. Soak the foot twice daily in warm water and an antibacterial soap for 20 minutes. While the foot is soaking, massage outward the swollen part of the cuticle.

Antibiotic Ointment. If your child's cuticle is just red and irritated, an antibiotic ointment is probably not needed. If the cuticle becomes swollen or oozes secretions, though, apply Neosporin ointment (no prescription needed) 5 or 6 times daily.

Cutting off the Corner of the Toenail. The pain is always caused by the corner of the toenail rubbing against the raw cuticle. Therefore we have to cut this corner off so that the irritated tissue can quiet down and heal. We need to do this only once. The main purpose of treatment is to help the nail grow over the nail cuticle rather than get stuck in it. Therefore during soaks try to bend the corners of the nail upward.

Shoes. Have your child wear sandals or go barefoot as much as possible to prevent pressure on the toenail. When she must wear closed shoes, protect the ingrown toenail as follows: If the inner edge is involved, tape a foam pad between the first and second toes to keep them from touching. If the outer edge is involved, tape a foam pad to the outside of the ball of the toe to keep the toenail from touching the side of the shoe.

PREVENTION

Prevent recurrences by making sure that your child's shoes are not too narrow. Get rid of any pointed or tight shoes. After the cuticle is healed, cut the toenails straight across, leaving the corners. Don't cut them too short. Cut the nail weekly to prevent pressure on the end of the nail, which can drive in the corners. Also, after every shower or bath, lift up the corners of the nail.

 CALL OUR OFFICE

IMMEDIATELY if
- Fever develops.
- A red streak spreads beyond the toe.

During regular hours if
- Any pus or yellow drainage is not cleared up after 48 hours on this home treatment.
- The problem is not totally resolved in 2 weeks.
- You have other concerns or questions.

Instructions for Pediatric Patients, 2nd Edition, ©1999 by WB Saunders Company.
Written by Barton D. Schmitt, MD, pediatrician and author of *Your Child's Health,* Bantam Books, a book for parents.

DEFINITION

- Raised, round, rough-surfaced growth on the skin
- Most commonly on the hands
- Not painful unless located on the bottom of the foot (called plantar warts)
- Brown dots within the wart (unlike a callus) and a clear boundary with the normal skin

Cause

Warts are caused by papillomaviruses.

Expected Course

Warts are harmless. Most warts disappear without treatment in 2 or 3 years. With treatment they resolve in 2 to 3 months. There are no shortcuts in treating warts.

HOME TREATMENT

Wart-Removing Acids

Your child's wart-removing acid is _____.

Apply it once per day, enough to cover the entire wart. Keep the lid on the container closed tightly so it won't evaporate.

The acid will turn the top of the wart into dead skin (it will look white). The acid will work faster if it is covered with adhesive tape or duct tape. Once or twice each week, remove the dead wart material by paring it down with a razor blade. If that is hard for you to do, rub the dead skin off with a washcloth instead. The dead wart will be easier to remove if you soak the area first in warm water for 10 minutes. If the cutting causes any pain or minor bleeding, you have cut into living wart tissue. Since you are using an acid, avoid getting any near the eyes or mouth.

Cover the Wart. Cover the wart with a piece of adhesive tape or duct tape. Warts deprived of air and sun exposure sometimes die without the need for treatment with acids. Remove the tape once a week and wash the skin. After it has dried thoroughly, re-apply the tape. The tape treatment may be needed for 8 weeks.

Contagiousness. Encourage your child not to pick at the wart because this may cause it to spread. If your child chews or sucks the wart, cover the area with a Band-Aid and change it daily. Encourage your child to give up this habit because chewing on warts can cause warts on the lips or face. Warts are not very contagious to other people.

 ## CALL OUR OFFICE

During regular hours if

- Warts develop on the feet, genitals, or face.
- A wart becomes open *and* looks infected.
- New warts develop after 2 weeks of treatment.
- The warts are still present after 8 weeks of treatment.
- You have other concerns or questions.

PART 6

MISCELLANEOUS PHYSICAL PROBLEMS

ANAL FISSURE
ANEMIA, IRON DEFICIENCY
ASTHMA
CONSTIPATION
EARWAX PROBLEMS
EYE ALLERGIES
FEBRILE SEIZURES (CONVULSIONS WITH FEVER)
HAY FEVER (ALLERGIC RHINITIS)
HEAD TRAUMA
MENSTRUAL CRAMPS (DYSMENORRHEA)
NOSEBLEED
PINWORMS
SKIN TRAUMA
SUTURED WOUND CARE
TONSIL AND ADENOID SURGERY
VENTILATION TUBES SURGERY

DEFINITION

An anal fissure is a shallow tear or crack in the skin at the opening of the anus. More than 90% of children with blood in their stools have an anal fissure. The main symptoms are as follows:

- The blood is bright red.
- The blood is only a few streaks or flecks.
- The blood is on the surface of the stool or on the toilet tissue after wiping.
- Your child usually passes a large or hard bowel movement just before the bleeding starts.
- You may see a shallow tear at the opening of the anus when the buttocks are spread apart, usually at 6 or 12 o'clock. (A tear cannot always be seen.)
- Touching the tear causes mild pain.

Cause

Trauma to the anal canal during constipation is the usual cause of anal fissures.

Expected Course

Bleeding from a fissure stops on its own in 5 or 10 minutes.

HOME CARE

Warm Saline Baths. Give your child warm baths for 20 minutes, 3 times each day. Have him sit in a basin or tub of warm water with about 2 ounces of table salt or baking soda added. Don't use any soap on the irritated area. Then gently dry the anal area.

Ointments. If the anus seems irritated, you can apply 1% hydrocortisone ointment (nonprescription). If the pain is severe, apply 2½% Xylocaine or 1% Nupercainal ointment (no prescription needed) 3 times each day for a few days to numb the area.

Diet. The most important aspect of treatment is to keep your child on a nonconstipating diet. Increase the amounts of fresh fruits and vegetables, beans, and bran products that your child eats. Reduce the amounts of milk products your child eats or drinks.

Occasionally, a stool softener (such as mineral oil) is needed temporarily.

 ## CALL OUR OFFICE

During regular hours if
- The bleeding increases in amount.
- The bleeding occurs more than two times after treatment begins.
- You have other concerns or questions.

ANEMIA, IRON DEFICIENCY

DEFINITION

- Anemia means that the number of red blood cells in your child's body is below normal. The red blood cells carry oxygen in the bloodstream, and iron is needed for the body to produce red blood cells.
- Iron deficiency anemia is caused by too little iron in the diet.
- This diagnosis must be confirmed by a physician.

HOME TREATMENT

Iron Medicines

The iron medicine for your child is _____.

Your child's dose is _____ mL given _____ times

each day for _____ weeks.

This medicine contains iron and will need to be taken for 2 to 3 months to get your child's red blood cells back to a normal level. It can occasionally cause an upset stomach and should be taken with food to prevent this. Mix the iron medicine with a juice containing vitamin C (orange juice, for example). This will improve iron absorption and prevent staining of the teeth. (*Note:* If the teeth become stained, the stain can be brushed off with baking soda. The iron may change the color of bowel movements to greenish black, but this is harmless. Too much iron can be dangerous and cause a serious poisoning. Treat iron like any medicine: Keep it out of your child's reach.

Diet. If your child's diet is well balanced, she won't get anemia again. The following foods contain iron:

- Meats, fish, and poultry have the most iron.
- Raisins, dried fruits, sweet potatoes, lima beans, kidney beans, chili beans, pinto beans, green peas, peanut butter, enriched cereals, and breads are other iron-rich foods. Spinach and egg yolks also contain iron, but it is in a form that is not readily available to the body.

Your child should not drink more than 24 ounces of milk each day (about three glasses) so that she has an adequate appetite for iron-containing foods. Milk doesn't contain any iron.

Follow-up Visits. We would like to see your child in 1 week and again in 2 months to be sure the level of red cells in the blood has returned to normal.

 CALL OUR OFFICE

During regular hours if
- Your child refuses the iron medicine.
- You have other concerns or questions.

Instructions for Pediatric Patients, 2nd Edition, ©1999 by WB Saunders Company.
Written by Barton D. Schmitt, MD, pediatrician and author of *Your Child's Health,* Bantam Books, a book for parents.

DEFINITION

- Wheezing: a high-pitched whistling sound produced during breathing out
- Recurrent attacks of wheezing, coughing, chest tightness, and difficulty in breathing
- Often associated with sneezing and a runny nose
- Usually no fever
- Also called reactive airway disease (RAD)
- This diagnosis must be confirmed by a physician

Causes

Asthma is an inherited type of "twitchy" lung. The airways go into spasm and become narrow when allergic or irritating substances enter them. Viral respiratory infections trigger most attacks, especially in younger children. If asthma is caused by pollens, the asthma only flares up during a particular season. Asthma often occurs in children who have other allergies such as eczema or hay fever. Although an emotional stress can occasionally trigger an attack, emotional problems are not the cause of asthma. Some common triggers are listed under "Prevention."

Expected Course

Although asthma attacks may be frightening, they are treatable. When medicines are taken as directed, the symptoms are reversible and there are no permanent lung changes. Although asthma can be a long-lasting disease, over half of children outgrow it during adolescence.

HOME CARE

Asthma is a chronic disease that requires close follow-up by a physician who coordinates your child's treatment program. If you have any doubt about whether your child is wheezing, start the following asthma medicines. The later medicines are begun, the longer it takes to stop the wheezing. Once medicine is begun, your child should keep taking it until he has not wheezed or coughed for 48 hours (take medicine for 7 days minimum). If your child has one or more attacks of wheezing each month, he probably needs to be on continuous medicines.

Asthma Inhalers. Your child's metered-dose inhaler is _____. Your child's dose is 2 puffs every _____ hours for _____ days.

Your child will need careful instructions on how to use the inhaler.

1. The canister must be shaken.
2. The inhaler should be held 2 inches in front of the open mouth.
3. Your child should breathe out completely.
4. The spray should be released at the start of slowly breathing in.
5. The breath should be held for 10 seconds after the lungs are filled.

6. Wait 10 minutes before taking the second puff.

Spacers. These inhalers usually can't be coordinated by children less than 6 years old unless you also use a plastic airway spacer (or chamber). The spacer (chamber) will trap the asthma medicine and give your child time to breathe it in. Some children need to use a spacer until they are teenagers.

Your child's spacer is _____.

Asthma Nebulizer Treatments. Children younger than 4 years old can't use inhalers. They need nebulized medicine treatment, using a machine. Even older children get more of the medicine delivered to their lungs using a nebulizer rather than an inhaler.

Your child's nebulizer should contain _____ mL of _____ mixed with _____ mL of _____.

Give a nebulizer treatment every _____ hours for _____ days.

Oral Steroids or Other Asthma Medicines. Although inhaled medicines work best for asthma, some children also need to take medicines by mouth.

Your child's oral asthma medicine is _____.

Give _____ every _____ hours for _____ days.

Begin Treatment Early. Many children wheeze soon after they get coughs and colds. For some children, itching of the neck or chest means an asthma attack will soon begin. If this is the case for your child, start the asthma medicine or inhaler at the first sign of any coughing, chest tightness, or itching. Don't wait for wheezing. The best "cough medicine" for a child with asthma is the asthma medicine. Always keep this medicine handy; take it with you on trips. If your supply runs low, obtain a refill.

Peak Flow Meters. Peak flow meters (PFM) measure how fast your child can move air out of the lungs. Every child over age 6 should use a PFM. These measurements will tell you when to increase medications (flow rate less than 20% of baseline) and when to see a doctor immediately (less than 50%).

Fluid Intake. Normal hydration keeps the normal lung mucus from becoming sticky. Encourage your child to drink a normal intake of clear fluids. Sipping warm fluids may improve the wheezing.

Exercise-Induced Asthma. Most people with asthma also get 20- to 30-minute attacks of coughing and wheezing with strenuous exercise. Running, especially in cold air or polluted air, is the main trigger. This problem should not interfere with participation in most sports nor require a physical education excuse. The symptoms can be prevented by using an oral asthma medicine 90 minutes before exercise *or* an inhaler 10 minutes before exercise. Children with asthma usually have no problems with swimming or sports not requiring rapid breathing.

Hay Fever. For hay fever symptoms, it's okay to give antihistamines. Poor control of hay fever can make asthma attacks worse. Recent research has shown that although antihistamines can dry the airway, they don't make asthma worse.

Going to School. Asthma is not contagious. Your child should go to school during mild asthma attacks but avoid gym and sports on these days. Arrange to have the asthma medicines available at school. If your child uses an inhaler, he should be permitted to keep it with him so he can use it readily. For continued wheezing, your child should be seeing a physician on a daily basis.

Common Mistakes. The most common mistake is delaying the start of asthma medicines or not replacing them when they run out. Nonprescription inhalers and medicines are not helpful. Another common error is keeping a cat that your child is allergic to. Also, prohibit all smoking in your home; tobacco smoke can persist for up to a week. In addition, don't panic during asthma attacks. Fear can make tight breathing worse, so try to remain calm and reassuring to your child. Finally, don't let asthma restrict your child's activities, sports, or social life.

PREVENTION BY AVOIDING ASTHMA TRIGGERS

Try to discover and avoid the substances that trigger attacks in your child. Second-hand tobacco smoke is the biggest offender. If someone in your household smokes, your child will have more asthma attacks, take more medication, and require more emergency room visits. Try to keep pets outside or at least out of your child's bedroom. Learn how to dustproof the bedroom. Avoid feather pillows. Change the filters on your hot air heating system or air conditioner regularly. For allergies to molds or carpet dust mites, try to keep the house humidity less than 50%. Consider using a dehumidifier. If there has been any recent contact with grass, pollen, weeds, or animals that your child might be allergic to, the pollen remaining in the hair and clothing is probably keeping the wheezing going. Have your child shower, wash his hair, and put on clean clothes.

 CALL OUR OFFICE

IMMEDIATELY if
- The wheezing is severe.
- The breathing is difficult or tight.
- The peak flow rate is less than 50% of normal.
- The wheezing or breathing is not improved after the second dose of asthma medicine.
- Your child starts acting very sick.

During regular hours if
- The wheezing is not completely cleared by 5 days.
- You have other questions or concerns.

Instructions for Pediatric Patients, 2nd Edition, ©1999 by WB Saunders Company.
Written by Barton D. Schmitt, MD, pediatrician and author of *Your Child's Health,* Bantam Books, a book for parents.

DEFINITION

- Painful passage of stools: The most reliable sign of constipation is discomfort with the passage of a bowel movement.
- Inability to pass stools: These children feel a desperate urge to have a bowel movement (BM), have discomfort in the anal area, but are unable to pass a BM after straining and pushing for more than 10 minutes.
- Infrequent movements: Going 3 or more days without a BM can be considered constipation, even though this may cause no pain in some children and even be normal for a few. (*Exception:* After the second month or so of life, many breast-fed babies pass normal, large, soft BMs at infrequent intervals [up to 7 days is not abnormal] without pain.)

Common Misconceptions in Defining Constipation

Large or hard BMs unaccompanied by any of the conditions just described are usually normal variations in BMs. Some normal people have hard BMs daily without any pain. Children who eat large quantities of food pass extremely large BMs. Babies less than 6 months of age commonly grunt, push, strain, draw up the legs, and become flushed in the face during passage of BMs. However, they don't cry. These behaviors are normal and should remind us that it is difficult to have a BM while lying down.

Causes

Constipation is often due to a diet that does not include enough fiber. Drinking or eating too many milk products can cause constipation. It's also caused by repeatedly waiting too long to go to the bathroom. If constipation begins during toilet training, usually the parent is applying too much pressure.

Expected Course

Changes in the diet usually relieve constipation. After your child is better, be sure to keep her on a nonconstipating diet so that it doesn't happen again.

Sometimes the trauma to the anal canal during constipation causes an anal fissure (a small tear). This is confirmed by finding small amounts of bright red blood on the toilet tissue or the stool surface.

HOME CARE

Diet Treatment for Infants (Less than 1 Year Old)

- If your baby is under 2 months of age, try 1 teaspoon of dark Karo syrup twice a day.
- If over 2 months old, give fruit juices (such as apple or prune juice) twice each day.
- If over 4 months old, add strained foods with a high fiber content, such as cereals, apricots, prunes, peaches, pears, plums, beans, peas, or spinach twice daily.
- Strained bananas and apples are neither helpful nor constipating.

Diet Treatment for Older Children (More than 1 Year Old)

- Make sure that your child eats fruits or vegetables at least three times each day (raw unpeeled fruits and vegetables are best). Some examples are prunes, figs, dates, raisins, peaches, pears, apricots, beans, celery, peas, cauliflower, broccoli, and cabbage. (*Warning:* Avoid any foods your child can't chew easily.)
- Increase bran. Bran is an excellent natural stool softener because it has a high fiber content. Make sure that your child's daily diet includes a source of bran, such as one of the new "natural" cereals, unmilled bran, bran flakes, bran muffins, shredded wheat, graham crackers, oatmeal, high-fiber cookies, brown rice, or whole wheat bread. Popcorn is one of the best high-fiber foods for children over 4 years old.
- Decrease consumption of constipating foods, such as milk, ice cream, yogurt, cheese, and cooked carrots.
- Increase the amount of fruit juices your child drinks. (*Exception:* Orange juice is not as helpful as others.)

Sitting on the Toilet (Children Who Are Toilet Trained). Encourage your child to establish a regular bowel pattern by sitting on the toilet for 10 minutes after meals, especially breakfast. Some children and adults repeatedly get blocked up if they don't do this. If your child is resisting toilet training by holding back, stop the toilet training for a while and put her back in diapers or Pull-ups.

Stool Softeners. If a change in diet doesn't relieve the constipation, give your child a stool softener with dinner every night for 1 week. Stool softeners are not habit forming. They work 8 to 12 hours after they are taken. Examples of stool softeners that you can buy at your drug store without a prescription are Haley's M-O (1 tablespoon), Metamucil or Citrucel (1 tablespoon), or plain mineral oil (1 tablespoon).

Measures for Acute Rectal Pain. If your child has acute rectal pain needing immediate relief, one of the following will usually provide quick relief: sitting in a warm bath to relax the anal sphincter, a glycerine suppository, gentle rectal stimulation for 10 seconds using a thermometer, or a gentle rectal dilation with a lubricated finger (covered with plastic wrap).

 ## CALL OUR OFFICE

IMMEDIATELY for advice about an enema if
- Your child develops severe rectal or abdominal pain.

During regular hours if
- Your child does not have a bowel movement after 3 days on this nonconstipating diet.
- You have other concerns or questions.

Instructions for Pediatric Patients, 2nd Edition, ©1999 by WB Saunders Company.
Written by Barton D. Schmitt, MD, pediatrician and author of *Your Child's Health,* Bantam Books, a book for parents.

DESCRIPTION

Everyone has earwax. The color can normally vary from light yellow to dark brown. Earwax is not dirty or abnormal; in fact it contains natural chemicals that can kill germs. It also keeps dust off the eardrum and protects the lining of the ear canal. The ear canal is designed to clean itself. Earwax is produced in the outer third of the ear canal. Earwax moves outward naturally during chewing and the normal growth of the ear canal's lining. Every day or two, you may notice a little earwax at the opening of the ear canal. If you do nothing, this earwax will fall out on its own.

Unless there is a blockage, it is best to leave earwax alone. If you push the earwax back into the ear, as usually happens when you try to remove the wax from the inside of the ear canal, it becomes more difficult for the wax to come out naturally.

Proceed with this guideline if earwax is completely blocking one of the ear canals and your child can't hear on that side. If the hearing seems normal on that side, that means the blockage is only partial and you can leave it alone.

HOME CARE

Flushing Out Packed Earwax

- If the wax is hard, soften it first. Mineral oil or baby oil is a good earwax softener. Put in 5 drops. Leave the oil in for 1 to 2 hours.
- When the wax is soft, wash it out with a rubber ear syringe or Water-Pik at the lowest setting. The water must be at body temperature to prevent dizziness. If the earwax doesn't seem to be coming out, flush it with the head tilted so that the involved ear is down. Gravity will help the water wash it out (the waterfall effect).

- Flush out the ear several times, until the water that comes out is clear and the ear canal seems open when you look in with a light.

Caution: Never put water in your child's ear if there is any chance the eardrum has a hole in it or if your child has ventilation tubes.

Prevention. Nothing should be put inside the ear canal to try to hurry the earwax process along. Using cotton swabs just ends up packing the wax deeper. Earwax doesn't need any help getting out. Cotton swabs also carry the risk of damaging your child's eardrum if he turns his head suddenly. Tell everyone in your family that the most common cause of earwax buildup is putting cotton swabs into the ear canal. Another common cause is wearing earplugs of any type.

Removing Visible Earwax. In general, leave it alone. On special occasions if earwax is right at the opening of the ear canal and you feel compelled to remove it for cosmetic reasons, flick it out with a bent paper clip or little folded piece of paper.

 CALL OUR OFFICE

During regular hours if

- Flushing out the ear canal doesn't return the hearing to normal.
- Any discharge other than earwax comes from the ear canal.
- Blockage from earwax recurs after you stop using cotton swabs.
- You have other concerns or questions.

Instructions for Pediatric Patients, 2nd Edition, ©1999 by WB Saunders Company.
Written by Barton D. Schmitt, MD, pediatrician and author of *Your Child's Health,* Bantam Books, a book for parents.

DEFINITION

- Itchy eyes with frequent rubbing
- Increased tearing
- Red or pink eyes (without pus)
- Mild swelling of the eyelids
- No pain or fever
- Similar symptoms during the same month of the previous year
- Often associated with allergic symptoms of the nose (hay fever)

Cause

Eye allergies that occur during the same season each year are caused by pollens. Allergies that are not seasonal may be caused by pets (e.g., cats), feathers, perfumes, mascara, and eyeliner, to name a few.

Expected Course

Most eye allergies due to a pollen last 4 to 6 weeks, which is the length of most pollen seasons. If the allergic substance (e.g., from a cat) can be identified *and* avoided, the symptoms will not recur.

HOME CARE

Remove Pollen. First wash the pollen off your child's face. Then use a clean washcloth and cool water to clean off the eyelids. (Tears will wash the pollen out of the eyes.) This rinse of the eyelids may need to be repeated every time your child comes inside on a windy day. Pollen also collects in the hair and on exposed body surfaces. This pollen can easily be reintroduced into the eyes. Therefore, give your

child a shower and shampoo every night before bedtime. Encourage your child not to touch her eyes unless her hands have been washed recently.

Vasoconstrictive Eye Drops. Usually, the eyes will feel much better after the pollen is washed out and a cold compress (e.g., a cold washcloth) is applied. If they are still itchy or bloodshot, put some long-acting vasoconstrictive eye drops in your child's eyes.

Your child's eye drops are _____. Use 2 drops every 6 to 8 hours as necessary.

Oral Antihistamines. If these measures aren't effective, your child probably also has hay fever (i.e., allergic symptoms of the nose) and needs an oral antihistamine.

Your child's medicine is _____. Give _____,

_____ times a day until the pollen season is over.

Prevention. Don't let your child touch her eyes unless her hands are washed. The hands may contain pollen, animal substances, or other irritants. For young women, mascara or eyeliner may be the cause.

 ## CALL OUR OFFICE

During regular hours if
- This treatment and an antihistamine do not relieve most of the symptoms in 2 or 3 days.
- You have other concerns or questions.

FEBRILE SEIZURES (CONVULSIONS WITH FEVER)

DEFINITION

Febrile convulsions are seizures triggered by high fever. They are the most common type of convulsion (occurring in 4% of children) and in general are harmless. The children are usually between 6 months and 4 years of age. Most first seizures occur by 2 years of age. The average temperature at which they occur is 104°F (40°C). The fever itself can be caused by an infection in any part of the body. Each febrile seizure usually lasts 1 to 10 minutes without any treatment.

Most of these children (60%) have just one febrile seizure in a lifetime. The other 40% have one to three recurrences over the next few years. Febrile seizures usually stop occurring by 5 or 6 years of age. They do not cause any brain damage; however, a few children (3%) will later have seizures without fever.

FIRST AID

Reduce the Fever. Bringing your child's fever down as quickly as possible will shorten the seizure. Remove your child's clothing and apply cold washcloths to the face and neck. Sponge the rest of the body with cool water. As the water evaporates, your child's temperature will fall. When the seizure is over and your child is awake, give him the usual dose of acetaminophen or ibuprofen. Encourage cool fluids.

Protect Your Child's Airway. If your child has anything visible in his mouth, clear it with a finger to prevent choking. Place your child on his side or abdomen (face down) to help drain secretions. If your child vomits, help clear his mouth. Use a suction bulb if available. If your child's breathing becomes noisy, pull the jaw and chin forward.

Common Mistakes in First Aid of Convulsions. During the seizure, don't try to restrain your child or stop the seizure movements. Once started, the seizure will run its course no matter what you do. Don't try to force anything into your child's mouth. This is unnecessary and can cut his mouth, injure a tooth, cause vomiting, or result in a serious bite of your finger. Don't try to hold his tongue. Although children may rarely bite the tongue during a convulsion, they can't "swallow the tongue."

Emergencies. Call a rescue squad (911) IMMEDIATELY if the febrile convulsion continues more than 5 minutes.

Driving In. If you are told to drive to a medical facility, keep the fever down during the drive. Dress your child lightly and continue applying a cold washcloth to the forehead. (*Warning:* Prolonged seizures caused by persistent fever have been caused by bundling up sick infants during a long drive.)

HOME CARE

If your physician decides the seizure can be treated safely at home, the following information may help you.

Oral Fever-Reducing Medicines. Febrile convulsions usually occur during the first day of an illness. Try to control fever more closely than is necessary for children who do not have febrile seizures. Begin acetaminophen or ibuprofen at the first sign of any fever (a rectal temperature over 100.4°F [38°C]) and give it continuously for the first 48 hours of the illness. If your child has a fever at bedtime, awaken her once during the night to give the fever medicine.

Because fever is common after diphtheria-tetanus-pertussis (DTP) immunizations, begin acetaminophen or ibuprofen in the physician's office when your child is immunized and continue it for at least 24 hours.

Fever-Reducing Suppositories. Have some acetaminophen suppositories on hand in case your child ever has another febrile seizure (same dosage as oral medicine). These suppositories may be kept in a refrigerator at the pharmacy, so you may have to ask for them.

Light Covers or Clothing. Avoid covering your child with more than one blanket. Bundling during sleep can push the temperature up 1 or 2 extra degrees.

Lots of Fluids. Keep your child well hydrated by offering plenty of fluids.

PREVENTION

The only way to completely prevent future febrile convulsions is for your child to take an anticonvulsant medicine on a daily basis until 3 or 4 years of age. Since anticonvulsants have side effects and febrile seizures are generally harmless, anticonvulsants are rarely prescribed unless your child has other neurologic problems. Your physician will discuss this decision with you.

 ## CALL OUR OFFICE

IMMEDIATELY if
- Your child has a febrile convulsion.
- The neck becomes stiff.
- Your child becomes confused or delirious.
- Your child becomes difficult to awaken.
- Your child starts to act very sick.

Instructions for Pediatric Patients, 2nd Edition, ©1999 by WB Saunders Company.
Written by Barton D. Schmitt, MD, pediatrician and author of *Your Child's Health*, Bantam Books, a book for parents.

DEFINITION

- There is a clear nasal discharge with sneezing, sniffing, and nasal itching.
- Symptoms occur during pollen season.
- Similar symptoms occurred during the same month of the previous year.
- Previous confirmation of this diagnosis by a physician is helpful.
- Itchy, watery eyes (eye allergies) are commonly associated.
- Sinus or ear congestion is sometimes associated.

Cause

Hay fever is an allergic reaction of the nose (and sinuses) to an inhaled substance. This allergic sensitivity is often inherited. During late April and May the most common offending pollen is from trees. From late May to mid-July, the offending pollen is usually grass. From late August to the first frost, the leading cause of hay fever is ragweed pollen. Although the inhaled substance is usually a pollen, it can also be animal dander or other agents your child is allergic to. Hay fever is the most common allergy; more than 15% of the population have it.

Expected Course

This is a chronic condition that will probably recur every year, perhaps for a lifetime. Therefore it is important to learn how to control it.

HOME TREATMENT

Oral Antihistamine Medicines. The best drug for hay fever is an antihistamine. It will relieve nose and eye symptoms.

Your child's antihistamine is _____.

Give_____, _____ times each day.

(There are many effective nonprescription antihistamines such as chlorpheniramine and brompheniramine.)

Symptoms clear up faster if antihistamines are given at the first sign of sneezing or sniffing. For children with occasional symptoms, antihistamines can be taken on days when symptoms are present or expected. For children with daily symptoms the best control is attained if antihistamines are taken continuously (several times each day) throughout the pollen season.

The main side effect of antihistamines is drowsiness. If your child becomes drowsy, switch to a combination product that contains an antihistamine with a decongestant (such as pseudoephedrine or phenylpropanolamine). If your child remains drowsy, continue the drug, but temporarily decrease the dosage. Tolerance of the regular dosage should occur in 1 to 2 weeks. Newer prescription antihistamines cause much less drowsiness and are approved by the Food and Drug Administration for use in children over age 6.

Nasal Sprays. Severe hay fever can now usually be controlled by new cromolyn or steroid nasal sprays rather than allergy shots. Since these sprays must be used when the nose is not dripping, antihistamines must be given first to stop the drainage.

If indicated, your child's nasal spray is _____.

Give _____ puff in each nostril _____ times per day.

Nasal sprays do not help eye symptoms. Therefore they are usually used with oral antihistamines.

Pollen Removal to Decrease Symptoms of Hay Fever. Pollen tends to collect on the exposed body surfaces and especially in the hair. Shower your child and wash her hair every night before going to bed. Avoid handling pets that have been outside and are probably covered with pollen.

Prevention of Hay Fever Symptoms. Your child's exposure to pollen can be reduced by not going on drives in the country, not sitting by an open car window on necessary drives, not being near someone cutting the grass during pollen season, staying indoors when it is windy or the pollen count is especially high, and closing the windows that face the prevailing winds. If your child's hay fever is especially bad and you don't have air-conditioning, you may wish to take her to an air-conditioned store or theater for a few hours. Avoid feather pillows, pets, farms, stables, and tobacco smoke if any of them seem to bring on symptoms of nasal allergy.

Eye Allergies Associated with Hay Fever. If your child also has itchy watery eyes, wash her face and eyelids to remove pollen. Then apply a cold compress to her eyelids for 10 minutes. An oral antihistamine will usually bring the eye symptoms under control. If not, instill 2 drops of long-acting vasoconstrictor eye drops (a nonprescription item) every 8 to 12 hours for a few days. Ask your pharmacist for help in choosing a reliable product.

Common Mistakes. Vasoconstrictive nose drops or nasal sprays usually do not help hay fever because they are washed out by nasal secretions as soon as they have been instilled. Also, when used for more than 5 days, they can irritate the nose and make it more congested.

 ## CALL OUR OFFICE

During regular hours if
- Symptoms aren't controlled in 2 days with antihistamines.
- Your child develops sinus pain or pressure.
- You have other concerns or questions.

Instructions for Pediatric Patients, 2nd Edition, ©1999 by WB Saunders Company.

Written by Barton D. Schmitt, MD, pediatrician and author of *Your Child's Health,* Bantam Books, a book for parents.

137

DEFINITION

- History of a blow to the head
- Scalp trauma (cut, scrape, bruise, or swelling)

Cause

Every child sooner or later strikes his head. Falls are especially common when your child is learning to walk. Most bruises occur on the forehead. Sometimes black eyes appear 3 days later because the bruising spreads downward by gravity.

Expected Course

Most head trauma simply results in a scalp injury. Big lumps can occur with minor injuries because the blood supply to the scalp is so plentiful. For the same reason small cuts here can bleed profusely. Only 1% to 2% of injured children get a skull fracture. Usually there are no associated symptoms except for a headache at the site of impact. Your child has not had a concussion unless there is temporary unconsciousness, confusion, and amnesia.

HOME CARE

Wound Care. If there is a scrape, wash it off with soap and water. Then apply pressure with a clean cloth (sterile gauze if you have it) for 10 minutes to stop any bleeding. For swelling, apply ice for 20 minutes.

Rest. Encourage your child to lie down and rest until all symptoms are gone (or at least 2 hours). Your child can be allowed to sleep; you don't have to try to keep him awake. Just have him sleep nearby so you can periodically check on him. Don't give any pain medicine. If the headache is bad enough to need acetaminophen, your child probably should be checked by a physician.

Diet. Only give clear fluids (ones you can see through) until your child has gone 2 hours without vomiting. Vomiting is common after head injuries, and there is no need to have him vomit up his dinner.

Pain Medicines. Don't give any pain medicine. If the headache is bad enough to require acetaminophen or aspirin, your child should be checked by a physician.

Special Precautions and Awakening. Although your child is probably fine, close observation for 48 hours will ensure that no serious complication is missed.

- Awakening your child twice during the night: Do this once at your bedtime and once 4 hours later. Awakening him every hour is unnecessary and next to impossible. Arouse him until he is walking and talking normally. Do this for two nights. Sleep in his room or have him sleep in your room for those two nights. If his breathing becomes abnormal or his sleep is otherwise unusual, awaken him to be sure a coma is not developing. After two nights, return to a normal sleep routine.

 CALL OUR OFFICE

IMMEDIATELY if
- The headache becomes severe.
- Vomiting occurs three or more times.
- Vision becomes blurred or double.
- Your child becomes difficult to awaken or confused.
- Walking or talking becomes difficult.
- Your child's neurological condition worsens in any other way.

Instructions for Pediatric Patients, 2nd Edition, ©1999 by WB Saunders Company.
Written by Barton D. Schmitt, MD, pediatrician and author of *Your Child's Health,* Bantam Books, a book for parents.

DEFINITION

- Cramps during the first 1 or 2 days of a period
- Pain in lower midabdomen
- Pain may radiate to the lower back or both thighs
- Similar cramps in the past with menstrual periods
- Associated symptoms of nausea, vomiting, diarrhea, or dizziness in some girls

Cause

Menstrual cramps are experienced by more than 50% of girls and women during menstrual periods. They are caused by strong contractions (even spasms) of the muscles in the womb (uterus) as it tries to expel menstrual blood. Menstrual periods usually are not painful during the first 1 to 2 years after a girl has started having periods. However, once ovulation (the release of an egg from the ovary) begins, the level of progesterone in the bloodstream increases and leads to stronger contractions and some cramps.

Expected Course

Cramps last 2 or 3 days and usually occur with each menstrual period. There are some drugs that can keep the pain to a very mild level. The cramps often disappear permanently after the first pregnancy and delivery, probably because the opening of the womb (cervical os) is stretched.

HOME CARE

Ibuprofen. Ibuprofen (Advil and Motrin are two brand names) is an excellent drug for menstrual cramps. It not only decreases the pain but also decreases contractions of the uterus.

Your daughter can take 2 or 3 200-mg tablets 4 times per day. Always give 3 tablets as the first dosage. The drug should be started as soon as there is any menstrual flow or the day before, if possible. Don't wait for the onset of menstrual cramps. Ibuprofen should make your daughter feel good enough not to miss anything important.

If you don't have ibuprofen, give aspirin until you can obtain ibuprofen.

Local Heat. A heating pad or warm washcloth applied to the area of pain may be helpful. A 20-minute warm bath twice daily may reduce the pain.

Aggravating Factors. Any type of pain will seem more severe in people who are tired or upset. Your daughter should try to avoid exhaustion and inadequate sleep during menstrual periods. If your daughter has troubles or worries, encourage her to share them with someone.

Full Activity During Menstrual Cramps. Your daughter should not miss any school, work, or social activities because of menstrual cramps. If the pains are limiting your daughter's activities even though she is using ibuprofen, ask your physician about stronger medication.

Common Mistakes. A common mistake is to go to bed, but people who are busy usually notice their pain less. There are absolutely no restrictions; your daughter can go to school, take physical education classes, swim, take a shower or bath, wash her hair, go outside in bad weather, date, and so on during her menstrual periods.

 ## CALL OUR OFFICE

IMMEDIATELY if

- The pain becomes severe and not relieved by ibuprofen.
- An unexplained fever (over 100°F [37.8°C]) occurs.
- Your daughter starts acting very sick.

During regular hours if

- Ibuprofen doesn't provide adequate pain relief.
- The menstrual cramps cause your daughter to miss school or other important activities.
- You have other concerns or questions.

NOSEBLEED

DEFINITION

Nosebleeds (epistaxes) are very common throughout childhood. They are usually caused by dryness of the nasal lining plus the normal rubbing and picking that all children do when the nose becomes blocked or itchy. Vigorous nose blowing can also cause bleeding. All of these behaviors are increased in children with nasal allergies.

HOME CARE

Lean Forward and Spit Out Any Blood. Have your child sit up and lean forward so he does not have to swallow the blood. Have a basin available so he can spit out any blood that drains into his throat. Blow his nose free of any large clots that might interfere with applying pressure.

Squeeze the Soft Part of the Nose. Tightly pinch the soft parts of the nose against the center wall for 10 minutes. Don't release the pressure until 10 minutes are up. If the bleeding continues, you may not be pressing on the right spot. During this time, your child will have to breathe through his mouth.

If Bleeding Continues, Use Vasoconstrictor Nose Drops and Squeeze Again. If the nosebleed hasn't stopped, insert a piece of gauze covered with vasoconstrictor nose drops (e.g., Neo-Synephrine) or petroleum jelly into the nostril. Squeeze again for 10 minutes. Leave the gauze in for another 10 minutes before removing it. If bleeding persists, call our office but continue the pressure in the meantime.

Swallowed blood is irritating to the stomach. Don't be surprised if it is vomited up.

Common Mistakes in Treating Nosebleed
- A cold washcloth applied to the forehead, back of the neck, bridge of the nose, or under the upper lip does not help to stop a nosebleed.
- Pressing on the bony part of the nose does not stop a nosebleed.
- Avoid packing the nose with anything, because when the packing is removed, bleeding usually recurs.

PREVENTION

- A small amount of petroleum jelly applied twice each day to the center wall (septum) inside the nose is often helpful for relieving dryness and irritation.
- Increasing the humidity in the room at night by using a humidifier may also be helpful.
- Get your child into the habit of putting 2 or 3 drops of warm water in each nostril before blowing a stuffy nose.
- Avoid aspirin. One aspirin can increase the tendency of the body to bleed easily for up to a week and can make nosebleeds last much longer.
- If your child has nasal allergies, treating them with antihistamines will help break the itching-bleeding cycle.

 CALL OUR OFFICE

IMMEDIATELY if
- The bleeding does not stop after 20 minutes of direct pressure.

During regular hours if
- Nosebleeds occur frequently, even after petroleum jelly and humidification are used.
- You have other concerns or questions.

Instructions for Pediatric Patients, 2nd Edition, ©1999 by WB Saunders Company.
Written by Barton D. Schmitt, MD, pediatrician and author of *Your Child's Health,* Bantam Books, a book for parents.

DEFINITION

A pinworm is a white, very thin worm about ¼ inch long that moves. If it doesn't wiggle it's probably lint or a thread. Pinworms usually are seen in the anal and buttock area, especially at night or early in the morning. Occasionally one is found on the surface of a bowel movement. More than 10% of children have them. They do not cause any serious health problems, but they can cause considerable itching and irritation of the anal area and buttocks.

HOME TREATMENT WHEN PINWORM IS SEEN

Antipinworm Medicine. If you have definitely seen a pinworm, your child needs to be treated.

The pinworm medicine is called _____.

The dose is _____, given _____.

Treatment of Other Family Members for Pinworm. Children are usually infected by children outside the family. If anyone else in your family has anal symptoms or anyone sleeps with your child, call our office during office hours for instructions. Physicians do not agree on whether to treat everyone in the family or only those with symptoms. If any of your child's friends have similar symptoms, be sure to tell their parents to get them tested. Dogs and cats do not carry pinworms.

SUSPICIOUS SYMPTOMS BUT PINWORM NOT SEEN

If your child has itching or irritation of the anal area, she could have pinworms. Keep in mind that many children get itching in this area just from washing their anal area too frequently or vigorously with soap.

Check your child for pinworms as follows: First, look for a ½ inch, white, threadlike worm that moves. Examine the area around the anus using a flashlight. Do this a few hours after your child goes to bed and first thing in the morning for two consecutive nights. If no adult pinworm is seen, do a cellophane tape test for pinworm eggs.

Instructions for Cellophane Tape Test. Pick up glass slides at our office (two for each child) and mark your child's name on the slides. Touch the sticky side of a piece of clear cellophane tape to the skin on both sides of the anus. Do this in the morning soon after your child has awakened and definitely before any bath or shower. Do this two mornings in a row. Apply one piece of tape to each slide. Bring the slides to our office for examination with a microscope. We will call you to give you the results. If pinworm eggs are seen, we will prescribe a medication.

PINWORM EXPOSURE OR CONTACT

If your child has had recent contact with a child who has pinworms but has no symptoms, your child probably won't get them. Pinworms are harmless and are never present very long without causing some anal itching. If you want to be sure your child doesn't have them, wait for at least 1 month. The swallowed egg will not mature into an adult pinworm for 3 to 4 weeks. Then contact our office about doing a cellophane tape test for pinworm eggs.

PREVENTION OF PINWORMS

Infection is caused by swallowing pinworm eggs. Your children can get pinworms no matter how carefully you keep them and your house clean. The following hygiene measures, however, can help to reduce the chances of reinfection of your child or new infections in other people.

- Have your child scrub her hands and fingernails thoroughly before each meal and after each use of the toilet. Keep the fingernails cut short because eggs can collect here. Thumb sucking and nail biting should be discouraged.
- Vacuum or wet mop your child's entire room once every week because any eggs scattered on the floor are infectious for 1 to 2 weeks.
- Machine washing at regular temperature will kill any eggs present in clothing or bedding.

 ## CALL OUR OFFICE

During regular hours if
- The skin around the anus becomes red or tender. (*Streptococcus* bacteria and infections have a special affinity for this site.)
- The anal itching is not resolved within 1 week after treatment.
- You have other concerns or questions.

The following four skin injuries are covered. Go directly to the type of injury that pertains to your child.

1. Cuts and scratches
2. Scrapes (abrasions)
3. Puncture wounds
4. Bruises

1. CUTS AND SCRATCHES

DEFINITION

Most cuts are superficial and extend only partially through the skin. They are caused by sharp objects. The cuts that need sutures are deep and leave the skin edges separated. Another rule of thumb is that cuts need sutures if they are longer than ½ inch (¼ inch if on the face).

HOME CARE

Treatment
- Apply direct pressure for 10 minutes to stop any bleeding.
- Wash the wound with soap and water for 5 minutes.
- Cut off any pieces of loose skin using a small scissors (for torn skin with scrapes).
- Apply an antibiotic ointment and cover it with a Band-Aid or gauze. Wash the wound, apply the ointment, and change the Band-Aid or gauze daily.
- Give acetaminophen or ibuprofen as needed for pain relief.

Common Mistakes in Treating Cuts and Scratches
- Don't use alcohol or Merthiolate on open wounds. They sting and damage normal tissue.
- Don't kiss an open wound because the wound will become contaminated by the many germs in a normal person's mouth.
- Let the scab fall off by itself; picking it off may cause a scar.

 ## CALL OUR OFFICE

IMMEDIATELY if
- Bleeding won't stop after 10 minutes of direct pressure.
- The skin is split open and might need sutures. *Note:* Lacerations must be sutured within 12 hours of the time of injury, and the infection rate is far lower if they are closed within 4 hours.
- There is any dirt in the wound that you can't get out.
- The cut looks infected (yellow pus, spreading redness, red streaks).

During regular hours if
- Your child hasn't had a tetanus booster in more than 10 years (5 years for dirty cuts).
- The wound doesn't heal by 10 days.
- You have other questions or concerns.

2. SCRAPES (ABRASIONS)

DEFINITION

An abrasion is an area of superficial skin that has been scraped off during a fall (e.g., a floor burn or skinned knee).

HOME CARE

Cleaning the Scrape. First, wash your hands. Then wash the wound vigorously for at least 5 minutes with warm water and liquid soap. The area will probably need to be scrubbed several times with a wet piece of gauze to get out all the dirt. You may have to remove some dirt particles (e.g., gravel) with a pair of tweezers. If there is tar in the wound, it can often be removed by rubbing it with petroleum jelly, followed by soap and water again. Pieces of loose skin should be cut off with sterile scissors, especially if the pieces of skin are dirty. Rinse the wound well.

Antibiotic Ointments and Dressing
- Apply an antibiotic ointment and cover the scrape with a Band-Aid or gauze dressing. This is especially important for scrapes over joints (such as the elbow, knee, or hand) that are always being stretched. Cracking and reopening at these sites can be prevented with an antibiotic ointment, which keeps the crust soft (no prescription is needed). Cleanse the area once a day with warm water and then reapply the ointment and dressing until the scrape is healed.

Pain Relief. Because abrasions can hurt badly, give acetaminophen or ibuprofen for the first day.

 ## CALL OUR OFFICE

IMMEDIATELY if
- There is any dirt or grime in the wound that you can't get out.
- Skin loss involves a very large area.
- The scrape looks infected (yellow pus, spreading redness, red streaks).

During regular hours if
- Your child hasn't had a tetanus booster in over 10 years.
- The scrape doesn't heal by 2 weeks.
- You have other questions or concerns.

Instructions for Pediatric Patients, 2nd Edition, ©1999 by WB Saunders Company.
Written by Barton D. Schmitt, MD, pediatrician and author of *Your Child's Health,* Bantam Books, a book for parents.

3. PUNCTURE WOUNDS

DEFINITION

The skin has been completely punctured by an object that is narrow and sharp, such as a nail. The wound is not wide enough to need sutures. Since puncture wounds usually seal over quickly, there is a greater chance of wound infection with this type of skin injury. Puncture wounds of the upper eyelid are especially dangerous and can lead to a brain abscess. A deep infection of the foot can begin with swelling of the top of the foot 1 to 2 weeks after the puncture. Another risk is tetanus if your child is not immunized.

HOME CARE

Cleansing. Soak the wound in warm water and soap for 15 minutes. Scrub the wound with a washcloth to remove any debris. If the wound rebleeds a little, that may help remove germs.

Trimming. Cut off any flaps of loose skin that cover the wound and interfere with drainage or removing debris. Use a fine scissors after cleaning them with rubbing alcohol.

Antibiotic Ointment. Apply an antibiotic ointment and a Band-Aid to reduce the risk of infection. Resoak the area and reapply antibiotic ointment every 12 hours for 2 days.

Pain Relief. Give acetaminophen or ibuprofen for any pain.

 CALL OUR OFFICE

IMMEDIATELY if
- Dirt in the wound remains after you have soaked the wound.
- The tip of the object could have broken off in the wound.

- The sharp object or place where the injury occurred was very dirty (e.g., a barnyard).
- The wound looks infected (yellow pus, spreading redness, red streaks).

During regular hours if
- It has been at least 5 years since your child last had a tetanus booster.
- Pain, redness, or swelling increases after 48 hours.
- You have other questions or concerns.

4. BRUISES

DEFINITION

Bleeding into the skin from damaged blood vessels gives a black and blue mark. Since the skin is not broken, there is no risk of infection. Bruises usually follow injury caused by blunt objects. Unexplained bruises can indicate a bleeding tendency. (***Exception:*** "Unexplained" bruises overlying the shins are usually not a sign of a bleeding tendency: children often bump this area and then forget about it.)

HOME CARE

Bruises. Apply ice for 20 to 30 minutes. No other treatment should be necessary. Give acetaminophen or ibuprofen for pain. Avoid aspirin because it may prolong the bleeding. After 48 hours apply a warm washcloth for 10 minutes 3 times a day to help the skin reabsorb the blood. Bruises clear in about 2 weeks.

Blood Blisters. Do not open blisters; it will only increase the possibility of infection. They will dry up and peel off in 1 to 2 weeks.

 CALL OUR OFFICE

IMMEDIATELY if
- Bruises are unexplained *and* several in number.

SUTURED WOUND CARE

DEFINITION

Most contaminated wounds that are going to become infected do so 24 to 72 hours after the initial injury. Keep in mind that a 2- to 3-mm rim of pinkness or redness confined to the edge of a wound can be normal, especially if the wound is sutured. However, the area of redness should not spread. Pain and tenderness also occur normally, but the pain and swelling should be greatest during the second day and should thereafter diminish.

HOME CARE

Do not wash the area for 24 hours. Then begin gently washing it with warm water and liquid soap 1 or 2 times each day. Apply an antibiotic ointment afterward to keep a thick scab from forming over the sutures. Swimming and baths are safe after 48 hours.

SUTURE REMOVAL

Sutures are ready for removal at different times, depending on the site of the wound. The following table can serve as a guide:

Area of Body	Number of Days
Face	3-4
Neck	5
Scalp	6
Anterior chest or abdomen	7
Arms and back of hands	7
Legs and top of feet	10
Back	10
Palms and soles	14

Have your child's stitches removed on the correct day. Stitches removed too late can leave unnecessary skin marks or even scarring. If any sutures come out too early, call your child's physician. In the meantime, reinforce the wound with tape or butterfly Band-Aids. Continue the tape until the date when the sutures would have been removed.

Protection. After removal of sutures:

- Protect the wound from injury during the following month.
- Avoid sports that could reinjure the wound. If a sport is essential, apply tape before playing.

SCARS

If your child needed sutures, he will develop a scar. All wounds heal by scarring. The scar can be kept to a minimum by taking the sutures out at the right time, preventing wound infections, and protecting the wound from being reinjured during the following month. The healing process continues for 6 to 12 months, and only then will the scar assume its final appearance.

 ## CALL OUR OFFICE

IMMEDIATELY if
- An unexplained fever (over 100°F [37.8°C]) occurs.
- A red streak or red area spreads from the wound.

Within 24 hours if
- The wound looks infected (pus or a pimple).
- The wound becomes more painful than it was on the second day.
- A stitch comes out early.
- You have other concerns or questions.

Instructions for Pediatric Patients, 2nd Edition, ©1999 by **WB Saunders Company**.
Written by Barton D. Schmitt, MD, pediatrician and author of *Your Child's Health*, Bantam Books, a book for parents.

DEFINITION

Surgical removal of the tonsils and adenoids (known as a T&A) is one of the most common operations performed on children in the United States. Only 2% or 3% of children have adequate medical indications for this procedure. Parents need to be armed with enough facts to prevent unnecessary surgery.

The tonsils are not just some worthless pieces of tissue that block our view of the throat. They have a purpose. They produce antibodies that fight nose and throat infections. They confine the infection to the throat, rather than allowing it to spread to the neck or bloodstream.

RISKS OF T&A SURGERY

T&A procedures are not without risk. Under ideal conditions, the death rate is 1 child per 250,000 operations. Approximately 5% of children bleed on the fifth to eighth postoperative day and a few require a transfusion or additional surgery. All children experience throat discomfort for several days.

ERRONEOUS REASONS FOR T&A SURGERY

Some T&As are performed for unwarranted reasons. By all means, don't pressure a physician to remove your child's tonsils.

"Large" Tonsils. Large tonsils do not mean "bad" tonsils or infected tonsils. The tonsils are normally large during childhood (called "physiological tonsillar hypertrophy"). They can't be "too large" unless they touch each other. The peak size is reached between 8 and 12 years of age. Thereafter, they spontaneously shrink in size each year, as do all of the body's lymph tissues.

Recurrent Colds and Viral Sore Throats. Several studies have shown that T&As do not decrease the frequency of viral upper respiratory infections (URIs). These URIs are unavoidable. Eventually your child develops immunity to these viruses and experiences fewer colds per year.

Recurrent Strep Throats. Recent studies have shown that a child does not have fewer streptococcal infections of the throat after the tonsils are removed unless the child experiences seven or more strep infections per year (a rare occurrence). For children with seven or more severe throat infections per year, some physicians would recommend daily penicillin for 6 months instead of a T&A, since penicillin can almost always eradicate the strep bacteria from the tonsils. The strep carrier state (which causes no symptoms and is harmless and not contagious) is not an indication for a T&A.

Recurrent Ear Infections. This reason for a T&A was formerly controversial, but more recent studies have shown that removal of the adenoids will not open the eustachian tube and decrease the frequency of ear infections or fluid in the middle ear. The exceptions are children who also have persistent nasal obstruction and mouth breathing caused by large adenoids. Recurrent ear infections usually respond to a 3-month course of antibiotics. Persistent middle-ear fluid may require the insertion of ventilation tubes in the eardrums.

School Absence. If your child misses school for vague reasons (including sore throats), removing the tonsils will not improve attendance.

Miscellaneous Conditions. A T&A will not help a poor appetite, hay fever, asthma, febrile convulsions, or bad breath. There are few medical conditions that have not at one time or another been blamed on the tonsils.

MEDICAL INDICATIONS FOR T&A SURGERY

Yes, sometimes the tonsils should come out. But the benefits must outweigh the risks. All but the first three of the following valid reasons are rare.

Persistent Mouth Breathing. Mouth breathing during colds or hay fever is common. Continued mouth breathing is less common and deserves an evaluation to see if it is due to large adenoids. The open-mouth appearance results in teasing, and the mouth breathing itself leads to changes in the facial bone structure (including an overbite that could require orthodontics).

Abnormal Speech. The speech can be muffled by large tonsils or made hyponasal (no nasal resonance) by large adenoids. Although other causes are possible, an evaluation is in order.

Severe Snoring. Snoring can have many causes. If the adenoids are the cause, they should be removed. In severe cases, the loud snoring is associated with retractions (pulling in of the spaces between the ribs) and is interrupted by 30- to 60-second bouts of stopped breathing (sleep apnea).

Heart Failure. Rarely, large tonsils and adenoids interfere so much with breathing that blood oxygen is reduced and the right side of the heart goes into failure. Children with this condition are short of breath and have limited exercise tolerance.

Persistent Swallowing Difficulties. During a throat infection, the tonsils may temporarily swell enough to cause swallowing problems. Some children refuse solid foods. If the problem is persistent and the tonsils are seen to be touching, an evaluation is in order.

Recurrent Abscess (Deep Infection) of the Tonsil. Your child's physician will make this decision.

Recurrent Abscess of a Lymph Node Draining the Tonsil. Your child's physician will make this decision.

Suspected Tumor of the Tonsil. These rare tumors cause one tonsil to be much larger than the other. The tonsil is also quite firm to the touch.

VENTILATION TUBES SURGERY

DEFINITION

- Ventilation tubes are tiny plastic tubes that are inserted through the eardrum by an ear, nose, and throat surgeon. They are also called tympanostomy tubes, because they are placed in the tympanic membrane (eardrum).
- At least 1 million children in the United States (most of them 1 to 3 years of age) have ventilation tubes placed each year.
- The operation costs about $300 if done in the office (only possible with older, cooperative children) and about $1000 if it needs to be done in the hospital with the child under brief anesthesia.

The ventilation tubes are used to drain fluid out of the middle ear space and ventilate the area with air. The eardrum normally vibrates with sound because the space behind it (the middle ear) is filled with air. If it is filled with fluid, the hearing is muffled. This happens with ear infections. Sometimes after the infection clears, the fluid remains. This occurs if the eustachian tube (which runs from the back of the nose to the middle ear) has become blocked and no longer allows air in and fluid out. Following an ear infection, approximately 30% of children still have fluid in the middle ear at 1 month, 20% at 2 months, and 5% at 4 months. The main concern about prolonged fluid in the middle ear is that the associated hearing deficit may have an impact on speech development. By 5 years of age, the eustachian tube is wider and fluid usually doesn't persist long after ear infections are treated.

BENEFITS

Ventilation tubes allow secretions to drain out of the middle ear space and air to reenter. The risk of recurrent ear infections is greatly reduced. The hearing returns to normal with the tube in place and speech development can get back on track. Tubes also prevent the fluid from becoming thicker (a "glue ear") and damaging the middle ear. The ventilation tubes also buy time while the child matures and the eustachian tubes begin to function better.

RISKS

First, approximately 10% of children with ventilation tubes continue to have ear infections with drainage and pain. These bouts of infection, which require antibiotics, probably would have occurred anyway. Second, complications may occur around the tubes falling out too early or too late. Normally the tubes come out and fall into the ear canal after about 1 year. Sometimes they come out too quickly and need to be replaced by another set. If they remain in the eardrum for over 2 years, the ear, nose, and throat specialist may need to remove them. Third, after they come out, some leave scarring of the eardrum or a small hole (perforation) that doesn't heal. These both can cause a small hearing loss. Because of these possible complications and the requirement for an anesthetic, physicians recommend ventilation tubes only for children who definitely need them.

DEALING WITH TEMPORARY HEARING LOSS

As described earlier, most children with a hearing loss caused by fluid in their middle ear have it on just a temporary basis. During this time when you talk with your child, get close to him, get eye contact, get his full attention, and occasionally check that he understands what you have said. If not, speak in a louder voice than you normally use. A common mistake is to assume your child is ignoring you when actually he doesn't hear you. Reduce any background noise from radio or television while talking with your child. If your child goes to school, be sure he sits in front near the teacher. (Middle ear fluid interferes with the ability to hear in a crowd or classroom.) Keep in mind that most children's speech will catch up following a brief period of partial hearing.

MEDICAL INDICATIONS FOR TUBES

The surgical placement of ventilation tubes is usually indicated if several of the following conditions are met:

- The fluid has been present continuously for over 4 months.
- Both ears are involved.
- The fluid has caused a documented hearing loss. (Although a loss greater than 20 decibels (dB) can significantly affect speech, many children with fluid in their ears have nearly normal hearing.)
- The fluid has caused a speech delay (e.g., child is not using 3 words by 18 months or 20 words by 2 years).
- Recurrent ear infections have failed to respond to treatment with continuous antibiotics.

PREVENTION OF CHRONIC EAR FLUID

Chronic ear fluid and recurrent ear infections are usually due to a blocked eustachian tube. If any of the following triggers are present, treat or eliminate them before considering ventilation tubes.

- Exposure to tobacco smoke.
- Drinking a bottle while lying down (or bottle propping) can cause milk to enter the middle ear space.
- Children with nasal allergies have more frequent ear fluid buildup. Consider this if your child has associated hay fever, eczema, asthma, or food allergies.
- Children with nightly snoring caused by large adenoids may also have ear problems.

Instructions for Pediatric Patients, 2nd Edition, ©1999 by WB Saunders Company.
Written by Barton D. Schmitt, MD, pediatrician and author of *Your Child's Health,* Bantam Books, a book for parents.

PART 7

BEHAVIOR PROBLEMS

Instructions for Pediatric Patients, 2nd Edition, ©1999 by WB Saunders Company.
Written by Barton D. Schmitt, MD, pediatrician and author of *Your Child's Health,* Bantam Books, a book for parents.

DEFINITION

- Unexplained crying
- Intermittent crying one or two times per day
- Healthy child (not sick or in pain)
- Well-fed child (not hungry)
- Bouts of crying usually last 1 to 2 hours
- Child fine between bouts of crying
- Child usually consolable when held
- Onset under 4 weeks of age
- Resolution by 3 months of age
- This diagnosis must be confirmed by a physician

Cause

Normally infants do some crying during the first months of life. When babies cry without being hungry, overheated, or in pain, we call it "colic." About 10% of babies have colic. Although no one is certain what causes colic, these babies seem to want to be cuddled or to go to sleep. Colic tends to occur in high-needs babies with a sensitive temperament. Colic is not the result of bad parenting, so don't blame yourself. Colic is also not due to excessive gas, so don't bother with extra burping or special nipples. Cow's milk allergy may cause crying in a few babies, but only if your baby also has diarrhea or vomiting.

Colic is not caused by abdominal pain. The reason the belly muscles feel hard is that a baby needs these muscles to cry. Drawing up the legs is also a normal posture for a crying baby, as is flexing the arms.

Expected Course

This fussy crying is harmless for your baby. The hard crying spontaneously starts to improve at 2 months and is gone by 3 months. Although the crying can't be eliminated, the minutes of crying per day can be dramatically reduced with treatment. In the long run, these children tend to remain more sensitive and alert to their surroundings.

COPING WITH COLIC

1. **Hold and soothe your baby whenever she cries without a reason.** A soothing, gentle activity is the best approach to helping a baby relax, settle down, and go to sleep. You can't spoil a baby during the first 3 or 4 months of life. Consider using the following:

   - Cuddling your child in a rocking chair
   - Rocking your child in a cradle
   - Placing your child in a baby carrier or sling (which frees your hands for housework)
   - A windup swing or a vibrating chair
   - A stroller (or buggy) ride outdoors or indoors
   - Anything else you think may be helpful (e.g., a pacifier, a warm bath, or massage)

   If all else fails, Sleep Tight is a new device that attaches under the crib and simulates the motion and sound of a moving car. This gadget has lessened colicky behavior in over 90% of babies. It costs about $90. For more information call 1-800-662-6542.

2. **A last resort: Let your baby cry herself to sleep.** If none of these measures quiets your baby after 30 minutes of trying and she has been fed recently, your baby is probably trying to go to sleep. She needs you to minimize outside stimuli while she tries to find her own way into sleep. Wrap her up and place her in her crib. She will probably be somewhat restless until she falls asleep. Close the door, go into a different room, turn up the radio, and do something you want to do. Even consider earplugs or earphones. Save your strength for when your baby definitely needs you. If she cries for over 15 minutes, however, pick her up and again try the soothing activities.

3. **Prevent later sleep problems.** Although babies need to be held when they are crying, they don't need to be held all the time. If you overinterpret the advice for colic and rock your baby every time she goes to sleep, you will become indispensable to your baby's sleep process. Your baby's colic won't resolve at 3 months of age. To prevent this from occurring, when your baby is drowsy but not crying, place her in the crib and let her learn to self-comfort and self-induce sleep. Don't rock or nurse her to sleep at these times. Although colic can't be prevented, secondary sleep problems can be.

4. **Promote nighttime sleep (rather than daytime sleep).** Try to keep your infant from sleeping excessively during the daytime. If your baby has napped 3 hours, gently awaken your baby, and entertain or feed her, depending on her needs. In this way the time when your infant sleeps the longest (often 5 hours) will occur during the night.

5. **Try these feeding strategies.** Don't feed your baby every time she cries. Being hungry is only one of the reasons babies cry. It takes about 2 hours for the stomach to empty, so wait that long between feedings or you may cause cramps from bloating. For breast-fed babies, however, nurse them every time they cry until your milk supply is well established and your baby is gaining weight (usually 2 weeks). Babies who feed too frequently during the day become hungry at frequent intervals during the night. If you are breast-feeding, avoid drinking coffee, tea, and colas and avoid taking other stimulants. Suspect a cow's milk allergy if your child also has diarrhea, vomiting, eczema, wheezing, or a strong family history of milk allergy. If any of these factors are present, try a soy formula for 1 week. Soy formulas are nutritionally complete and no more expensive than regular formula. If you are breast-feeding, avoid all forms of cow's milk in your diet for 1 week. If the crying dramatically improves when your child is on the soy formula, call us for additional advice about keeping her on the formula.

Also, if you think your child is allergic, but she doesn't improve with soy formula, call us about the elemental formulas.

6. **Get rest and help for yourself.** Although the crying can be reduced, what's left must be endured and shared. Avoid fatigue and exhaustion. Get at least one nap each day in case the night goes badly. Ask your husband, a friend, or a relative for help with other children and chores. Caring for a colicky baby is a two-person job. Hire a babysitter so you can get out of the house and clear your mind. Talk to someone every day about your mixed feelings. The screaming can drive anyone to desperation.

7. **Avoid these common mistakes.** If you are breast-feeding, don't stop. If your baby needs extra calories, talk with a lactation consultant about ways to increase your milk supply. The available medicines are ineffective and many (especially those containing phenobarbital) are dangerous for children of this age. The medicines that slow intestinal activity (the anticholinergics) can cause fever or constipation. The ones that remove gas bubbles are not helpful according to recent research, but they are harmless. Inserting a thermometer or suppository into the rectum to "release gas" does nothing ex-

cept irritate the anal sphincter. Don't place your baby face down on a waterbed, sheepskin rug, bead-filled pillow, or other soft pillow. While these surfaces can be soothing, they also increase the risk of suffocation and crib death. A young infant may not be able to lift the head adequately to breathe. Stay with TLC (tender loving care) for best results.

 CALL OUR OFFICE

IMMEDIATELY if
- Your baby cries constantly for more than 2 hours.
- You are afraid you might hurt your baby.
- You have shaken your baby.
- Your baby starts acting very sick.

During regular hours if
- You can't find a way to soothe your baby's crying.
- The crying continues after your baby reaches 4 months of age.
- Your baby is not gaining weight and may be hungry.
- You have other questions or concerns.

Instructions for Pediatric Patients, **2nd Edition,** ©1999 by WB Saunders Company.
Written by Barton D. Schmitt, MD, pediatrician and author of *Your Child's Health,* Bantam Books, a book for parents.

DEFINITION

Parents want their children to go to bed without resistance and to sleep through the night. They look forward to a time when they can again have 7 or 8 hours of uninterrupted sleep. Newborns, however, have a limit to how many hours they can go without a feeding (usually 4 or 5 hours). By 2 months of age, some 50% of bottle-fed infants can sleep through the night. By 4 months, most bottle-fed infants have acquired this capacity. Most breast-fed babies can sleep through the night by 5 months of age.

Good sleep habits may not develop, however, unless you have a plan. Consider the following guidelines if you want to teach your baby that nighttime is a special time for sleeping, that his crib is where he stays at night, and that he can put himself back to sleep. It is far easier to prevent sleep problems before 6 months of age than it is to treat them later.

Newborns

1. **Place your baby in the crib when he is drowsy but awake.** This step is very important. Without it, the other preventive measures will fail. Your baby's last waking memory should be of the crib, not of you or of being fed. He must learn to put himself to sleep without you. Don't expect him to go to sleep as soon as you lay him down. It often takes 20 minutes of restlessness for a baby to go to sleep. If he is crying, rock him and cuddle him; but when he settles down, try to place him in the crib before he falls asleep. Handle naps in the same way. This is how your child will learn to put himself back to sleep after normal awakenings. Don't help your infant when he doesn't need any help.

2. **Hold your baby for all fussy crying during the first 3 months.** All new babies cry some during the day and night. If your baby cries excessively, the cause is probably colic. Always respond to a crying baby. Gentle rocking and cuddling seem to help the most. Babies can't be spoiled during the first 3 or 4 months of life, but even colicky babies have a few times each day when they are drowsy and not crying. On these occasions, place the baby in his crib and let him learn to self-comfort and self-induce sleep.

3. **Carry your baby for at least 3 hours each day when he isn't crying.** This practice will reduce fussy crying.

4. **Do not let your baby sleep for more than 3 consecutive hours during the day.** Attempt to awaken him gently and entertain him. In this way, the time when your infant sleeps the longest will occur during the night. (**Note:** Many newborns can sleep 5 consecutive hours and you can teach your baby to take this longer period of sleep at night.)

5. **Keep daytime feeding intervals to at least 2 hours for newborns.** More frequent daytime feedings (such as hourly) lead to frequent awakenings for small feedings at night. Crying is the only form of communication newborns have. Crying does not always mean your baby is hungry. He may be tired, bored, lonely, or too hot. Hold your baby at these times or put him to bed. Don't let feeding become a pacifier. For every time you nurse your baby, there should be four or five times that you snuggle your baby *without* nursing. Don't let him get into the bad habit of eating every time you hold him. That's called "grazing."

6. **Make middle-of-the-night feedings brief and boring.** You want your baby to think of nighttime as a special time for sleeping. When he awakens at night for feedings, don't turn on the lights, talk to him, or rock him. Feed him quickly and quietly. Provide extra rocking and playtime during the day. This approach will lead to longer periods of sleep at night.

7. **Don't awaken your infant to change diapers during the night.** The exceptions to this rule are soiled diapers or times when you are treating a bad diaper rash. If you must change your child, use as little light as possible (e.g., a flashlight), do it quietly, and don't provide any entertainment.

8. **Don't let your baby sleep in your bed.** Once your baby is used to sleeping with you, a move to his own bed will be extremely difficult. Although it's not harmful for your child to sleep with you, you probably won't get a restful night's sleep. So why not teach your child to prefer his own bed? For the first 2 or 3 months, you can keep your baby in a crib or box next to your bed.

9. **Give the last feeding at your bedtime (10 or 11 PM).** Try to keep your baby awake for the 2 hours before this last feeding. Going to bed at the same time every night helps your baby develop good sleeping habits.

Two-Month-Old Babies

1. **Move your baby's crib to a separate room.** By 3 months of age, your baby should be sleeping in a separate room. This will help parents who are light sleepers sleep better. Also, your baby may forget that his parents are available if he can't see them when he awakens. If separate rooms are impractical, at least put up a screen or cover the crib railing with a blanket so that your baby cannot see your bed.

2. **Try to delay middle-of-the-night feedings.** By now, your baby should be down to one feeding during the night (two for some breast-fed babies). Before preparing a bottle, try holding your baby briefly to see if that will satisfy him. If you must feed him, give 1 or 2 ounces less formula than you would during the day. If you are breast-feeding, nurse for less time at night. As your baby gets close to 4 months of age, try nursing on just one side at night. Never awaken your baby at night for a feeding except at your bedtime.

Four-Month-Old Babies

1. **Try to discontinue the 2 AM feeding before it becomes a habit.** By 4 months of age, your bottle-fed baby does not need to be fed more than four times per day. Breast-fed babies do not need more than five nursing sessions per day. If you do not eliminate the night feeding at this time, it will become more difficult to stop as your child gets older. Remember to give the last feeding at 10 or 11 PM. If your child cries during the night, comfort him with a back rub and some soothing words instead of with a feeding. (*Note:* Some breast-fed babies will continue to need to be nursed once during the night.)

2. **Don't allow your baby to hold his bottle or take it to bed with him.** Babies should think that the bottle belongs to the parents. A bottle in bed leads to middle-of-the-night crying because your baby will inevitably reach for the bottle and find it empty or on the floor.

3. **Make any middle-of-the-night contacts brief and boring.** All children have four or five partial awakenings each night. They need to learn how to go back to sleep on their own at these times. If your baby cries for more than a few minutes, visit him but don't turn on the light, play with him, or take him out of his crib. Comfort him with a few soothing words and stay for less than 1 minute. If your child is standing in the crib, don't try to make him lie down. He can do this himself. If the crying continues for more than 10 minutes, calm him and stay in the room until he goes to sleep. (*Exceptions:* You feel your baby is sick, hungry, or afraid.)

Six-Month-Old Children

1. **Provide a friendly soft toy for your child to hold in his crib.** At the age of 6 months, children start to be anxious about separation from their parents. A stuffed animal, doll, or blanket can be a security object that will give comfort to your child when he wakes up during the night.

2. **Leave the door open to your child's room.** Children can become frightened when they are in a closed space and are not sure that their parents are still nearby.

3. **During the day, respond to separation fears by holding and reassuring your child.** This lessens nighttime fears and is especially important for mothers who work outside the home.

4. **For middle-of-the-night fears, make contacts**

prompt and reassuring. For mild nighttime fears, check on your child promptly and be reassuring, but keep the interaction as brief as possible. If your child panics when you leave or vomits with crying, stay in your child's room until he is either calm or goes to sleep. Do not take him out of the crib but provide whatever else he needs for comfort, keeping the light off and not talking too much. At most, sit next to the crib with your hand on him.

These measures will calm even a severely upset infant.

One-Year-Old Children

1. **Establish a pleasant and predictable bedtime ritual.** Bedtime rituals, which can start in the early months, become very important to a child by 1 year of age. Children need a familiar routine. Both parents can be involved at bedtime, taking turns with reading or making up stories. Both parents should kiss and hug the child "good night." Be sure that your child's security objects are nearby. Finish the bedtime ritual before your child falls asleep.

2. **Once put to bed, your child should stay there.** Some older infants have temper tantrums at bedtime. They may protest about bedtime or even refuse to lie down. You should ignore these protests and leave the room. You can ignore any ongoing questions or demands your child makes and enforce the rule that your child can't leave the bedroom. If your child comes out, return him quickly to the bedroom and avoid any conversation. If you respond to his protests in this way every time, he will learn not to try to prolong bedtime.

3. **If your child has nightmares or bedtime fears, reassure him.** Never ignore your child's fears or punish him for having fears. Everyone has four or five dreams every night. Some of these are bad dreams. If nightmares become frequent, try to determine what might be causing them, such as something your child might have seen on television.

4. **Don't worry about the amount of sleep your child is getting.** Different people need different amounts of sleep at different ages. The best way you can know that your child is getting enough sleep is that he is not tired during the day. Naps are important to young children but keep them less than 2 hours long. Children stop taking morning naps between 18 months and 2 years of age and give up their afternoon naps between 3 and 6 years of age.

Instructions for Pediatric Patients, 2nd Edition, ©1999 by WB Saunders Company.
Written by Barton D. Schmitt, MD, pediatrician and author of *Your Child's Health,* Bantam Books, a book for parents.

DEFINITION

- Your child is over 4 months old and wakes up and cries one or more times at night to be fed.
- Your child wakes up to be fed most nights.
- Your child is bottle-fed or breast-fed until asleep.
- Your child has awakened to be fed at night since birth.
- The child's parents are tired, but the child is not.

Note: From birth to the age of 2 months, most babies awaken twice each night for feedings. Between the ages of 2 and 3 months, most babies need one feeding in the middle of the night. By 4 months of age, most bottle-fed babies sleep more than 7 hours without feeding. Most breast-fed babies can sleep through by 5 months of age. Normal children of this age do not need calories during the night to stay healthy.

Causes

1. **Nursing or bottle-feeding the baby until asleep.** If the last memory before sleep is sucking the breast or bottle, the bottle or breast becomes the baby's security object. The child does not learn to comfort herself and fall asleep without the breast or bottle. Therefore, when the child normally wakes up at night, she has the habit of not being able to go back to sleep without feeding. Being brought to the parents' bed for a feeding makes the problem far worse.
2. **Leaving a bottle in the bed.** Periodically during the night the child sucks on a bottle. When it becomes empty, the child awakens fully and cries for a refill. Bottles in bed, unless they contain only water, also can lead to severe tooth decay.
3. **Feeding often during the day.** Some mothers misinterpret "demand feedings" to mean that they should feed the baby every time she cries. This misunderstanding can lead to feeding the baby every 30 to 60 minutes. The baby becomes used to being fed small amounts often instead of waiting at least 2 hours between feedings following birth and at least 4 hours between feedings at the age of 4 months. A pattern of feeding every hour or so is called "grazing." This problem occurs more often in breast-fed babies if nursing is used as a pacifier. Bottle dependency leads to the bad habit of carrying a bottle around during the day. Also, giving a child a lot of liquid at night means your child will wake up more often because her diapers are soaked.

Expected Outcome

If you try the following recommendations, your child's behavior will probably improve in 2 weeks. The older your child is, the harder it will be to change your child's habits. Children over 1 year old will fight sleep even when they are tired. They will vigorously protest any change and may cry for hours. However, if you don't take these steps, your child won't start sleeping through the night until 3 or 4 years of age, when busy daytime schedules finally exhaust your child.

HELPING A TRAINED NIGHT FEEDER

1. **Gradually lengthen the time between daytime feedings to 3 or 4 hours.** You can't lengthen the time between nighttime feedings if the time between daytime feedings is short. If a baby is used to frequent feedings during the day, she will get hungry during the night. Grazing often happens to mothers who don't separate holding from nursing. For every time you nurse your baby, there should be four or five times that you snuggle your baby *without* nursing.

   Gradually postpone daytime feeding times until they are more normal for your baby's age. If you currently feed your baby hourly, increase the time between feedings to 1½ hours. When your baby accepts the new schedule, go to 2 hours between feedings. When your baby cries, cuddle her or give her a pacifier. Your goal for a formula-fed baby is to give her four bottles a day by 4 months of age. Breast-fed babies often need five feedings each day until they are 6 months old, when solid foods are added to their diet. If your child is over 6 months old, also introduce cup feedings.

2. **At naps and bedtime, place your baby in the crib drowsy but awake.** When your baby starts to act sleepy, place her in the crib. If your baby is very fussy, rock her until she settles down or is almost asleep, but stop before she's fully asleep. If your baby falls asleep at the breast or bottle, it is best to wake her up. To help your baby not think of feeding at bedtime, consider feeding her 1 hour before bedtime or before a nap. Your baby's last waking memory needs to be of the crib and mattress, not of the breast or bottle. She needs to learn to put herself to sleep. Your baby needs to develop this skill so she can put herself to sleep when she wakes up at night.

3. **If your baby is crying at bedtime or naptime, visit your baby briefly every 5 to 15 minutes.** Visit your baby before she becomes too upset. You may need to check babies younger than 1 year or more sensitive babies every 5 minutes. Gradually lengthen the time between your visits. Make your visits brief and boring but supportive. Don't stay in the room longer than 1 minute. Don't turn on the lights. Act sleepy. Whisper, "Shhh, everyone's sleeping." Do not remove your child from the crib. Do not feed, rock, or play with your baby, or bring her to your bed. This brief contact will not reward your baby enough for her to want to continue the behavior.

4. **For crying during the middle of the night, temporarily hold your baby until asleep.** Until

Instructions for Pediatric Patients, 2nd Edition, ©1999 by WB Saunders Company.
Written by Barton D. Schmitt, MD, pediatrician and author of *Your Child's Health,* Bantam Books, a book for parents.

your child learns how to put herself to sleep at naps and bedtime, make the middle-of-the-night awakenings as easy as possible. If she doesn't fuss for more than 5 or 10 minutes, respond as you do at bedtime. Otherwise, take your crying child out of the crib and hold her until she falls asleep. However, don't turn on the lights or take her out of the room. Try not to talk to her very much. Often this goes better if Dad goes in.

After the last feeding of the day at 9 to 10 PM, feed your baby only once during the night. Provide this nighttime feeding only if 4 or more hours have passed since the last feeding. Make this nighttime feeding boring and brief (no longer than 20 minutes). Stop it before your child falls asleep, and replace it with holding only.

5. **Stop giving your baby any bottle in bed.** If you feed your child at bedtime, don't let her hold the bottle. Also feed your child in a different room than the bedroom. Try to separate mealtime and bedtime. If your baby needs to suck on something to help her go to sleep, offer a pacifier or help her find her thumb.

6. **Help your child attach to a security object.** A security (transitional) object is something that helps a waking child go to sleep. It comforts your child and helps your child to separate from you. A cuddly stuffed animal or doll, other soft toy, or blanket can be a good security object. Sometimes covering a stuffed animal with one of the mother's T-shirts helps a child accept it.

Include the security object whenever you cuddle or rock your child during the day. Also include it in your ritual before bedtime by weaving it into your storytelling. Tuck it into the crib next to your child. Eventually, your child will hold and cuddle the stuffed animal or doll at bedtime in place of you.

7. **Later, phase out the nighttime feeding.** Phase out the nighttime feeding only after the time between daytime feedings is more than 3 hours *and* your child can put herself to sleep without feeding or rocking. Gradually reduce the amount you feed your baby at night. Decrease the amount of formula you give a bottle-fed baby by 1 ounce every two to three nights. Nurse a breast-fed baby on just one side and reduce the time by 2 minutes every two

to three nights. After 1 to 2 weeks, your baby will no longer crave food at night and should be able to go back to sleep without holding or rocking.

8. **Other helpful hints for sleep problems.**

- **Move the crib to another room.** If the crib is in your bedroom, move it to a separate room. If this is impossible, cover one of the side rails with a blanket so your baby can't see you when she wakes up.
- **Avoid long naps during the day.** If your baby has napped for more than 2 hours, wake her up. If she has the habit of taking three naps during the day, try to change the habit to two naps each day.
- **Don't change wet diapers during the night.** Change the diaper only if it is soiled or you are treating a bad diaper rash. If you must change your child's diaper, use as little light as possible (e.g., a flashlight), do it quickly, and don't provide any entertainment.
- **If your child is standing up in the crib at bedtime, you can leave her in that position.**
- **Try to get your child to settle down and lie down.** If she refuses or pulls herself back up, leave her that way. She can lie down without your help. Encouraging your child to lie down soon becomes a game.

9. **Keep a sleep diary.** Write down the times when your baby is awake and asleep. Bring this record with you on your office follow-up visit.

 ## CALL OUR OFFICE

During regular hours if
- Your child is not gaining enough weight.
- You think the crying has a physical cause.
- Your child acts fearful.
- Someone in your family cannot tolerate the crying.
- The steps outlined here do not improve your child's sleeping habits within 2 weeks.
- You have other questions or concerns.

Instructions for Pediatric Patients, **2nd Edition,** ©1999 by **WB Saunders Company.**
Written by Barton D. Schmitt, MD, pediatrician and author of *Your Child's Health,* Bantam Books, a book for parents.

DEFINITION

- Your child is over 4 months old and wakes up and cries one or more times a night.
- The crying occurs most nights.
- Your child is held, rocked, or walked until asleep.
- Your child doesn't need to be fed in the middle of the night. (Until the age of 2 or 3 months, most babies need to be fed during the night.)
- Your child has awakened and cried at night since birth.
- The child's parents are tired, but the child is not.

Causes

1. **Holding or rocking your baby until asleep.** All children normally wake up four or five times each night after dreams. Because they usually do not wake up fully at these times, most children can get back to sleep by themselves. However, children who have not learned how to comfort and quiet themselves cry for a parent. If your custom at naps and bedtime is to hold, rock, or lie down with your baby until asleep, your child will not learn how to go back to sleep without your help. Babies who are not usually placed in their cribs while they are still awake expect their mothers to help them go back to sleep when they wake up at night. Because they usually fall asleep away from their cribs, they don't learn to associate the crib and mattress with sleep. This is called poor sleep-onset association.

2. **Providing entertainment during the night.** Children may awaken and cry more frequently if they realize they gain from it, for example, if they are walked, rocked, or played with, or enjoy other lengthy contact with their parents. Being brought to the parents' bed makes the problem far worse.

   Trained night crying can also begin after situations that required the parents to give more nighttime attention to their baby for a while. Examples of such problems are colds, discomfort during hot summer nights, or traveling. Many babies quickly settle back into their previous sleep patterns after such situations. However, some enjoy the nighttime contact so much that they begin to demand it.

3. **Believing any crying is harmful.** All young children cry when confronted with a change in their schedule or environment (called normal protest crying). Crying is their only way to communicate before they are able to talk. Crying for brief periods is not physically or psychologically harmful. The thousands of hours of attention and affection you have given your child will easily offset any unhappiness that may result from changing a bad sleep pattern.

Expected Outcome

If you try the following recommendations, your child's behavior will probably improve in 2 weeks. The older your child is, the harder it will be to change your child's habits. Children over 1 year old will fight sleep even when they are tired. They will vigorously protest any change and may cry for hours. However, if you don't take these steps, your child won't start sleeping through the night until 3 or 4 years of age, when busy daytime schedules finally exhaust your child.

HELPING A TRAINED NIGHT CRIER

1. **Place your baby in the crib when he is drowsy but awake for naps and bedtime.** It's good to hold babies and to provide pleasant bedtime rituals. However, when your baby starts to look drowsy, place him in the crib. Your child's last waking memory needs to be of the crib and mattress, not of you. If your baby is very fussy, rock him until he settles down or is almost asleep, but stop before he's fully asleep. He needs to learn to put himself to sleep. Your baby needs to develop this skill so he can put himself back to sleep when he normally wakes up at night.

2. **If your baby is crying at bedtime or naptime, visit your baby briefly every 5 to 15 minutes.** Visit your baby before he becomes too upset. You may need to check younger or more sensitive babies every 5 minutes. You be the judge. Gradually lengthen the time between your visits. Babies cannot learn how to comfort themselves without some crying. This crying is not harmful.

3. **Make the visits brief and boring but supportive.** Don't stay in your child's room longer than 1 minute. Don't turn on the lights. Keep the visit supportive and reassuring. Act sleepy. Whisper, "Shhh, everyone's sleeping." Add something positive, such as "You're a wonderful baby," or "You're almost asleep." Never show your anger or punish your baby during these visits. If you hug him, he probably won't let go. Touch your baby gently and help him find his security object, such as a doll, stuffed animal, or blanket.

4. **Do not remove your child from the crib.** Do not rock or play with your baby or bring him to your bed. Brief contact will not reward your baby enough for him to want to continue the behavior. Most young babies cry for 30 to 90 minutes and then fall asleep.

5. **For crying during the middle of the night, temporarily hold your baby until asleep.** Until your child learns how to put himself to sleep at naps and bedtime, make the middle-of-the-night awakenings as easy as possible for everyone. If he doesn't fuss for more than 5 or 10 minutes, respond as you do at bedtime. Otherwise, take your crying child out of the crib and hold him until he falls asleep. Don't turn on the lights or take him out of the room. Try not to talk to him very much. Often this goes better if Dad goes in.

6. **Help your child attach to a security object.** A security (transitional) object is something that helps

a waking child go to sleep. It comforts your child and helps your child separate from you. A cuddly stuffed animal or doll, other soft toy, or blanket can be a good security object. Sometimes covering a stuffed animal with one of the mother's T-shirts helps a child accept it.

Include the security object whenever you cuddle or rock your child during the day. Also include it in your ritual before bedtime by weaving it into your storytelling. Tuck it into the crib next to your child. Eventually, your child will hold and cuddle the stuffed animal or doll at bedtime in place of you.

7. **Later, phase out the nighttime holding.** Phase out nighttime holding only after your child has learned to quiet himself and put himself to sleep for naps and at bedtime. Then you can expect him to put himself back to sleep during normal middle-of-the-night awakenings. Go to him every 15 minutes while he is crying, but make your visits brief and boring. After your child learns to put himself to sleep at bedtime, awakening with crying usually stops in a few nights.

8. **Other helpful hints for sleep problems.**

   • **Move the crib to another room.** If the crib is in your bedroom, move it to a separate room. If this is impossible, cover one of the side rails with a blanket so your baby can't see you when he wakes up.

   • **Avoid long naps during the day.** If your baby has napped for more than 2 hours, wake him up. If he has the habit of taking three naps during the day, try to change his habit to two naps each day.

   • **Don't change wet diapers during the night.** Change the diaper only if it is soiled or you are treating a bad diaper rash. If you must change your child's diaper, use as little light as possible (e.g., a flashlight), do it quickly, and don't provide any entertainment.

   • **If your child is standing up in the crib at bedtime, you can leave him in that position.**

   • **Try to get your child to settle down and lie down.** If he refuses or pulls himself back up, leave him that way. He can lie down without your help. Encouraging your child to lie down can soon become a game.

9. **Keep a sleep diary.** Keep a record of when your baby is awake and asleep. Bring it with you on your office follow-up visit.

 CALL OUR OFFICE

During regular hours if
• You think the crying has a physical cause.
• Your child acts fearful.
• Someone in your family cannot tolerate the crying.
• The steps outlined here do not improve your child's sleeping habits within 2 weeks.
• You have other questions or concerns.

Instructions for Pediatric Patients, 2nd Edition, ©1999 by WB Saunders Company.
Written by Barton D. Schmitt, MD, pediatrician and author of *Your Child's Health,* Bantam Books, a book for parents.

DEFINITION

- These children are over 2 years old and refuse to go to bed or stay in the bedroom.
- These children can come out of the bedroom many times because they no longer sleep in a crib.
- In the usual form, the child eventually goes to sleep while watching television with the parent or in the parents' bed.
- In a milder form, the child stays in his or her bedroom but prolongs the bedtime interaction with ongoing questions, unreasonable requests, protests, crying, or temper tantrums.
- In the morning, these children sleep late or have to be awakened because they went to bed so late.

Cause

These are unreasonable attempts to test the limits, not expressions of fear. Your child has found a good way to postpone bedtime and receive extra entertainment. Your child is stalling and taking advantage of your good nature. If given a choice, over 90% of children would stay up until their parents' bedtime. These children also often try to share the parents' bed at bedtime or sneak into their parents' bed during the middle of the night. By contrast, the child who comes to the parents' bed if she is frightened or not feeling well should be supported at these times.

DEALING WITH BEDTIME RESISTANCE

The following recommendations apply to children who are manipulative at bedtime, not fearful.

1. **Clarify what a good sleeper does.** Tell your child what you want her to do: At bedtime a good sleeper stays in her bed and doesn't scream. During the night, a good sleeper doesn't leave her bedroom or wake up her parents unless it's an emergency. A good sleeper gets a sticker and a special treat for breakfast. A bad sleeper loses a privilege for the following day (e.g., all television shows or access to a favorite toy).

2. **Start the night with a pleasant bedtime ritual.** Provide a bedtime routine that is pleasant and predictable. Most prebedtime rituals last about 30 minutes and include taking a bath, brushing teeth, reading stories, talking about the day, saying prayers, and other interactions that relax your child. Try to keep the same sequence each night because familiarity is comforting for children. Try to have both parents take turns in creating this special experience. Never cancel this ritual because of misbehavior earlier in the day. Before you give your last hug and kiss and leave your child's bedroom, ask, "Do you need anything else?" Then leave and don't return. It's very important that you are *not* with your child at the moment of falling asleep. (Reason: she will then need you to be present following normal awakenings at night.)

3. **Establish a rule that your child can't leave the bedroom at night.** Enforce the rule that once the bedtime ritual is over and your child is placed in the bedroom, she cannot leave that room. Your child needs to learn to put herself to sleep for naps and at bedtime in her own bed. Do not stay in the room until she lies down or falls asleep. Establish a set bedtime and stick to it. Make it clear that your child is not allowed to leave the bedroom between 8:00 at night and 7:00 in the morning (or whatever sleep time you decide on). Obviously, this change won't be accomplished without some crying or screaming for a few nights.

   If your child has been sleeping with you, tell her "Starting tonight, we sleep in separate beds. You have your room, we have our room. You have your bed, we have our bed. You are too old to sleep with us anymore."

4. **Ignore verbal requests.** For ongoing questions or demands from the bedroom, ignore them and do not engage in any conversation with your child. All of these requests should have been dealt with during your prebedtime ritual. Don't return or talk with your child unless you think she is sick. (*Some Exceptions:* If your child says she needs to use the toilet, tell her to take care of it herself. If your child says her covers have fallen off and she is cold, promise her you will cover her up after she goes to sleep. You will usually find her well covered.)

5. **Close the bedroom door for screaming.** For screaming from the bedroom, tell your child, "I'm sorry I have to close your door. I'll open it as soon as you're quiet." If she pounds on the door, you can open it after 1 or 2 minutes and suggest that she go back to bed. If she does, you can leave the door open. If she doesn't, close the door again. For continued screaming or pounding on the door, reopen it approximately every 15 minutes, telling your child that if she quiets down, the door can stay open. Never spend more than 30 seconds reassuring her. Although you may not like to close the door, you don't have many options. Rest assured, if your child is over 2 years old and has no daytime separation fears, it's quite reasonable to do this.

6. **Close the bedroom door for coming out.** If your child comes out of the bedroom, return her immediately to her bed. During this process, avoid any lectures and skip the hug and kiss. Get good eye contact and remind her again that she cannot leave her bedroom during the night. Warn her that if she comes out again, you're sorry but you will need to close the door. If she comes out, close the door. Tell her, "I'll be happy to open your door as soon as you're in your bed." If your child says she's in her bed, open the door. If she screams, every 15 minutes, open the door just enough to ask your child if she's in her bed now.

7. **Lock the bedroom door or put up a barricade for repeated coming out.** If your child is very determined and continues to come out of the bedroom, consider putting a barricade in front of her door, such as a strong gate. A half-door or plywood plank may also serve this purpose. If your child makes a ruckus at night, you can go to her without taking her out of her bedroom and say, "Everyone is sleeping, I'll see you in the morning."

   If your child learns to climb over the barricade, a full door may need to be kept closed until morning with a push-button lock, hook and eyelet screw, piece of rope, or chain lock. Although you may consider this step extreme, it can be critical for protecting children less than 5 years old who wander through the house at night without an understanding of dangers (such as the stove, hot water, electricity, knives, and going outdoors).

   If your child does not get into trouble at night, you can open the door as soon as she falls asleep. Reassure her that you will do this. Also, each night give her a fresh chance to stay in the bedroom with the door open. (***Caution:*** If your child has bedtime fears, don't close her door. Get her some counseling.)

8. **If your child comes into your bed at night, return her to her own bed.** For middle-of-the-night attempts to crawl into your bed, unless your child is fearful, sternly order your child back to her own bed. If she doesn't move, escort her back immediately without any physical contact or pleasant conversation. If you are asleep when your child crawls into your bed, return her as soon as you discover her presence. If she attempts to come out again, lock her door until morning. If you are a deep sleeper, consider using some signaling device that will awaken you if your child enters your bedroom (such as a chair placed against your door or a loud bell attached to your doorknob). For children over age 5, some parents simply lock their bedroom door or put a stop sign poster on the outside of it. Remind your child that it is not polite to interrupt other people's sleep. Tell her that if she awakens at night and can't go back to sleep, she can read or play quietly in her room, but she is not to bother her parents.

9. **If your child awakens you at night with screaming or demands, visit her briefly.** Reassure her that she is safe. If she needs her blankets readjusted, help her do this. Then leave. On the following day teach her how to solve independently any complaints she makes during the night. (Remind your child that it is not polite to awaken people at night. Tell her that if she awakens at night and can't go back to sleep, she can read or play quietly in her room.)

10. **Help the roommate.** If the bedtime screaming wakes up a roommate, have the well-behaved sibling sleep in a separate room until the nighttime behavior has improved. Tell your child with the sleep problem that her roommate cannot return until she stays in her room quietly for three consecutive nights. If you have a small home, have the sibling sleep in your room temporarily and this will be an added incentive for your other child to improve.

11. **Awaken your child at the regular time each morning.** Even if she fought bedtime and fell asleep late, wake her up at the regular time so she will be tired earlier the next evening.

12. **Start bedtime later if you want to minimize bedtime crying.** The later the bedtime, the more tired your child will be and the less resistance she will offer. For most children, you can pick the bedtime hour. For children who are very stubborn and cry a lot, you may want to start the bedtime at 10 PM (or whenever your child naturally falls asleep). If the bedtime is at 10 PM, start the bedtime ritual at 9:30 PM. After your child learns to fall asleep without fussing at 10 PM, move the bedtime back by 15 minutes every week. In children who can't tell time, you can gradually (over 8 weeks or so) achieve an 8 PM bedtime in this way with many fewer tantrums (this technique was described by Adams and Rickert in 1989). However, don't let your child sleep late in the morning or you won't be able to advance the bedtime.

 CALL OUR OFFICE

During regular hours if
- Your child is not sleeping well after trying this program for 2 weeks.
- Your child needs to be locked in the bedroom for more than 7 nights.
- Your child is frightened at bedtime (she probably needs some counseling).
- Your child has lots of nightmares.
- Your child also has several discipline problems during the day.
- You have other questions or concerns.

Instructions for Pediatric Patients, 2nd Edition, ©1999 by WB Saunders Company.
Written by Barton D. Schmitt, MD, pediatrician and author of *Your Child's Health,* Bantam Books, a book for parents.

PROS AND CONS

In general, bed sharing is not recommended. Although it's not harmful for your children to sleep with you, it's unnecessary and it may cause problems for you. Once begun, it's a rather hard habit to undo; so don't start until you have all the facts.

1. **Your child doesn't need this arrangement to be secure and happy.** Children's fears and insecurities can be dealt with during the day. Children can turn out fine either way. The majority of children in the United States sleep happily in their own bed. In poor countries, families sleep together by necessity.
2. **Bed sharing is not quality time.** If your child is asleep in your bed, it is neutral time. If your child is crying and keeping you awake, it is aggravating time. So there is really no quality time here.
3. **Neither parents nor child get a good night's sleep.** Several studies have shown that over 50% of children who sleep with parents resist going to bed and awaken several times at night. Most parents who bed-share have to lie down with their child for 30 to 60 minutes to get them to sleep. Most of these parents also do not get a good night's sleep and become sleep deprived. Sleeping with your child is a bad choice if you are a light sleeper and also need your sleep because you work outside the home.
4. **Bed sharing is never a long-term solution to sleep problems.** Your child will not learn to sleep well in your bed and then decide on his own to start sleeping in his bed. With every passing month, the habit becomes harder to change. Your child can no longer sleep alone.
5. **There is no evidence that bed sharing produces children who are more spoiled or dependent.**

PREVENTION OF BED SHARING

- During infancy, place your child in the crib when he is drowsy but awake. In this way he will learn to put himself back to sleep following normal awakenings.
- Make middle-of-the-night feedings brief and boring. This is hard to do if you are sleeping with your child.

- Put your child in his own room by 3 or 4 months of age. Have a rule that he does not leave the crib at night, and after 2 years old, that he does not leave the bedroom. Most children in the United States follow these guidelines and do just fine.
- If you must sleep in the same room with your infant, don't allow him to see you during his normal awakenings. If he does, it's an invitation to wake you to play. Instead, cover the side of his crib with something (e.g., a firmly attached blanket).
- After 6 months of age, encourage a soft toy or stuffed animal as a security object. Otherwise he may select you as his security object.

PUTTING AN END TO BED SHARING

If you are sleeping with your child and want to stop it, here are some suggestions:

- Tell your child the new rule. "You are too old to sleep with us anymore. You have your bed, and we have our bed. Starting tonight, we want you to stay in your bed during the night."
- For being a "good sleeper" who sleeps in his bedroom all night, give him a treat with breakfast.
- If your child leaves the bedroom, return him immediately. If he does it again, close the door until he's in his bed.
- If your child crawls into your bed during the night, order him back to his own bed using a stern voice. If he doesn't move, escort him back immediately without any conversation.
- If you are asleep when your child crawls into your bed, return him as soon as you discover him. If he attempts to come out again, temporarily close his door. If you are a deep sleeper, consider using some signaling device that will awaken you if your child enters your bedroom (such as a chair placed against your door or a loud bell attached to your doorknob). Some parents simply lock their bedroom door. Remind your child that "it is not polite to wake people who are sleeping unless it's an emergency."
- Expect some crying. Young children normally cry when they don't get their way. But continue to be firm and you will win back the privacy of your bed.

NIGHTMARES

DEFINITION

Nightmares are scary dreams that awaken a child. Occasional bad dreams are normal at all ages after about 6 months of age. When infants have a nightmare, they cry and scream until someone comes to them. When preschoolers have a nightmare, they usually cry and run into their parents' bedroom. Older children begin to understand what a nightmare is and put themselves back to sleep without waking their parents.

Cause

Everyone dreams four or five times each night. Some dreams are good, and some are bad. Dreams help the mind process complicated events or information. The content of nightmares usually relates to developmental challenges: Toddlers have nightmares about separation from their parents; preschoolers, about monsters or the dark; and school-age children, about death or real dangers. Frequent nightmares may be caused by violent television shows or movies.

DEALING WITH NIGHTMARES

1. **Reassure and cuddle your child.** Explain to your child that she was having a bad dream. Sit on the bed until your child is calm. Offer to leave the bedroom door open (never close the door on a fearful child). Provide a night-light, especially if your child has fears of the dark. Most children return to sleep fairly quickly.
2. **Help your child talk about the bad dreams during the day.** Your child may not remember what the dream was about unless you can remind her of something she said about it when she woke up. If your child was dreaming about falling or being chased, reassure her that lots of children dream about that. If your child has the same bad dream over and over again, help her imagine a good ending to the bad dream. Encourage your child to use a strong person or a magic weapon to help her overcome the bad person or event in the dream. You may want to help your child draw pictures or write stories about the new happier ending for the dream. Working through a bad fear often takes several conversations about it.
3. **Protect your child against frightening movies and television shows.** For many children, violent or horror movies cause bedtime fears and nightmares. These fears can persist for months or years. Absolutely forbid these movies before 13 years of age. Between 13 and 17 years, the maturity and sensitivity of your child must be considered carefully in deciding when she is ready to deal with the uncut versions of R-rated movies. Be vigilant about slumber parties or Halloween parties. Tell your child to call you if the family she is visiting is showing scary movies.

 CALL OUR OFFICE

During regular hours if
- The nightmares become worse.
- The nightmares are not minimal after using this approach for 2 weeks.
- The fear interferes with daytime activities.
- Your child has several fears.
- You have other concerns or questions.

Instructions for Pediatric Patients, 2nd Edition, ©1999 by WB Saunders Company.
Written by Barton D. Schmitt, MD, pediatrician and author of *Your Child's Health,* Bantam Books, a book for parents.

DEFINITION

- Your child is agitated and restless but cannot be awakened or comforted.
- Your child may sit up or run helplessly about, possibly screaming or talking wildly.
- Although your child appears to be anxious, he doesn't mention any specific fears.
- Your child doesn't appear to realize that you are there. Although the eyes are wide open and staring, your child looks right through you.
- Your child may mistake objects or persons in the room for dangers.
- The episode begins 1 to 2 hours after going to sleep.
- The episode lasts from 10 to 30 minutes.
- Your child cannot remember the episode in the morning (amnesia).
- The child is usually 1 to 8 years old.
- This diagnosis must be confirmed by a physician.

Cause

Night terrors are an inherited disorder in which a child tends to have dreams during deep sleep from which it is difficult to awaken. They occur in 2% of children and usually are not caused by psychological stress. Being overtired can trigger night terrors.

Expected Course

Night terrors usually occur within 2 hours of bedtime. Night terrors are harmless and each episode will end of its own accord in deep sleep. The problem usually disappears by 12 years of age or sooner.

DEALING WITH NIGHT TERRORS

1. **Try to help your child return to normal sleep.** Your goal is to help your child go from agitated sleep to a calm sleep. You won't be able to awaken your child, so don't try. Turn on the lights so that your child is less confused by shadows. Make soothing comments such as "You are all right. You are home in your own bed. You can rest now." Speak calmly and repetitively. Such comments are usually better than silence and may help your child refocus. Some children like to have their hand held during this time, but most will pull away. Hold your child only if it seems to help him feel better. There is no way to abruptly shorten the episode. Shaking your child or shouting at him will just cause the child to become more agitated and will prolong the attack.
2. **Protect your child against injury.** During a night terror, a child can fall down a stairway, run into a

wall, or break a window. Try to gently direct your child back to bed.
3. **Prepare babysitters or overnight leaders for these episodes.** Explain to people who care for your child what a night terror is and what to do if one happens. Understanding this will prevent them from overreacting if your child has a night terror.

PREVENTION OF NIGHT TERRORS

1. **Keep your child from becoming overtired.** Sleep deprivation is the most common trigger for night terrors. For preschoolers, restore the afternoon nap. If your child refuses the nap, encourage a 1-hour "quiet time." Also avoid late bedtimes because they may trigger a night terror. If your child needs to be awakened in the morning, that means he needs an earlier bedtime. Move lights-out time to 15 minutes earlier each night until your child can self-awaken in the morning.
2. **Use prompted awakenings for frequent night terrors.** If your child has frequent night terrors, Dr. B. Lask of London has found a new way to eliminate this distressing sleep pattern in 90% of children. For several nights, note how many minutes elapse from falling asleep to the onset of the night terror. Then awaken your child 15 minutes before the expected time of onset. (Remind your child at bedtime that when you do this, his job is "to wake up fast." Keep your child fully awake and out of bed for 5 minutes. Carry out these prompted awakenings for seven consecutive nights. If the night terrors return, repeat this seven-night training program.

 CALL OUR OFFICE

During regular hours if
- Any drooling, jerking, or stiffening occurs.
- The episodes occur two or more times per week after doing the seven prompted awakenings.
- Episodes last longer than 30 minutes.
- Your child does something dangerous during an episode.
- Episodes occur during the second half of the night.
- Your child has several daytime fears.
- You feel family stress may be a factor.
- You have other questions or concerns.

DEFINITION

- Your child walks while asleep.
- Your child's eyes are open but blank.
- Your child is not as well coordinated as when awake.
- Your child may perform semipurposeful acts such as dressing and undressing, opening and closing doors, or turning lights on and off.
- The episode begins 1 to 2 hours after going to sleep.
- The episode may last 5 to 20 minutes.
- During this time your child cannot be awakened no matter what the parent does.
- The child is usually 4 to 15 years old.

Cause

Sleepwalking is an inherited tendency to wander during deep sleep. About 15% of normal children sleepwalk.

Expected Course

Sleepwalking usually occurs within 2 hours of bedtime. Children stop sleepwalking during adolescence.

DEALING WITH SLEEPWALKING

1. **Gently lead your child back to bed.** First, steer your child into the bathroom because she may be looking for a place to urinate. Then guide her to her bedroom. The episode may end once she's in bed. Don't expect to awaken her, however, before she returns to normal sleep.

2. **Protect your child from accidents.** Although accidents are rare, they do happen, especially if the child wanders outside. Sleepwalkers can be hit by a car or bitten by a dog, or they may become lost. Put gates on your stairways and special locks on your outside doors (above your child's reach). Do not let your child sleep in a bunk bed.

3. **Help your child avoid exhaustion.** Fatigue and a lack of sleep can lead to more frequent sleepwalking. So be sure your child goes to bed at a reasonable hour, especially when ill or exhausted. If your child needs to be awakened in the morning, that means she needs an earlier bedtime. Move lights-out time to 15 minutes earlier each night until your child can self-awaken in the morning.

4. **Try prompted awakenings to prevent sleepwalking.** If your child has frequent sleepwalking, try to eliminate this distressing sleep pattern. For several nights, note how many minutes elapse from falling asleep to the onset of the sleepwalking. Then awaken your child 15 minutes before the expected time of onset. Remind your child at bedtime that when you do this, her job is "to wake up fast." Keep your child fully awake for 5 minutes. Carry out these prompted awakenings for 7 consecutive nights. If the sleepwalking returns, repeat this seven-night training program.

Instructions for Pediatric Patients, 2nd Edition, ©1999 by WB Saunders Company.
Written by Barton D. Schmitt, MD, pediatrician and author of *Your Child's Health,* Bantam Books, a book for parents.

Some children awaken before their parents do, usually between 5 and 6 AM. These 1 to 3 year olds are well rested and raring to go. They come out of their room or call out from the crib and want everyone to wake up. They are excited about the new day and want to share it with you. If people don't respond, they make a racket. Such a child is a morning person.

Causes

Most of these children have received plenty of sleep. They are no longer tired. They are not awakening early on purpose. Most of them were put to bed too early the night before, had too many naps, or had naps that were too long. (*Note:* Early morning naps that begin within 2 hours after breakfast also contribute to early morning awakening.) Some of them have a reduced sleep requirement—one that is below the average of 10 to 12 hours per night that most children 1 to 10 years old need. This is a genetic trait. Such children often have a parent who only needs 6 hours or so of sleep at night. Other children may begin awakening early in the springtime because of sunlight streaming through their window. (This scenario is easily remedied with dark shades or curtains.) Finally, those children who are given a bottle in their crib, fed an early breakfast, or allowed to come into their parents' bed early in the morning may develop a bad habit that persists after the original cause (e.g., too much nap time) is removed.

HELPING YOUR CHILD SLEEP LATER

1. **Reduce naps.** Assume your child is getting too much sleep during the day. Many children over 1 year of age and most over 18 months of age need only one nap (unless they are sick). If your child needs two naps, be sure the first nap doesn't begin before 9 AM. If cutting back to one 2-hour nap after lunch doesn't help, shorten the nap to 1½ hours maximum. Also make sure your child gets plenty of exercise after his nap, so he'll be tired at night.
2. **Delay bedtime until 8 or 9 PM.** These two steps should cure your child unless he has a below-average sleep requirement. In that case, proceed with the following limit-setting suggestions.
3. **Establish a rule.** "You can't leave your bedroom until your parents are up. You can play quietly in your bedroom until breakfast." Also, tell your child, "It's not polite to wake up someone who is sleeping. Your parents need their sleep."
4. **If your child is in a crib, leave him there until 6 AM.** Put some toys in a bag in his crib the night before (but not ones he can stand on). If you put them in before he goes to sleep, he may play with them for a while, fall asleep later, and sleep longer.

If he cries, go in once to reassure him and remind him of the toys. Don't include any surprises or treats in his toy bag or he'll awaken early as children do on holiday mornings. If he makes loud noises with the toys, remove those particular toys. If he cries, ignore it. If crying continues, visit him briefly every 15 minutes to reassure him that all is well and most people are sleeping. Don't turn on the lights, talk much, give him a bottle, remove him from the crib, or stay more than 1 minute.
5. **If your child is in a floor-level bed, keep him in his bedroom until 6 AM.** Get him a clock radio and set it for 6 AM. Tell him he can't leave his bedroom until the music comes on. Tell him he can play quietly until then. Help him put out special toys or books the night before. If he comes out of his room, put up a gate or close the door. Tell him that you'll be happy to open the door as soon as he is back in his bed. If this is a chronic problem, put up the gate the night before.
6. **If you meet strong resistance from your child, change his wake-up time gradually.** Some children protest a great deal about the new rule, especially if they have been coming into your bed in the morning. In that case, move ahead a little more gradually. If he's been awakening at 5 AM, help him to wait until 5:15 for 3 days. Set the clock radio for that time. After your child has adjusted to 5:15, change the clock radio to 5:30. Move the wake-up time forward every 3 or 4 days.
7. **Praise your child for not waking other people in the morning.** A star chart or special treat at breakfast may help your child wait more cooperatively.
8. **Change your tactics for weekends.** Many parents want their child to sleep in on Saturday and Sunday mornings. If this is your preference, keep your early morning riser up an hour later the night before. If you are using a clock radio with your program, turn it off or reset the times for an hour later. As a last resort, put a breakfast together for your child the night before and allow him to watch a preselected videotape.

 ## CALL OUR OFFICE

During regular hours if
- Your child's sleep doesn't improve after trying this approach for 4 weeks.
- Your child has several other behavior problems.
- You have other questions or concerns.

DEFINITION

Negativism is a normal phase most children go through between 18 months and 3 years of age. It begins when children discover they have the power to refuse other people's requests. They respond negatively to many requests, including pleasant ones. In general, they are stubborn rather than cooperative. They delight in refusing a suggestion, whether it's about getting dressed or taking off their clothes, taking a bath or getting out of the bathtub, going to bed or getting up. Unless understood, this behavior can become extremely frustrating for parents. Handled appropriately, it lasts about 1 year.

DEALING WITH A NEGATIVE, STUBBORN TODDLER

Consider the following guidelines for helping you and your child through this phase.

1. **Don't take this normal phase too personally.** By "no" your child means "Do I have to?" or "Do you mean it?" A negative response should not be confused with disrespect. Also, it is not meant to annoy you. This phase is critical to the development of independence and identity. Try to look at it with a sense of humor and amazement.

2. **Don't punish your child for saying "no."** Punish your child for what she does, not what she says. Since saying "no" is not something you control, ignore it. If you argue with your child about saying "no," you will probably prolong this behavior.

3. **Give your child plenty of choices.** This is the best way to increase your child's sense of freedom and control, so that she will become more cooperative. Examples of choices are letting your child choose between a shower or a bath; which book to read; which toys to take into the tub; which fruit to eat for a snack; which clothes or shoes to wear; which breakfast cereal to eat; and which game to play, whether inside or outside, in the park or in the yard. For tasks your child doesn't like, give her a say in the matter by asking, "Do you want to do it slowly or fast?" or "Do you want me to do it, or you?" The more quickly your child gains a feeling that she is a decision maker, the sooner she will become cooperative.

4. **Don't give your child a choice when there is none.** Safety rules, such as sitting in the car seat, are not open to discussion, although you can explain why the rule must be followed. Going to bed or to day care also is not negotiable. Don't ask a question when there's only one acceptable answer, but direct your child in as kind a way as possible (e.g., "I'm sorry, but now you have to go to bed."). Commands such as "do this or else" should be avoided.

5. **Give transition time when changing activities.** If your child is having fun and must change to another activity, she probably needs a transition time. For example, if your child is playing with trucks as dinnertime approaches, give her a 5-minute warning. A kitchen timer sometimes helps a child accept the change better.

6. **Eliminate excessive rules.** The more rules you have, the less likely it is that your child will be agreeable about following them. Eliminate unnecessary expectations and arguments about wearing socks or cleaning her plate. Help your child feel less controlled by having more positive interactions than negative contacts each day.

7. **Avoid responding to your child's requests with excessive "no's."** Be for your child a model of agreeableness. When your child asks for something and you are unsure, try to say "yes" or postpone your decision by saying "Let me think about it." If you are going to grant a request, do so right away, before your child whines or begs for it. When you must say "no," tell your child that you're sorry and give your child a reason.

 CALL OUR OFFICE

During regular hours if
- You or your spouse can't accept your child's need to say "no."
- You or your spouse have trouble controlling your temper.
- Your child has several other discipline problems.
- This approach doesn't bring improvement within 1 month.
- You have other questions or concerns.

Instructions for Pediatric Patients, 2nd Edition, ©1999 by WB Saunders Company.
Written by Barton D. Schmitt, MD, pediatrician and author of *Your Child's Health*, Bantam Books, a book for parents.

The first goal of discipline is to protect your child from danger. Another important goal is to teach your child an understanding of right from wrong. Reasonable limit setting keeps us from raising a "spoiled" child. To teach respect for the rights of others, first teach your child to respect your rights. Begin *external* controls by 6 months of age. Children don't start to develop *internal* controls (self-control) until 3 or 4 years of age. They continue to need external controls, in gradually decreasing amounts, through adolescence.

GUIDELINES FOR SETTING RULES

1. **Begin discipline after 6 months of age.** Young infants don't need any discipline. By the time they crawl, all children need rules for their safety.
2. **Express each misbehavior as a clear and concrete rule.** Examples of clear rules are "Don't push your brother" and "Don't interrupt me on the telephone."
3. **Also state the acceptable or appropriate behavior.** Your child needs to know what is expected of him. Examples are "Play with your brother," "Look at books when I'm on the telephone," or "Walk, don't run."
4. **Ignore unimportant or irrelevant misbehavior.** Avoid constant criticism. Behavior such as swinging the legs, poor table manners, or normal negativism is unimportant during the early years.
5. **Use rules that are fair and attainable.** A child should not be punished for behavior that is part of normal emotional development, such as thumb sucking, fears of being separated from the parents, and toilet-training accidents.
6. **Concentrate on two or three rules initially.** Give highest priority to issues of safety, such as not running into the street, and to the prevention of harm to others. Of next importance is behavior that damages property. Then come all the annoying behavior traits that wear you down (such as tantrums or whining).
7. **Avoid trying to change "no-win" behavior through punishment.** Examples are wetting pants, pulling their own hair, thumb sucking, body rocking, masturbation, not eating enough, not going to sleep, and refusal to complete schoolwork. The first step in resolving such a power struggle is to withdraw from the conflict and stop punishing your child for the misbehavior. Then give your child positive feedback when he behaves as you'd like.
8. **Apply the rules consistently.** After the parents agree on the rules, it may be helpful to write them down and post them.

DISCIPLINE TECHNIQUES (INCLUDING CONSEQUENCES)

1. **Techniques to use for different ages are summarized here.** The techniques mentioned here are further described after this list.

- From birth to 6 months: no discipline necessary
- From 6 months to 3 years: structuring the home environment, distracting, ignoring, verbal and nonverbal disapproval, physically moving or escorting, and temporary time-out
- From 3 years to 5 years: the preceding techniques (especially temporary time-out) plus natural consequences, restricting places where the child can misbehave, and logical consequences
- From 5 years to adolescence: the preceding techniques plus delay of a privilege, "I" messages, and negotiation via family conferences
- Adolescence: logical consequences, "I" messages, and family conferences about house rules; time-out and manual guidance (see below) can be discontinued

2. **Structure the home environment.** You can change your child's surroundings so that an object or situation that could cause a problem is eliminated. Examples are installing gates, locks, and fences to protect the child.
3. **Distracting your child from misbehavior.** Distracting a young child from temptation by attracting his attention to something else is especially helpful when the child is in someone else's house or a store (e.g., distract with toys, food, or games).
4. **Ignore the misbehavior.** Ignoring helps to stop unacceptable behavior that is harmless—such as tantrums, sulking, whining, quarreling, or interrupting.
5. **Use verbal and nonverbal disapproval.** Mild disapproval is often all that is required to stop a young child's misbehavior. Get close to your child, get eye contact, look stern, and give a brief "no" or "stop."
6. **Physically move or escort ("manual guidance").** Manual guidance means that you move a child from one place to another (e.g., to bed, bath, car, or time-out chair) against his will and help him as much as needed (e.g., carrying).
7. **Use temporary time-out or social isolation.** Time-out is the most effective discipline technique available to parents. Time-out is used to interrupt unacceptable behavior by removing the child from the scene to a boring place, such as a playpen, corner of a room, chair, or bedroom. Time-outs should last about 1 minute per year of age and not more than 5 minutes.
8. **Restrict places where a child can misbehave.** This technique is especially helpful for behavior problems that can't be eliminated. Allowing nose picking and masturbation in your child's room prevents an unnecessary power struggle.
9. **Use natural consequences.** Your child can learn good behavior from the natural laws of the physical world; for example, not dressing properly for the weather means your child will be cold or wet,

or breaking a toy means it isn't fun to play with anymore.

10. **Use logical consequences.** These should be logically related to the misbehavior, making your child accountable for his problems and decisions. Many logical consequences are simply the temporary removal of a possession or privilege if your child has misused the object or right.

11. **Delay a privilege.** Examples of work before play are "After you clean your room, you can go out and play" or "When you finish your homework, you can watch television."

12. **Use "I" messages.** When your child misbehaves, tell your child how you feel. Say, "I am upset when you do such and such." Your child is more likely to listen to this than a message that starts with "you." "You" messages usually trigger a defensive reaction.

13. **Negotiate and hold family conferences.** As children become older they need more communication and discussion with their parents about problems. A parent can begin such a conversation by saying, "We need to change these things. What are some ways we could handle this? What do you think would be fair?"

14. **Temporarily discontinue any physical punishment.** Most out-of-control children are already too aggressive. Physical punishment teaches them that it's acceptable to be aggressive (e.g., hit or hurt someone else) to solve problems.

15. **Discontinue any yelling.** Yelling and screaming teach your child to yell back; you are thereby legitimizing shouting matches. Your child will respond better in the long run to a pleasant tone of voice and words of diplomacy.

16. **Don't forget to reward acceptable (desired) behaviors.** Don't take good behavior for granted. Watch for behavior you like, and then praise your child. At these times, move close to your child, look at him, smile, and be affectionate. A parent's attention is the favorite reward of most children.

GUIDELINES FOR GIVING CONSEQUENCES (PUNISHMENTS)

1. **Be unambivalent.** Mean what you say and follow through.

2. **Correct with love.** Talk to your child the way you want people to talk to you. Avoid yelling or using a disrespectful tone of voice. Correct your child in a kind way. Sometimes begin your correction with "I'm sorry I can't let you . . ."

3. **Apply the consequence immediately.** Delayed punishments are less effective because young children forget why they are being punished. Punishment should occur very soon after the misbehavior and be administered by the adult who witnessed the misdeed.

4. **Make a one-sentence comment about the rule when you punish your child.** Also restate the preferred behavior, but avoid making a long speech.

5. **Ignore your child's arguments while you are correcting him.** This is the child's way of delaying punishment. Have a discussion with your child at a later, more pleasant time.

6. **Make the punishment brief.** Take toys out of circulation for no more than 1 or 2 days. Time-outs should last no longer than 1 minute per year of the child's age and 5 minutes maximum.

7. **Follow the consequence with love and trust.** Welcome your child back into the family circle and do not comment on the previous misbehavior or require an apology for it.

8. **Direct the punishment against the misbehavior, not the person.** Avoid degrading comments such as "You never do anything right."

 ## CALL OUR OFFICE

During regular hours if
- Your child's misbehavior is dangerous.
- The instances of misbehavior seem too numerous to count.
- Your child is also having behavior problems at school.
- Your child doesn't seem to have many good points.
- Your child seems depressed.
- The parents can't agree on discipline.
- You can't give up physical punishment. (*Note:* Call immediately if you are afraid you might hurt your child.)
- The misbehavior does not improve after 1 month of using this approach.

RECOMMENDED READING

Edward R. Christophersen: Little People. Westport Publishers, Kansas City, Mo., 1988.
Don Dinkmeyer and Gary D. McKay: Parenting Young Children. American Guidance Service, Circle Pines, Minn., 1990.
Michael Popkin: Active Parenting. Harper and Row Publishers, San Francisco, 1987.
Jerry Wyckoff and Barbara C. Unell: Discipline Without Spanking or Shouting. Meadowbrook, Deephaven, Minn., 1984.

Instructions for Pediatric Patients, **2nd Edition**, ©1999 by **WB Saunders Company.**
Written by Barton D. Schmitt, MD, pediatrician and author of *Your Child's Health*, Bantam Books, a book for parents.

DEFINITION

Time-out consists of immediately isolating a child in a boring place for a few minutes whenever she misbehaves. Time-out is also called quiet time, thinking time, or cooling-off time. Time-out has the advantage of providing a cooling-off period to allow both child and parent to calm down and regain control of their emotions.

Used repeatedly and correctly, the time-out technique can change almost any childhood behavior. Time-out is the most effective consequence for toddlers and preschoolers who misbehave—much better than threatening, shouting, or spanking. Every parent needs to know how to give time-out.

Time-out is most useful for aggressive, harmful, or disruptive behavior that cannot be ignored. Time-out is unnecessary for most temper tantrums. Time-out is not needed until a child is at least 8 months old and beginning to crawl. Time-out is rarely needed for children younger than 18 months because they usually respond to verbal disapproval. The peak ages for using time-out are 2 to 4 years. During these years children respond to action much better than to words.

CHOOSING A PLACE FOR TIME-OUT

- **A time-out chair.** When a chair is designated for time-out, it gives time-out a destination. The chair should be in a boring location, facing a blank wall or a corner. Don't allow your child to take anything with her to time-out, such as a toy, pacifier, security blanket, or pet. The child shouldn't be able to see television or other people from the location. A good chair is a heavy one with side arms. Placed in a corner, such a chair surrounds the child with boundaries, leaves a small space for the legs, and reduces thoughts of escape. Alternatives to chairs are standing in a particular corner, sitting on a particular spot on the floor, or being in a playpen (if the child is not old enough to climb out of it).

  Usually the chair is placed in an adjacent hallway or room. Some children less than 2 years old have separation fears and need the time-out chair (or playpen) to be in the same room as the parent. When you are in the same room as your child, carefully avoid making eye contact with the child.

- **A time-out room.** Children who refuse to stay in a time-out chair need to be sent to a time-out room. Confinement to a room is easier to enforce. The room should be one that is safe for the child and contains no valuables. The child's bedroom is often the most convenient and safe place for time-out. Although toys are available in the bedroom, the child does not initially play with them because he or she is upset about being excluded from mainstream activities. Forbid turning on the radio, stereo, or video games during time-out in the bedroom. Avoid any room that is dark or scary (such as some basements), contains hot water (bathrooms), or has filing

cabinets or bookshelves that could be pulled down on the child.

- **Time-out away from home.** Time-out can be effectively used in any setting. In a supermarket, younger children can be put back in the grocery cart and older children may need to stand in a corner. In shopping malls, children can take their time-out sitting on a bench or in a restroom. Sometimes a child needs to be taken to the car and made to sit on the floor of the back seat for the required minutes. If the child is outdoors and misbehaves, you can ask her to stand facing a tree.

HOW TO ADMINISTER TIME-OUT

- **Deciding the length of time-out.** Time-out should be short enough to allow your child to have many chances to go back to the original situation and learn the acceptable behavior. A good rule of thumb is 1 minute per year of age (with a maximum of 5 minutes). After age 6, most children can be told they are in time-out "until you can behave," allowing them to choose how long they stay there. If the problem behavior recurs, the next time-out should last the recommended time for their age.

  Setting a portable kitchen timer for the required number of minutes is helpful. The best type ticks continuously and rings when the time is up. A timer can stop a child from asking the parents when he or she can come out.

- **Sending your child to time-out.** Older children will usually go to time-out on their own. Younger children often need to be led there by their wrist, or in some cases carried there protesting. If your child doesn't go to time-out within 5 seconds, take her there. Tell your child what she did wrong in one sentence (such as, "No hitting"). If possible, also clarify the preferred behavior (such as, "Be kind to George"). These brief comments give your child something to think about during the time-out.

- **Requiring quiet behavior in time-out.** The minimum requirement for time-out completion is that your child does not leave the chair or time-out place until the time-out is over. If your child leaves ahead of time, reset the timer.

  Some parents do not consider a time-out to be completed unless the child has been quiet for the entire time. However, until 4 years of age, many children are unwilling or unable to stay quiet. Ignore tantrums in time-out, just as you should ignore tantrums outside of time-out. After age 4, quiet time is preferred but not required. You can tell your child, "Time-out is supposed to be for thinking, and to think you've got to be quiet. If you yell or fuss, the time will start over."

- **Dealing with room damage.** If your child makes a mess in his room (e.g., empties clothing out of drawers or takes the bed apart), she must clean it up before she is released from time-out. Toys that were misused can be packed away. Some damage can be prevented by removing any scissors or crayons from the room before the time-out begins.

- **Releasing your child from time-out.** To be released, your child must have performed a successful time-out. This means she stayed in time-out for the required number of minutes. Your child can leave time-out when the timer rings. If you don't have a timer, she can leave when you tell her, "Time-out is over. You can get up now." Many parents of children over 4 years old require their children to be quiet at the end of time-out. If a child is still noisy when the timer rings, it can be reset for 1 minute.

BACK-UP PLANS

- **The younger child who refuses to stay in time-out.** In general, if a child escapes from time-out (gets up from the chair or spot), you should quickly take the child back to time-out and reset the timer. This approach works for most children. If a child refuses to stay in time-out, the parent should take action rather than arguing or scolding the child. You may temporarily need to hold a strong-willed, 2- or 3-year-old child in time-out. Holding your child in time-out teaches your child that you mean what you say and that she must obey you. Place your child in the time-out chair and hold her by the shoulders from behind. Tell your child that you will stop holding her when she stops trying to escape. Then avoid eye contact and any more talking. Pretend that you don't mind doing this and are thinking of something else or listening to music. Your child will probably stop trying to escape after a week of this approach.

A last resort for young children who continue to resist sitting in a chair is putting them in the bedroom with a gate blocking the door. Occasionally a parent with carpentry skills can install a half-door. If you cannot devise a barricade, then you can close the door. You can hold the door closed for the 3 to 5 minutes it takes to complete the time-out period. If you don't want to hold the door, you can put a latch on the door that allows it to be temporarily locked. Most children need their door closed only two or three times.

- **The older child who refuses to stay in time-out.** An older child can be defined in this context as one who is too strong for the parent to hold in a time-out chair. In general, any child older than 5 years who does not take time-out quickly should be considered a refuser. In such cases the discipline should escalate to a consequence that matters to the child. First, you can make the time-out longer, adding 1 extra minute for each minute of delay. Second, if 5 minutes pass without your child going to time-out, your child can be grounded. "Grounded" is defined as no television, radio, stereo, video games, toys, telephone access, outside play, snacks, or visits with friends. After grounding your child, walk away and no longer talk to her. Your child becomes "ungrounded" only after she takes her regular time-out plus the 5 minutes of penalty time. Until then, her day is very boring. If your child refuses the conditions of grounding, she can be sent to bed 15 minutes earlier for each time she breaks the grounding requirements. The child whose behavior doesn't improve with this approach usually needs to be evaluated by a mental health professional.

PRACTICING TIME-OUT WITH YOUR CHILD

If you have not used time-out before, go over it with your child before you start using it. Tell your child it will replace spanking, yelling, and other forms of discipline. Review the kinds of negative behavior that will lead to placement in time-out. Also review the positive behavior that you would prefer. Then pretend with your child that he has broken one of the rules. Take him through the steps of time-out so he will understand your directions when you send him to time-out in the future. Also teach this technique to your babysitter.

Instructions for Pediatric Patients, **2nd Edition,** ©1999 by **WB Saunders Company.**
Written by Barton D. Schmitt, MD, pediatrician and author of *Your Child's Health,* Bantam Books, a book for parents.

DEFINITION

Some parents become discouraged with time-out. Their child repeats misbehavior immediately after release from time-out. Some children refuse to go to time-out or won't stay there. None of these examples means that time-out should be abandoned. It remains the best discipline technique for 2- to 5-year-old children. If you use time-out repeatedly, consistently, and correctly, your child will eventually improve. The following recommendations may help you fine-tune how you are using time-out.

1. **Give your child more physical affection each day.** Be sure your child receives two time-ins for every time-out each day. A time-in is a positive, close, brief human interaction. Try to restore the positive side of your relationship with your child. Catch him being good. Try to hold your child for 1 or 2 minutes every 15 minutes when he is not in time-out or misbehaving. Play with your child more. Children who feel neglected or overly criticized don't want to please their parents.

2. **Use time-out every time your child engages in the behavior you are trying to change (target behavior).** Use time-out more frequently. For the first 2 or 3 days you may need to use time-outs 20 or more times a day to gain a defiant toddler's attention. Brief time-outs are harmless and there is no upper limit on how many times you can use them as long as you offset them with positive interactions.

3. **Use time-out. Don't just threaten to use time-out.** For aggressive behaviors, give no warnings; just put your child in time-out. Better yet, intercept your child when you see him starting to raise his arm or clench his fist and before he makes others cry. For other behaviors, remind your child of the rule, count to three, and if he doesn't stop immediately, put him in time-out.

4. **Put your child in time-out earlier.** Put your child in time-out before his behavior worsens. Your child is more likely to accept a time-out calmly if he's put in early rather than if he's put in late (and screaming). Also, putting him in early means you will be more in control of your emotions. Try to put your child in time-out before you become angry. If you are still yelling when you put your child in time-out, it will not work.

5. **Put your child in time-out quickly.** Don't talk about it first. When your child breaks a rule, have him in time-out within 10 seconds.

6. **Don't talk to your child during time-out.** Don't answer his questions or complaints. Don't try to lecture your child.

7. **Ignore tantrums in time-out.** Don't insist on quietness during time-out because it makes it harder to finish the time-out.

8. **Return your child to time-out if he escapes.** Have a back-up plan for further discipline, for example, holding a young child in the time-out chair or grounding an older child.

9. **Consider increasing the length of time-out.** If your child is over 3 years old and needs to be placed in time-out more than 10 times each day, a longer time-out may be needed to get his attention. A preschooler with a strong-willed temperament may temporarily need a time-out that lasts 2 or 3 minutes per year of his age. Children younger than 3 years should receive only brief time-outs (1 minute per year of age) because it is difficult for them to stay in time-out any longer.

10. **Make the time-out place more boring.** If your child doesn't seem to mind the time-outs, eliminate sources of entertainment. Move the time-out chair to a more boring location. If you use your child's bedroom, close the blinds or shades. Temporarily remove all toys and games from the bedroom and store them elsewhere.

11. **Use a portable timer for keeping track of the time.** Your child is more likely to obey a timer than to obey you.

12. **Be kinder in your delivery of time-out.** This will help reduce your child's anger. Say you're sorry he needs a time-out, but be firm about it. Try to handle your child gently when you take him to time-out.

13. **Praise your child for taking a good time-out.** Forgive your child completely when you release him from time-out. Don't give lectures or ask for an apology. Give your child a clean slate and don't tell his father or relatives how many time-outs he needed that day.

14. **Don't punish your child for the normal expression of anger.** If he is saying angry things or looking angry, don't be too alarmed. Don't try to control your child too much.

15. **Give your child more choices about how he takes his time-out.** Ask, "Do you want to take a time-out by yourself or do you want me to hold you in your chair? It doesn't matter to me." (For older children, the choice can be, "By yourself or do you want to be grounded?")

16. **Give your child the option of coming out of time-out as soon as he is under control rather than taking the specified number of minutes.** Some children feel overly controlled.

17. **Use a variety of consequences for misbehavior.** Ignore harmless behaviors. Also use distraction for bad habits. Use logical consequences—such as removal of toys, other possessions, or privileges—for some misbehavior.

18. **Clarify with your child what you want him to do.** Also clarify the house rules. Review this at a time when your child is in a good mood. This will help him be more successful.

19. **Use time-out with siblings when appropriate.** If siblings touch the timer or tease the child in time-out, they should also be placed in time-out.

20. **Teach all caretakers to use time-out correctly and consistently.**

PHYSICAL PUNISHMENT (SPANKING)

The place of physical punishment in discipline is controversial. There are several good arguments for not using corporal punishment at all. We can raise children to be agreeable, responsible, productive adults without ever spanking them. All children need discipline on hundreds of occasions, but there are alternatives to spanking, such as redirecting (distracting) the child, taking away a privilege, or sending a child to her room. Spanking carries the risk of triggering the unrelated pent-up anger that many adults carry inside them. This anger could escalate the well-intentioned spanking and end in child abuse. Parents who turn to spanking as a last resort for "breaking their child's will" may find that they have underestimated their child's determination. In addition, physical punishment worsens aggressive behavior because it teaches a child to lash out when she is angry. Other forms of discipline can be more constructive, leaving a child with some sense of guilt and contributing to the formation of a conscience.

SAFE SPANKING

We would prefer that you not use spanking to discipline your children.

If you occasionally feel the need to spank your child, follow these guidelines for safe physical punishment:

- Always use other techniques (such as time-out) first. Use spanking only for behaviors that are dangerous or deliberately defiant of your instructions.
- Hit only with an open hand. Hit through clothing. It is difficult to judge how hard you are hitting your child if you hit her with an object other than your hand. Paddles and belts may cause bruises.
- Spanking should never leave more than temporary redness of the skin.
- Hit only on the buttocks, legs, or hands. Hitting a child on the face is demeaning as well as dangerous; in fact, slapping the face is inappropriate at any age. Your child could suddenly turn her head and the slap could damage her vision or hearing.

- Give only one swat; that is enough to change behavior. Hitting your child more than once may relieve your anger but will probably not teach your child anything additional.
- Don't spank children less than 18 months of age. Spanking is absolutely inappropriate before your child has learned to walk. Spanking should be unnecessary after the age of 6 years because you can use negotiation and discussion to resolve most differences with school-age children.
- Avoid shaking children, because of the serious risk of causing blood clots on the brain (subdural hematomas).
- Don't use physical punishment more than once each day. The more your child is spanked, the less effect it will have.
- Learn alternatives to physical discipline. Isolating a child in a corner or bedroom for a time-out is much more civilized and effective. Learn how to use other forms of discipline. Spanking should never be the main form of discipline a child receives.
- Never spank your child when you are out of control, scared, or drinking. A few parents can't stop hitting their child once they start. They can't control their rage and need help for themselves, such as from Parents Anonymous groups. They must learn to walk away from their children and never use physical punishment.
- Don't use physical punishment for aggressive misbehavior, such as biting, hitting, or kicking. Physical punishment under such circumstances teaches a child that it is all right for a bigger person to strike a smaller person. Aggressive children need to be taught restraint and self-control. They respond best to time-outs, which give them an opportunity to think about the pain they have caused. If you are not using time-outs, read more on how to make them work for you.
- Don't allow babysitters, child-care staff, and teachers to spank your children.

Instructions for Pediatric Patients, **2nd Edition,** ©1999 by **WB Saunders Company.**
Written by Barton D. Schmitt, MD, pediatrician and author of *Your Child's Health,* Bantam Books, a book for parents.

DEFINITION

A spoiled child is undisciplined, manipulative, and unpleasant to be with much of the time. He has many of the following behaviors by age 2 or 3:

- Doesn't follow rules or cooperate with suggestions
- Doesn't respond to "no," "stop," or other commands
- Protests everything
- Doesn't know difference between his needs and wants
- Insists on having his own way
- Makes unfair or excessive demands on others
- Doesn't respect other people's rights
- Tries to control other people
- Has a low frustration tolerance
- Frequently whines or throws tantrums
- Constantly complains about being bored

Causes

The main cause of spoiled children is a lenient, permissive parent who doesn't set limits and gives in to tantrums and whining. If the parent gives the child too much power, he will become more self-centered. Such parents also rescue the child from normal frustrations (such as waiting and sharing). Occasionally, the child of working parents is left with a nanny or babysitter who spoils the child by providing constant entertainment and giving in to unrealistic demands.

The reason some parents are overly lenient is that they confuse the child's needs (e.g., for demand feeding) with the child's wants or whims (e.g., for demand play). They do not want to hurt their child's feelings or to cause any crying. In the process, they may take the short-term solution of doing whatever prevents crying, which in the long run causes more crying. The child's ability to deliberately cry and fuss to get something usually doesn't begin before 5 or 6 months of age. There may be a small epidemic of spoiling in the United States because some working parents come home feeling guilty about not having enough total time for their children and so spend their free time together trying to avoid any friction or limit setting.

Confusion exists about the differences between giving attention to children and spoiling children. In general, attention is good for children. Indeed, it is essential for normal development. Attention can become harmful if it is excessive, given at the wrong time, or always given immediately. Attention from you is excessive if it interferes with your child's learning to do things for himself and deal with life's frustrations. An example of giving attention at the wrong time is when you are busy and your child is demanding attention. Another wrong time is when a child has just misbehaved and needs to be ignored.

Expected Outcome

Without changes in child rearing, spoiled children run into trouble by school age. Other children do not like them because they are too bossy and selfish. Adults do not like them because they are rude and make excessive demands on them. Eventually they become hard for even the parent to love because of their behaviors. As a reaction to not getting along well with other children and adults, spoiled children eventually become unhappy. Spoiled children may show reduced motivation and perseverance in schoolwork. Because of poor self-control they may become involved with adolescent risk-taking behaviors, such as drug abuse. Overall, spoiling a child prepares that child poorly for life in the real world.

HOW TO PREVENT A SPOILED CHILD

1. **Provide age-appropriate limits or rules for your child.** Parents have the right and responsibility to take charge and make rules. Adults must keep their child's environment safe. Age-appropriate discipline must begin by the age of crawling. Saying "no" occasionally is good for children. Children need external controls until they develop self-control and self-discipline. Your child will still love you after you say "no." If your children like you all the time, you are not being a good parent.

2. **Require cooperation with your important rules.** It is important that your child be in the habit of responding properly to your directions long before entering school. Important rules include staying in the car seat, not hitting other children, being ready to leave on time in the morning, going to bed, and so forth. These adult decisions are not open to negotiation. Do not give your child a choice when there is none.

   Child decisions, however, involve such things as which cereal to eat, book to read, toys to take into the tub, and clothes to wear. Make sure that your child understands the difference between areas in which he has choices (control) and your rules. Try to keep your important rules to no more than 10 or 12 items and be willing to go to the mat about these. Also, be sure that all adult caretakers consistently enforce these rules.

3. **Expect your child to cry.** Distinguish between needs and wants. Needs include crying from pain, hunger, or fear. In these cases, respond immediately. Other crying is harmless. Crying usually relates to your child's wants or whims. Crying is a normal response to change or frustration. When the crying is part of a tantrum, ignore it. Don't punish him for crying, tell him he's a crybaby, or tell him he shouldn't cry. Although not denying your child his feelings, don't be moved by his crying. To compensate for the extra crying your child does during a time when you are tightening up on the rules, provide extra cuddling and enjoyable activities at a time when he is not crying or having a tantrum. There are times when it is necessary to temporarily withhold attention and comforting to help your child learn something

that is important (such as that he can't pull on your earrings).

4. **Do not allow tantrums to work.** Children throw temper tantrums to get your attention, to wear you down, to change your mind, and to get their way. The crying is to change your "no" vote to a "yes" vote. Tantrums may include whining, complaining, crying, breath holding, pounding the floor, shouting, or slamming a door. As long as your child stays in one place and is not too disruptive or in a position to harm himself, you can leave him alone at these times. By all means, don't give in to tantrums.

5. **Don't overlook discipline during quality time.** If you are working parents, you will want to spend part of each evening with your child. This special time spent with your child needs to be enjoyable but also reality based. Don't ease up on the rules. If your child misbehaves, remind him of the existing limits. Even during fun activities, you occasionally need to be the parent.

6. **Don't start democratic child rearing until your child is 4 or 5 years old.** Don't give away your power as a parent. At 2 years of age, be careful not to talk too much with your toddler about the rules. Toddlers don't play by the rules. By 4 or 5 years of age, you can begin to reason with your child about discipline issues, but he still lacks the judgment necessary to make the rules. During the elementary school years, show a willingness to discuss the rules. By 14 to 16 years old, an adolescent can be negotiated with as an adult. At that time you can ask for his input about what rules or consequences would be fair.

The more democratic the parents are during the first 2 or 3 years, the more demanding the children tend to become. Generally, young children do not know what to do with power. Left to their own devices, they usually spoil themselves. If they are testing everything at age 3, it is abnormal. If you have given away your power, take it back (i.e., set new limits and enforce them). You don't have to explain the reason for every rule. Sometimes the only reason needed is just because "I said so."

7. **Teach your child to get herself unbored.** Your job is to provide toys, books, and art supplies. Your child's job is to play with them. Assuming you talk and play with your child several hours each day, you do not need to become your child's constant playmate, nor do you need to constantly provide him with an outside friend. When you're busy, expect your child to amuse himself. Even 1-year-olds can keep themselves occupied for 15-minute blocks of time. By 3 years, most children can entertain themselves half the time. Sending your child outside to "find something to do" is doing him a favor. Much good creative play, thinking, and daydreaming come out of solving boredom. If you can't seem to resign as social director, enroll your child in a preschool.

8. **Teach your child to wait.** Waiting helps children better deal with frustration. All jobs in the adult world carry some degree of frustration. Delaying immediate gratification is a trait your child must gradually learn and it takes practice. Don't feel guilty if you have to make your child wait a few minutes now and then (e.g., don't allow your child to interrupt your conversations with others). Waiting doesn't hurt him as long as he doesn't become overwhelmed or unglued by waiting. His perseverance and emotional fitness will be enhanced.

9. **Don't rescue your child from normal life challenges.** Changes such as moving and starting school are normal life stressors. These are opportunities for learning and problem solving. Always be available and supportive, but don't help your child if he can handle it for himself. Overall, make your child's life as realistic as he can tolerate for his age, rather than going out of your way to make it as pleasant as possible. His coping skills and self-confidence will benefit from this practice.

10. **Don't overpraise your child.** Children need praise, but it can be overdone. Praise your child for good behavior and following the rules. Encourage him to try new things and work on difficult tasks, but teach him to do things for his own reasons too. Self-confidence and a sense of accomplishment come from doing and completing things that he is proud of. Praising your child while he is in the process of doing something may make him stop at each step and want more praise. Avoid the tendency (common with the first-born child) to overpraise your child's normal development.

11. **Teach your child to respect parents' rights and time together.** The needs of your children for love, food, clothing, safety, and security obviously come first. However, your needs should come next. Your children's wants (e.g., for play) and whims (e.g., for an extra bedtime story) should come after your needs are met and as time is available on that day. This is especially important for working parents where family time is limited. It is both the quality and quantity of time that you spend with your children that are important. Quality time is time that is enjoyable, interactive, and focused on your child. Children need some quality time with their parents every day. Spending every free moment of every evening and weekend with your child is not good for your child or your marriage. You need a balance to preserve your mental health. Scheduled nights out with your mate will not only nurture your marriage but also help you to return to parenting with more to give. Your child needs to learn to trust other adults and that he can survive separations from you. If your child isn't taught to respect your rights, he may not respect the rights of other adults.

Instructions for Pediatric Patients, **2nd Edition,** ©1999 by WB Saunders Company.
Written by Barton D. Schmitt, MD, pediatrician and author of *Your Child's Health,* Bantam Books, a book for parents.

DEFINITION

A temper tantrum is an immature way of expressing anger. No matter how calm and gentle a parent you are, your child will probably throw some tantrums. Try to teach your child that temper tantrums don't work and that you don't change your mind because of them. By 3 years of age, you can begin to teach your child to verbalize his feelings ("You feel angry because . . ."). We need to teach children that anger is normal but that it must be channeled appropriately. By school age, temper tantrums should be rare. During adolescence, tantrums reappear, but your teenager can be reminded that blowing up creates a bad impression and that counting to 10 can help her regain control.

RESPONSES TO TEMPER TANTRUMS

Overall, praise your child when she controls her temper, verbally expresses her anger, and is cooperative. Be a good model by staying calm and not screaming or having adult tantrums. Try using the following responses to the different types of temper tantrums.

1. **Support and help children having frustration- or fatigue-related tantrums.** Children often have temper tantrums when they are frustrated with themselves. They may be frustrated because they can't put something together. Young children may be frustrated because their parents don't understand their speech. Older children may be frustrated with their inability to do their homework.

   At these times your child needs encouragement and a parent who listens. Put an arm around her and say something brief that shows understanding such as "I know it's hard, but you'll get better at it. Is there something I can do to help you?" Also give praise for not giving up. Some of these tantrums can be prevented by steering your child away from tasks that she can't do well.

   Children tend to have more temper tantrums when they are tired (e.g., when they've missed a nap) because they are less able to cope with frustrating situations. At these times put your child to bed. Hunger can contribute to temper tantrums. If you suspect this, give your child a snack. Temper tantrums also increase during sickness.

2. **Ignore attention-seeking or demanding-type tantrums.** Young children may throw temper tantrums to get their way. They may want to go with you rather than be left with the babysitter, want candy, want to empty a desk drawer, or want to go outside in bad weather. They don't accept rules for their safety. Tantrums for attention may include whining, crying, pounding the floor or wall, slamming a door, or breath holding. As long as your child stays in one place and is not too disruptive, you can leave her alone.

   If you recognize that a certain event is going to push your child over the edge, try to shift her attention to something else. However, don't give in to your child's demands. During the temper tantrum, if her behavior is harmless, ignore it completely. Once a tantrum has started, it rarely can be stopped.

   Move away, even to a different room; then your child no longer has an audience. Don't try to reason with your child—it will only make the tantrum worse. Simply state, "I can see you're very angry. I'll leave you alone until you cool off. Let me know if you want to talk." Let your child regain control. After the tantrum, be friendly and try to return things to normal. You can prevent some of these tantrums by saying "no" less often.

3. **Physically move children having refusal-type tantrums.** If your child refuses something unimportant (such as a snack or lying down in bed), let it go before a tantrum begins. However, if your child must do something important, such as go to bed or to day care, she should not be able to avoid it by having a tantrum. Some of these tantrums can be prevented by giving your child a 5-minute warning instead of asking her suddenly to stop what she is doing. Once a tantrum has begun, let your child have the tantrum for 2 or 3 minutes. Try to put her displeasure into words:"You want to play some more, but it's bedtime." Then take her to the intended destination (e.g., the bed), helping her as much as is needed (including carrying).

4. **Use time-outs for disruptive-type tantrums.** Some temper tantrums are too disruptive for parents to ignore. On such occasions send or take your child to her room for 2 to 5 minutes. Examples of disruptive behavior include

   - Clinging to you or following you around during the tantrum
   - Hitting you
   - Screaming or yelling for such a long time that it gets on your nerves
   - Having a temper tantrum in a public place such as a restaurant or church (Move your child to another place for her time-out. The rights of other people need to be protected.)
   - Throwing something or damaging property during a temper tantrum

5. **Hold children having harmful or rage-type tantrums.** If your child is totally out of control and screaming wildly, consider holding her. Her loss of control probably scares her. Also hold your child when she is having tantrums that carry a danger of self-injury (such as if she is violently throwing herself backward).

   Take your child in your arms, tell her you know she is angry, and offer her your sense of control. Hold her until you feel her body start to relax. This usually takes 1 to 3 minutes. Then let her go. This comforting response is rarely needed after 3 years of age.

DEFINITION

Biting another child is one of the more unacceptable aggressive behaviors in our society. The parent of the child who has been bitten is usually very upset and worried about the risk of infection. If it happens in a child-care setting, the other parents want the biter to be expelled. If it happens in another's home, the child is often told never to return. Adults tend to forget that some biting behavior in a group of toddlers is to be expected. Most children first learn to bite by doing it to their parents in a playful manner. It is important to try to interrupt this primitive behavior at this early stage.

Causes

Biting is usually a chance discovery around 1 year of age, at a time when teething and mouthing are normal behaviors. It often continues because the parents initially think it is cute and the child considers it a type of game to get attention. Later, children may use it when they are frustrated and want something from another child. At this age for children with minimal verbal skills, biting becomes a primitive form of communication. Only after 2 or 3 years of age can it become a deliberate way to express anger and intimidate others.

RECOMMENDATIONS FOR DEALING WITH BITING

1. **Establish a rule.** "We never bite people." Give your child a reason for the rule, namely, that biting hurts. Other reasons (that won't interest him at his age) are that bites can lead to infection or scarring.
2. **Suggest a safe alternative behavior.** Tell your child if he wants something he should come to you and ask for help or point to it, rather than bite the person who has it. If he bites when he is angry, tell him "If you are mad, come to me and tell me." If your child is at the chewing everything stage (usually less than 18 months), help him choose a toy that he can bite rather than telling him that he cannot bite anything. A firm toy or teething ring will do. Encourage him to carry his "chewy" with him for a few days.
3. **Interrupt biting with a sharp "no."** Be sure to use an unfriendly voice and look your child straight in the eye. Try to interrupt him when he looks like he might bite somebody, before he actually does it, leaving the victim hurt and screaming. Extra close supervision may be necessary until the biting has stopped.
4. **Give your child a time-out for biting others.** Send him to a boring place for approximately 1 minute per year of age. If he attempts to bite you while you are holding him, say "no," always put him down immediately, and walk away (a form of time-out). If time-out does not work, take away a favorite toy for the remainder of the day.
5. **Never bite your child for biting someone else.** Biting back will make your child upset that you hurt him and may teach him that it is okay to bite if you are bigger. Also do not wash his mouth out with soap, pinch his cheek, or slap his mouth. In fact, if your child tends to be aggressive, avoid physical punishment in general (e.g., spanking). Also eliminate "love bites," since your child will be unable to distinguish them from painful biting.
6. **Praise your child for not biting.** The most important time to praise him is when he is in situations or with particular children where he used to frequently bite. Initially give him a kind reminder just before these high-risk visits. Then praise him afterward for good behavior.
7. **Prevention.** The best time to stop a biting behavior from becoming a habit is when it first starts. Be sure that no one laughs when he bites and that no one treats it like a game. (This includes older siblings.) Also never "give in" to your child's demands because of biting. Since biting commonly occurs in child-care settings, be sure the providers understand your approach and are willing to apply it.
8. **Biting in child-care settings.** Biting behavior is common in child-care settings. The preceding approach should be used by day care staff to eliminate the behavior in their setting. Provide careful supervision and quickly place the biting child in time-out, even when he acts like he might bite someone. In general, biting is harmless since most bites by younger children don't puncture the skin. Calling the parent at work is pointless since the problem should be dealt with immediately by whoever witnesses it.

 CALL OUR OFFICE

IMMEDIATELY if
- Biting causes a puncture or a cut that completely breaks the skin.

During regular hours if
- Biting behavior lasts for more than 4 weeks with this approach.
- Your child bites or hurts himself.
- Your child has several other behavior problems.
- You have other questions or concerns.

Instructions for Pediatric Patients, 2nd Edition, ©1999 by WB Saunders Company.
Written by Barton D. Schmitt, MD, pediatrician and author of *Your Child's Health*, Bantam Books, a book for parents.

DEFINITION

Some aggressive behaviors that children experiment with are hitting, slapping, pinching, scratching, poking, hair pulling, biting, kicking, shoving, and knocking down. Since these behaviors are unacceptable in the adult world and potentially harmful, they should not be allowed between children.

Causes

Many children fight when they are angry. They do not like something another child did and they retaliate. They want something another child has and see force as the easiest way to get it. Most children try aggressive behaviors because they see this behavior in playmates or on television. If children get their way through hitting, it will only become more frequent. Occasionally children become excessively aggressive because they receive lots of spankings at home or witness spouse or sibling abuse.

RECOMMENDATIONS

1. **Establish a rule.** "Do not hit because it hurts. We do not hurt people."
2. **For aggressive behavior give your child a brief time-out in a boring place.** Being in time-out helps a child learn to cool down (rather than blow up) when she is angry. When it looks as if your child might hurt someone, intervene immediately. Stop the behavior at the early threatening or shoving stage. Do not wait until the victim is hurt or screams. If a time-out does not seem to be effective, also take away your child's favorite toy or television time for the remainder of the day.
3. **Suggest acceptable ways to express anger.** In the long run you want your child to be able to verbalize her anger in a calm but assertive way. Encourage your child to come to you when she's angry and talk about it until she feels better. A second option is to teach your child to stop and count to 10 before doing anything about her anger. A third option is to help her learn to walk away from a bad situation. Giving your child a time-out is one way of teaching her to walk away from anger.

   Younger children (less than 3 or 4 years old) with limited expressive language need time to develop these skills. When they are in time-out, don't be surprised if they pout, mutter to themselves, yell in their room, or pound on their door. If these physical outlets for anger are blocked, a more aggressive outburst may occur. As long as the behavior is not destructive, ignore it. Teaching your child how to control anger provides her with a valuable resource.
4. **Verbalize your child's feelings for her.** If your child can't talk about her anger, put it into words for her: "I know that you feel angry." It is unrealistic to expect your child not to feel anger. You may need to make an understanding statement such as "You wish you could punch your brother, but we cannot hurt other people."
5. **Teach your child acceptable ways to get what she wants.** Teach her how to negotiate (ask for) what she wants, rather than taking it. Teach her how to take turns or how to trade one of her toys to gain use of another child's toy.
6. **Give special attention to the victim.** After putting your child in time-out, pick up the child who has been injured and give him extra sympathy and attention. It is especially helpful if you can rescue the victim before he is hurt. In your child's mind the attention she wanted is now being given to the other person and that should give her some "food for thought." If fighting is a pattern with certain playmates or siblings, be sure the "victim" isn't "setting up" the "perpetrator" to gain attention.
7. **Never hit your child for hitting someone else.** Hitting your child only teaches her that it is fine to hit if you are bigger. If your child tends to be aggressive it's critical to eliminate all physical punishment (such as spanking). You can use many other consequences (such as time-out) to teach your child right from wrong.
8. **Praise your child for friendly behavior.** Praise her for being nice to people, playing with age mates in a friendly way, sharing things, and helping other children. Remind your child that people like to be treated kindly, not hurt. Some children respond to a system of receiving a treat or a star on a chart for each day they go without any "hitting" type of behavior.
9. **Prevention.** Set a good example. Show self-control and verbal problem solving. Avoid playmates who often tease or other situations in which your child frequently gets into fights. When your child becomes tired or hungry, leave the play setting until these needs are met.

 ## CALL OUR OFFICE

During regular hours if
- The aggressive behavior is very frequent.
- Your child has seriously hurt another child.
- Your child can't keep friends.
- Your child seems very angry.
- The misbehavior lasts more than 4 weeks with this approach.
- You have other questions or concerns.

SIBLINGS' ARGUMENTS AND QUARRELS

DEFINITION

Most siblings argue and bicker occasionally. They fight over possessions, space on the sofa, time in the bathroom, the last donut, and so on. Quarreling is an inevitable part of sibling relationships. On some days, brothers and sisters are rivals and competitors, but on most days they are friends and companions. The positive side of this sibling rivalry is that it gives children a chance to learn to give and take, share, and stand up for their rights.

COPING WITH SIBLING QUARRELS

1. **Encourage children to settle their own disagreements.** Have a rule: "Settle your own arguments but no hitting, property damage, or name calling." The more you intervene, the more you will be called on to intervene. When possible, stay out of disagreements as long as they remain verbal. Children can't go through life having a referee to resolve their differences. They need to learn how to negotiate with people and find the common ground. Arguing with siblings and peers provides this experience. The only exception is if they are both under 2 or 3 years of age and one of them is aggressive. At this age they do not understand the potential dangers of fighting and they need to be supervised more closely.

2. **If they come to you, try to stay out of the middle.** Try to keep your children from bringing their argument to you for an opinion. Remind them again to settle it themselves. If you do become involved, help them clarify what they are arguing about. To achieve this, try to teach them to listen better. Encourage each child to describe the problem for 1 or 2 minutes without being interrupted by the other. If they still don't understand the issue, reframe it for them. Unless there's an obvious culprit, do not try to decide who is to blame, who started it, or who is right. Interrogation in this area can be counterproductive because it may cause them to exaggerate or lie. Also do not impose a solution. Since it's their problem, let them find their own solution whenever possible.

3. **If an argument becomes too loud, do something about it.** If the arguing becomes annoying or interferes with your ability to think, go to your children and tell them "I do not want to hear your arguing. Please settle your differences quietly or find another place to argue." If they do not change at that point, send them to the basement, outdoors, or to time-out in separate rooms. If they are arguing over an object such as the television, take it away. If they are arguing over who gets to sit in the front seat of the car, have them both sit in the back seat. If they are arguing about going somewhere, cancel the trip for both.

4. **Do not permit hitting, breaking things, or name calling.** Under these circumstances punish both of your children. If they are hurting each other, send them both to time-out in separate places no matter who you see doing the hitting when you come on the scene. That may not be the person who took the first swing or provoked it. Name calling or teasing hurts people's feelings and should never be allowed (e.g., calling a child who is not good in school "dummy"; one who is not athletic "clumsy"; or one who wets the bed "smelly"). Derogatory comments such as these can be harmful to self-esteem and should not be permitted.

5. **Stop any arguing that occurs in public places.** If you are in a shopping mall, restaurant, or movie theater and your children begin arguing, you need to stop them because it is annoying to other people. If the arguing continues after a warning, separate them (e.g., by sitting between them). If that doesn't work, give them a brief (2- to 5-minute) time-out outside or at an out-of-the-way spot. If they are over 4 or 5 years old, you can sometimes tell them to stop or they will get a 30-minute time-out (or 30-minute loss of television time) on arrival at home. Sometimes you will have to leave the public setting and take them home.

6. **Protect each child's personal possessions, privacy, and friendships.** When children argue over toys, if the toy belongs to one of the children, return it to that child. Although children don't have to share their possessions, warn them that sharing works both ways. For family "toys" (such as video games or board games) teach taking turns. Also teach sharing toys when friends come over. Sharing is a skill they will need in order to have friends and get along in school. Younger siblings often intrude on older siblings' friendships and play. It is helpful if the younger sibling is provided with a playmate or special activity when your older child has a friend over. Your child's study time also deserves protection from interruption. Designating a study room often helps.

7. **Avoid showing favoritism.** It is critical that all punishment for arguing or fighting be "group punishment." Parents must avoid the myth that fighting is always started by the brother rather than the sister, by the older child rather than the younger one, or by one child who is the "troublemaker." Rivalry will be intense if the parent shows favoritism. Try to treat your children as unique and special individuals. Do not take sides. Do not compare them and do not polarize them into good ones and bad ones. Do not listen to tattling. If one of your children complains about your not being fair, either ignore this comment or restate the rule that has been broken. If you're feeling guilty, remind yourself that "it all balances out."

8. **Praise cooperative behavior.** Catch your children "being good," namely, playing together in a friendly way. Give "group praise" whenever possible. Compliment them for helping each other and settling disagreements politely.

Instructions for Pediatric Patients, **2nd Edition**, ©1999 by **WB Saunders Company**.
Written by Barton D. Schmitt, MD, pediatrician and author of *Your Child's Health*, Bantam Books, a book for parents.

CALENDAR FOR TRACKING TARGET BEHAVIORS

Fill in your calendar each day.
Please bring it with you at your next appointment.

Name _____

Date begun _____

	Monday	Tuesday	Wednesday	Thursday	Friday	Saturday	Sunday
1st Week							
2nd Week							
3rd Week							
4th Week							
5th Week							
6th Week							
7th Week							
8th Week							

SIBLING RIVALRY TOWARD A NEWBORN

DEFINITION

Sibling rivalry refers here to the natural jealousy of children toward a new brother or sister. Older siblings can feel jealous when a new baby arrives until they are 4 or 5 years old. Not surprisingly, most children prefer to be the only child at this age. Basically, they don't want to share your time and affection. The arrival of a new baby is especially stressful for the first-born child and for those less than 3 years old.

The most common symptom of sibling rivalry is lots of demands for attention: The older child wants to be held and carried about, especially when Mom is busy with the newborn. Other symptoms include acting like a baby again (regressive behavior), such as thumb sucking, wetting, or soiling. Aggressive behavior—for example, handling the baby roughly—can also occur. All of these symptoms are normal. Although some can be prevented, the remainder can be improved within a few months.

PREVENTION OF SIBLING RIVALRY

During Pregnancy

- Prepare the older sibling for the newcomer. Talk about the pregnancy. Have him feel your baby's movements.
- Try to find a hospital that provides sibling classes where children can learn about babies and sharing parents. Try to give your older child a chance to be around a new baby so that he has a better idea of what to expect.
- Encourage your older child to help you prepare the baby's room.
- Move your older child to a different room or new bed several months before the baby's birth so he won't feel pushed out by the new baby. If he will be enrolling in a play group or nursery school, start it well in advance of the delivery.
- Tell your child where he'll go and who will care for him when you go to the hospital, if he won't be home with his father.
- Read books together about what happens during pregnancy as well as after the baby is born.
- Look through family photographs and talk about your older child's first year of life.

In the Hospital

- Call your older child daily from the hospital.
- Try to have your older child visit you and the baby in the hospital. Many hospitals will allow this.
- If your older child can't visit you, send him a picture of the new baby.
- Encourage Dad to take your youngster on some special outings at this time (e.g., to the park, zoo, museum, or fire station).

Coming Home

- When you enter your home, spend your first moments with the older sibling. Have someone else carry the new baby into the house.
- Give the sibling a gift "from the new baby."
- Ask visitors to give extra notice to the older child. Have your older child unwrap the baby's gifts.
- From the beginning, refer to your newborn as "our baby."

The First Months at Home

- Give your older child the extra attention he needs. Help him feel more important. Try to give him at least 30 minutes every day of exclusive, uninterrupted time. Hire a babysitter and take your older child outside or look through his baby album with him. Make sure that the father and relatives spend extra time with him during the first month. Give him lots of physical affection throughout the day. If he demands to be held while you are feeding or rocking the baby, try to include him. At least talk with him when you are busy taking care of the baby.
- Encourage your older child to touch and play with the new baby in your presence. Allow him to hold the baby while sitting in a chair with arms. Avoid such warnings as "Don't touch the baby." Newborns are not fragile, and it is important to show your trust. However, you can't allow the sibling to carry the baby until he reaches school age.
- Enlist your older child as a helper. Encourage him to help with baths, dry the baby, get a clean diaper, or find toys or a pacifier. At other times encourage him to feed or bathe a doll when you are feeding or bathing the baby. Emphasize how much the baby "likes" the older sibling. Make comments such as "Look how happy she gets when you play with her" or "You can always make her laugh."
- Don't ask the older siblings to "be quiet for the baby." Newborns can sleep fine without the house being perfectly quiet. This request can lead to unnecessary resentment.
- Accept regressive behavior, such as thumb sucking or clinging, as something your child needs to do temporarily. Do not criticize him.
- Intervene promptly for any aggressive behavior. Tell him that "we never hurt babies." Send your child to time-out for a few minutes. Don't spank your child or slap his hand at these times. If you hit him, he will eventually try to do the same to the baby as revenge. For the next few weeks don't leave the two of them alone.
- If your child is old enough, encourage him to talk about his mixed feelings about the new arrival. Give him an alternative behavior: "When you're upset with the baby, come to me for a big hug."

Instructions for Pediatric Patients, 2nd Edition, ©1999 by WB Saunders Company.
Written by Barton D. Schmitt, MD, pediatrician and author of *Your Child's Health,* Bantam Books, a book for parents.

DEFINITION

- A child sucks on the thumb or fingers when not hungry.
- A security object, such as a blanket, may become part of the ritual.
- Thumb sucking begins before birth or by 3 months of age at the latest.

Causes

An infant's desire to suck on the breast or bottle is a drive that is essential for survival. More than 80% of babies also do some extra sucking when they are not hungry (non-nutritive sucking). Thumb sucking also helps a child comfort herself. It does not mean that a child is insecure or has emotional problems.

Expected Course

The sucking need is strongest during the first 6 months of a child's life. By 4 years of age, only 15% of children still suck their thumbs. Those children who continue sucking their thumbs after 4 years of age often have become involved in a power struggle with a parent who tried to stop their thumb sucking at too young an age. Occasionally the thumb sucking simply persists as a bad habit. Thumb sucking must be stopped before a child's permanent teeth erupt (6 or 7 years of age), because it can lead to an overbite ("buck teeth").

HOW TO OVERCOME THUMB SUCKING

1. **Before 4 years of age, distract or ignore.** Thumb sucking should be considered normal before the age of 4 years, especially when your child is tired. However, if the thumb sucking occurs when your child is bored and she is over 1 year old, try to distract her. Give her something to do with her hands without mentioning your concern about the thumb sucking. Occasionally praise your child for not thumb sucking. Until your child is old enough for you to reason with her, any pressure or punishment you apply to stop thumb sucking will only lead to increased thumb sucking.

2. **Daytime control.** After 4 years of age, help your child give up thumb sucking during the day. First get your child's commitment to giving up thumb sucking by showing her what thumb sucking is doing to her body. Show her the gap between her teeth with a mirror. Have her look at the wrinkled rough skin (callus) on her thumb. Appeal to her sense of pride. At this point most children will agree that they would like to stop thumb sucking.

   Ask your child if it will be all right if you remind her when she forgets. Do this gently with comments such as "Guess what?" and put an arm around your child as she remembers that she has been sucking on her thumb again. Encourage your child to remind herself by painting a star on her thumb with a Magic Marker, putting a Band-Aid on the thumb, or applying fingernail polish. Your child should put these reminders on herself. Praise your child whenever you notice she is not sucking her thumb in situations where she previously did. Also, give her a reward (such as a dime, a snack, or an extra story) at the end of any day during which she did not suck her thumb at all.

3. **Nighttime control.** After daytime control is established, help your child give up thumb sucking during sleep. Thumb sucking during naps and night is usually an involuntary process. Your child can be told that although the nighttime thumb sucking is not her fault, she can learn not to suck her thumb during sleep by putting something on her thumb to remind her. A glove, sock, splint (thumb guard), or piece of adhesive tape that runs up one side and down the other can be used. Your child should be in charge of putting on whatever material is used to prevent thumb sucking or asking you for assistance. Help your child look on this method as a clever idea rather than any kind of penalty.

4. **Bitter-tasting medicines.** Consider using bitter-tasting medicines if your child is over 4 years of age. A recent study by Dr. P. C. Friman demonstrated a high success rate in 1 to 3 nights using a bitter-tasting solution called Stop-zit (no prescription necessary) in combination with a reward system. Use Stop-zit only if your child is over 4 years old and agrees to use it. Don't use it as a punishment. Present it as a reminder that "other kids like to use it also." Help your child apply Stop-zit only to the thumbnail at the following times: (1) before breakfast, (2) before bedtime, and (3) whenever thumb sucking is observed day or night.

   Look to see whether your child is thumb sucking every 30 minutes after her bedtime until you retire. After 5 nights without thumb sucking, discontinue the morning Stop-zit. After 5 more nights without any thumb sucking, stop using Stop-zit at bedtime. If the thumb sucking recurs, repeat this program.

5. **Dental help.** Bring thumb sucking to the attention of your child's dentist at least by the time your child is 6 years old. Dentists have a variety of approaches to thumb sucking. By the time a child is 7 or 8 years old, dentists can place a reminder bar in the upper part of the mouth that interferes with the ability to suck. This helpful appliance does not cause any pain to your child but may spare you the later economic pain of $4000 worth of orthodontic treatment.

Instructions for Pediatric Patients, 2nd Edition, ©1999 by WB Saunders Company.
Written by Barton D. Schmitt, MD, pediatrician and author of *Your Child's Health,* Bantam Books, a book for parents.

Babies vary in how much extra sucking they do when they are not feeding. This extra sucking is a beneficial self-comforting behavior. Some babies almost constantly suck on their thumb or fingers. If you have a baby like this, you may want to try to interest him in a pacifier. The pacifier has to be introduced during the first month or two of life for it to be accepted as a substitute for the thumb. Although the orthodontic type of pacifier is preferred because it prevents tongue thrusting during sucking, the regular type usually causes no problems. By trial and error, let your baby find the shape he prefers.

ADVANTAGES OF A PACIFIER OVER THUMB SUCKING

The main advantage of a pacifier is that if you can get your child to use one, he usually won't be a thumb sucker. Thumb sucking can cause a severe overbite if it is continued after the permanent teeth come in. The pacifier exerts less pressure on the teeth and causes much less overbite than the thumb. In addition, the pacifier's use can be controlled as your child grows older. You can decide when it's reasonable to discontinue it. By contrast, thumb sucking can't be stopped when you want it to, because the thumb belongs to your child.

WHEN TO OFFER THE PACIFIER

The peak age for sucking is 2 to 4 months. During the following months, the sucking drive normally decreases. A good age to make the pacifier less available is when your child starts to crawl. A pacifier can interfere with normal babbling and speech development. This is especially important after 12 months of age when speech should develop rapidly. It's hard to talk with a pacifier in your mouth. To prevent problems with pacifiers, make sure your child doesn't become overly attached to one (e.g., walks around with one in his mouth.) Consider the following recommendations for preventing excessive use and a "pacifier habit":

- During the first 6 months of life, give it to your baby whenever he wants to suck, but don't offer it whenever your baby cries. Crying has a number of causes besides hunger and sucking.
- When your older infant is stressed, first try to hold and cuddle him rather than using the pacifier for this purpose. Some infants like massage. Try not to overuse the pacifier while you are comforting him.
- After 6 months of age (or when your infant starts crawling), keep the pacifier in your child's crib. He can use it for naptime and bedtime. After your infant falls asleep, remove it from his mouth if it doesn't fall out. If you allow him to use it all the time, his interest in it will increase rather than decrease. If your child seems to want a security object while awake, offer him alternatives such as a stuffed animal.

- *Reminder:* If your baby likes the pacifier, don't forget to take it with you when you travel. Keeping a spare pacifier in the car is helpful. For air travel, sucking or swallowing fluids during descent can prevent ear pain.

PACIFIER SAFETY

Some cautions regarding the pacifier should be observed.

- Use a one-piece commercial pacifier, not a homemade one. Don't try making one yourself by taping a nipple to a plastic bottle cap. A homemade pacifier can be pulled apart, become caught in your baby's throat, and cause choking.
- Don't put the pacifier on a string around your baby's neck. The string could strangle your baby. The new "catch-it-clips" that attach the pacifier to your child's clothing on a short ribbon are practical and safe.
- Don't use pacifiers with a liquid center. (Some have been found to be contaminated with germs.)
- Don't coat it with any sweets, which may cause dental cavities if teeth have erupted.
- Don't coat it with honey, which may cause a serious disease called botulism in children less than 1 year of age.
- Rinse off the pacifier each time your baby finishes using it or if it drops to the floor.
- Replace the pacifier if it becomes damaged.

STOPPING USE OF THE PACIFIER

If the pacifier's use has been restricted to naptime and bedtime, many toddlers lose interest in it between 12 and 18 months of age. If your child continues to need the pacifier, you can introduce the idea of giving it up completely by 3 or 4 years of age. Pick a time when your child is not coping with new stresses or fears. Sometimes giving it up on a birthday, holiday, or other celebration makes it easier.

Make the transition as pleasant as possible. Sometimes incentives are needed. If your child seems especially attached to it, help him give it up at naptime first. Use a star chart to mark his progress. When that goal is accomplished, offer to replace the nighttime pacifier with a new stuffed animal or encourage him to trade it for something else he wants. Never force him to give up the pacifier through punishment or humiliation. Abruptly removing the pacifier without preparation can be psychologically harmful.

Give your child a choice such as throwing it away or leaving it out for Santa Claus or the "pacifier fairy." Saving it somewhere in the house is usually not a good idea, because your child will be more likely to ask for it during periods of stress. At such times, offer to cuddle your child instead. Help your child talk about how he misses the pacifier. Praise your child for this sign of growing up.

Instructions for Pediatric Patients, 2nd Edition, ©1999 by WB Saunders Company.
Written by Barton D. Schmitt, MD, pediatrician and author of *Your Child's Health,* Bantam Books, a book for parents.

DEFINITION

- Breath holding is preceded by an upsetting event, such as being frustrated, angry, injured, or frightened.
- Your child gives out one or two long cries and then holds her breath in expiration until the lips become bluish.
- Your child then passes out. (Most children stiffen out and some have a few twitches or muscle jerks.)
- Your child then resumes normal breathing and becomes fully alert in less than 1 minute.
- Onset is between 6 months and 2 years old. These attacks occur only while the child is awake.
- This diagnosis must be confirmed by a physician.

Cause

Breath-holding spells are caused by an abnormal reflex that allows 5% of normal children to hold their breath long enough to actually pass out. It's not deliberate in most children. Holding the breath (when angry) and becoming bluish *without* passing out is a common reaction and not considered abnormal.

Expected Course

Breath-holding spells usually occur from one or two times daily to one or two times per month and are gone by 4 or 5 years of age. They are not dangerous, and they don't lead to epilepsy or brain damage.

HOME CARE

Treatment During Attacks of Breath Holding. These attacks are harmless and always stop by themselves. Since it's difficult to accurately estimate the length of an attack, time a few using a watch with a second hand. Have your child lie flat (rather than holding her upright) to increase blood flow to the brain (this position may prevent some of the muscle jerking). Apply a cold, wet washcloth to your child's forehead until she starts breathing again. Don't start resuscitation or call 911—it's unnecessary. Also don't put anything in your child's mouth; it could cause your child to choke or vomit.

Treatment After Attacks of Breath Holding. Give your child a brief hug and go about your business.

A relaxed attitude is best. If you are frightened, don't let your child know it. If your child had a temper tantrum because she wanted her way, don't give in to her after the attack.

PREVENTION OF BREATH-HOLDING SPELLS

Most attacks from falling down or a sudden fright can't be prevented; neither can most attacks that are triggered by anger. However, some children can be distracted from their breath holding if you intervene before they become blue. Tell your child to come to you for a hug or to look at something interesting. Ask her if she wants a drink of juice.

If your child is having daily attacks, she probably has learned to trigger some of the attacks herself. This can happen when parents run to the child and pick her up every time she starts to cry or when they give her her way as soon as the attack is over. Avoid these responses, and your child won't have an undue number of attacks.

PREVENTION OF INJURIES

The main risk of breath-holding spells is sustaining a head injury. If your child starts to have an attack while standing near a hard surface, go to her quickly and help lower her to the floor.

 CALL OUR OFFICE

IMMEDIATELY if
- Your child stops breathing for more than 1 minute (call 911).
- Your child was unconscious for more than 1 minute (by the clock).
- Your child turns white, not bluish.

During regular hours if
- More than one spell occurs per week.
- The attacks change.
- You have other questions about breath holding.

DEFINITION

Your child is toilet trained when, without any reminders, he walks to the potty, undresses, urinates or has a bowel movement, and pulls up his pants. Some children will learn to control their bladders first; others will start with bowel control. Both kinds of control can be worked on simultaneously. Bladder control through the night normally happens several years later than daytime control. The gradual type of toilet training discussed here can usually be completed in 2 weeks to 2 months.

TOILET-TRAINING READINESS

Don't begin training until your child is clearly ready. Readiness doesn't just happen; it involves concepts and skills you can begin teaching your child at 12 months of age. Reading some of the special toilet-learning books to your child can help. Most children can be made ready for toilet training by 24 months of age and many by 18 months. By the time your child is 3 years old, he will probably have trained himself. The following signs indicate that your child is ready.

- Your child understands what "pee," "poop," "dry," "wet," "clean," "messy," and "potty" mean. (Teach him these words.)
- Your child understands what the potty is for. (Teach this by having your child watch parents, older siblings, and children near his age use the toilet correctly.)
- Your child prefers dry, clean diapers. (Change your child frequently to encourage this preference.)
- Your child likes to be changed. (As soon as he is able to walk, teach him to come to you immediately whenever he is wet or dirty. Praise him for coming to you for a change.)
- Your child understands the connection between dry pants and using the potty.
- Your child can recognize the feeling of a full bladder and the urge to have a bowel movement; that is, he paces, jumps up and down, holds his genitals, pulls at his jeans, squats down, or tells you. (Clarify for him: "The poop [or pee] wants to come out. It needs your help.")
- Your child has the ability to briefly postpone urinating or having a bowel movement. He may go off by himself and come back wet or soiled, or he may wake up from naps dry.

METHOD FOR TOILET TRAINING

The way to train your child is to offer encouragement and praise, be patient, and make the process fun. Avoid any pressure or punishment. Your child must feel in control of the process.

1. **Buy supplies.**
   - Potty chair (floor-level type). If your child's feet can reach the floor while he sits on the potty, he has leverage for pushing and a sense of security. He also can get on and off whenever he wants to.
   - Favorite treats (such as fruit slices, raisins, animal crackers, and cookies) for rewards.
   - Stickers or stars for rewards.

2. **Make the potty chair one of your child's favorite possessions.** Several weeks before you plan to begin toilet training, take your child with you to buy a potty chair. Make it clear that this is your child's own special chair. Have your child help you put his name on it. Allow your child to decorate it or even paint it a different color. Then have your child sit on it fully clothed until he is comfortable with using it as a chair. Have your child use it while watching TV, eating snacks, playing games, or looking at books. Keep it in the room in which your child usually plays. Only after your child clearly has good feelings toward the potty chair (after at least 1 week), proceed to actual toilet training.

3. **Encourage practice runs on the potty.** Do a practice run whenever your child gives a signal that looks promising, such as a certain facial expression, grunting, holding the genital area, pulling at his pants, pacing, squatting, squirming, or passing gas. Other good times are after naps or 20 minutes after meals. Say encouragingly, "The poop [or pee] wants to come out. Let's use the potty." Encourage your child to walk to the potty and sit there with his diapers or pants off. Your child can then be told, "Try to go pee-pee in the potty." If your child is reluctant to cooperate, he can be encouraged to sit on the potty by doing something fun; for example, you might read a story. If your child wants to get up after 1 minute of encouragement, let him get up. Never force your child to sit there. Never physically hold your child there or strap him in. Even if your child seems to be enjoying it, end each session after 5 minutes unless something is happening.

4. **Praise or reward your child for cooperation or any success.** All cooperation with these practice sessions should be praised. For example, you might say, "You are sitting on the potty just like Mommy," or "You're trying real hard to put the pee-pee in the potty." If your child urinates into the potty, he can be rewarded with treats or stickers, as well as praise and hugs. Although a sense of accomplishment is enough for some children, others need treats to stay focused. Big rewards (such as going to the ice cream store) should be reserved for when your child walks over to the potty on his own and uses it or asks to go there with you and then uses it. Once your child uses the potty by himself two or more times, you can stop the practice runs. For the following week, continue to praise your child frequently for dryness and using the potty. (*Note:* Practice runs and reminders should not be necessary for more than 1 or 2 months.)

Instructions for Pediatric Patients, 2nd Edition, ©1999 by WB Saunders Company.
Written by Barton D. Schmitt, MD, pediatrician and author of *Your Child's Health*, Bantam Books, a book for parents.

5. **Change your child after accidents.** Change your child as soon as it's convenient, but respond sympathetically. Say something like, "You wanted to go pee-pee in the potty, but you went pee-pee in your pants. I know that makes you sad. You like to be dry. You'll get better at this." If you feel a need to be critical, keep it to mild verbal disapproval and use it rarely (e.g., "Big boys don't go pee-pee in their pants," or mention the name of another child whom he likes and who is trained); then change your child into a dry diaper or training pants in as pleasant and nonangry a way as possible. Avoid physical punishment, yelling, or scolding. Pressure or force can make a 2-year-old child completely uncooperative. Do not keep your child in wet or messy pants for punishment.

6. **Introduce training pants after your child starts using the potty.** Switch from diapers to training pants after your child is cooperative about sitting on the potty chair and passes about half of his urine and bowel movements there. He definitely needs training pants if he comes to you for help in taking off his diaper so he can use the potty. Take your child with you to buy the underwear and make it a reward for his success. Buy loose-fitting ones that he can easily lower and pull up by himself. Once you start using training pants, use diapers only for naps and nighttime.

PREVENTING PROBLEMS

Some Dos

- Change your child frequently.
- Teach your child to come to you when he needs to be changed.
- Help your child spend time with children who are trained and watch them use the toilet or potty chair.
- Read toilet-learning books to your child.
- Initially, keep the potty chair in the room your child usually plays in. This easy access markedly increases the chances that he will use it without your asking him. Consider owning two potty chairs.
- Teach him how the toilet works.
- Mention using the toilet or potty chair only if your child gives a cue that he needs to go.

- Give suggestions, not demands.
- Give your child an active role and let him do it his way.
- Be supportive.
- Keep a sense of humor.
- Keep the process fun and upbeat. Be positive about any interest your child shows.

Some Don'ts

- Don't start when your child is in a stubborn or negative phase.
- Don't use any punishment or pressure.
- Don't force your child to sit on a potty chair.
- Don't keep your child sitting on a potty chair against his will.
- Don't flush the toilet while your child is sitting on it.
- Don't lecture or remind your child.
- Avoid any friction.
- Avoid battles or showdowns.
- Don't try to control what you can't control.
- Never escalate your response; you will always lose.
- Don't act overconcerned about this normal body function. Try to appear casual and relaxed during the training.
- After your child uses the toilet, don't expect a perfect performance. Some accidents occur for months.

Request the Guideline on Toilet-Training Resistance if

- Your child won't sit on the potty or toilet.
- Your 2½-year-old child is negative about toilet training.
- You begin to use force or punishment.
- Your child is over 3 years old and not daytime toilet trained.
- The approach described here isn't working after 2 months.

RECOMMENDED READING

Joanna Cole: The Parents' Book of Toilet Teaching. Ballantine Books, New York, 1983.
Vicki Lansky: Koko Bear's New Potty. Bantam Books, New York, 1986.
Alison Mack: Toilet Learning. Little, Brown, Boston, 1983.
Katie Van Pelt: Potty Training Your Baby. Avery, New York, 1996.

DEFINITION

Children who refuse to be toilet trained either wet themselves, soil themselves, or try to hold back their bowel movements (thus becoming constipated). Many of these children also refuse to sit on the toilet or will use the toilet only if the parent brings up the subject and marches them into the bathroom. Any child who is over 2¹/₂ years old, healthy, and not toilet trained after several months of trying can be assumed to be resistant to the process, rather than untrained. Consider how capable your child is at delaying a bowel movement (BM) until she is off the toilet or you are on the telephone. More practice runs (as you used in toilet training) will not help. Instead, your child now needs full responsibility and some incentives to re-spark her motivation.

The most common cause of resistance to toilet training is that a child has been reminded or lectured too much. Some children have been forced to sit on the toilet against their will, occasionally for long periods of time. A few have been spanked or punished in other ways for not cooperating. Many parents make these mistakes, especially if they have a strong-willed child.

Most children younger than 5 or 6 years of age with soiling (encopresis) or daytime wetting (without any other symptoms) are simply engaged with you in a power struggle. These children can be helped with the following suggestions. If your child holds back BMs and becomes constipated, medicines will also be needed.

HELPING YOUR CHILD WITH DAYTIME WETTING OR SOILING

1. **Transfer all responsibility to your child.** Your child will decide to use the toilet only after she realizes that she has nothing left to resist. Have one last talk with her about the subject. Tell your child that her body makes "pee" and "poop" every day and it belongs to her. Explain that her "poop" wants to go in the toilet and her job is to help the "poop" come out. Tell your child you're sorry you punished her, forced her to sit on the toilet, or reminded her so much. Tell her from now on she doesn't need any help. Then stop all talk about this subject. When your child stops receiving conversation for nonperformance (not going), she will eventually decide to perform for attention.

2. **Stop all reminders about using the toilet.** Let your child decide when she needs to go to the bathroom. She should not be reminded to go to the bathroom nor asked if she needs to go. She knows what it feels like when she has to "poop" or "pee" and where the bathroom is. Reminders are a form of pressure, and pressure doesn't work. She should not be made to sit on the toilet against her will because this will foster a negative attitude about the whole process. Don't accompany your child into the bathroom or stand with her by the potty chair. She needs to get the feeling of success that comes from doing it on her own and then finding you to tell you what she did.

3. **Give incentives for using the toilet.** If your child stays clean and dry, she needs plenty of positive feedback, such as praise, smiles, and hugs. In general, this positive response should occur *every time* your child uses the toilet. If a child soils or wets herself on some days and not others, this recognition should occur only when she is clean for a complete day. On successful days consider taking 20 extra minutes to play a special game with your child or take her for a walk to the playground. Sometimes special incentives, such as favorite sweets or video time, can be invaluable. One of your main jobs is to find the right incentive. For using the toilet for BMs, initially err on the side of giving her too much (e.g., several sweets each time). The potency of these incentives is increased by reducing baseline access to them. Additional motivation can come from making a carefully orchestrated "fun trip" to the preschool, and then clarifying for the child that regular preschool attendance requires toilet training. If you want a breakthrough, make your child an offer she can't refuse.

4. **Give stars for using the toilet.** Get a calendar for your child and post it in a conspicuous location. Place a star on it every time she uses the toilet. Keep this record of progress until your child has gone 2 weeks without any accidents.

5. **Make the potty chair convenient.** Be sure to keep the potty chair in the room your child usually plays in. This gives her a convenient visual reminder about her options whenever she feels the need to urinate or defecate. For wetting, the presence of the chair and the promise of treats will usually bring about a change in behavior. For soiling, your child may need a pleasant reminder only if she is clearly holding back. You can say, "The poop wants to come out and go in the toilet. The poop needs your help." Tell your child that you want sitting on the potty to be lots of fun. What would she like to do? A few children temporarily may need treats for simply sitting on the toilet and trying.

6. **Diapers, pull-ups, or underwear.** Whenever possible, replace pull-ups or diapers with underwear. Help your child pick out some underwear with characters on them that "don't like poop or pee." This usually precipitates the correct decision on the part of the child. Even if your child wets the underwear, persist with this plan. If your child holds back BMs, allow selective access to diapers or pull-ups for BMs only.

7. **Remind your child to change her clothes if she wets or soils herself.** As soon as you notice that your child has wet or messy pants, tell her to clean herself up immediately. The main role you have in this program is to enforce this rule. If your

Instructions for Pediatric Patients, 2nd Edition, ©1999 by WB Saunders Company.
Written by Barton D. Schmitt, MD, pediatrician and author of *Your Child's Health,* Bantam Books, a book for parents.

child is wet, she can probably change into dry clothes by herself. If your child is soiled, she will probably need your help with cleanup. If your child refuses to let you change her, ground her until she is ready.

8. **Don't punish or criticize your child for accidents.** Respond gently to accidents, and do not allow siblings to tease the child. Do not put your child back into diapers unless she needs to be on laxatives. Pressure will only delay successful training, and it could cause secondary emotional problems.

9. **Ask the preschool or day care staff to use the same strategy.** Ask your child's teacher or day care provider for unlimited privileges to go to the bathroom any time your child wants to. Keep an extra set of clean underwear at the school or with the day care provider.

 CALL OUR OFFICE

During regular hours if
- Your child holds back her bowel movements or becomes constipated.
- Pain or burning occurs when she urinates.
- The resistance is not improved after 1 month on this program.
- The resistance has not stopped completely after 3 months.

DAYTIME FREQUENCY OF URINATION

DEFINITION

- Your child suddenly starts urinating every 10 to 30 minutes and as often as 30 to 40 times a day.
- Your child passes small amounts of urine each time.
- Your child has no pain with urination.
- Your child does not wet himself during the day.
- Your child does not drink excessive amounts of fluids.
- Your child has been toilet trained.
- The urinary frequency is not a problem during sleep.
- Daytime frequency of urination occurs most often when a child is 4 to 5 years old.

Causes

Frequent urination usually reflects emotional tension. It means your child is under pressure. The symptom is involuntary, not deliberate. The urinary frequency usually begins within 1 or 2 days of a stressful event. You can make the problem worse by worrying about disease. Punishment, criticism, or teasing also worsens the symptom. Although physical causes are rare, your child should be examined by a physician.

Expected Outcome

Overall, this is a harmless condition that eventually goes away by itself. If you can identify and deal with whatever is stressing your child, his frequent urination will disappear in 1 to 4 weeks. Without treatment, the symptom usually gets better on its own in 2 or 3 months.

A few children who also have small bladders and problems with bed-wetting may have this symptom more than once.

HOW TO HELP YOUR CHILD OVERCOME URINARY FREQUENCY

1. **Reassure your child that he is physically healthy.** Tell your child that his body, kidneys, urine, and any other aspects of his health that he is worried about are fine. Because the family (and also possibly physicians) have been concerned about the child's bladder and urine, he may fear there is something wrong with his urinary tract. Reassure him once or twice that he is quite healthy.
2. **Reassure your child that he can learn to wait longer to urinate.** Reassure him that he won't wet himself, which is a common fear. If he has wet himself before, encourage him to talk about his embarrassment and reassure him that it happens sometimes to many children. Tell him that he will gradually get back to urinating every 2 to 3 hours, or whatever his previous pattern was. If his frequency of urination has gotten worse during shopping trips or travel in general, don't take him with you to public places for a while.
3. **Help your child relax.** Frequency of urination can be a barometer of inner tension. Make sure your child has free time and fun time every day. If he is overscheduled with activities, try to lighten

the commitments. Relaxation exercises may help your child if he is over 8 years old.

Increasing the happiness and harmony within your home will usually restore your child's sense of security.

Ask the staff at your child's school or day care to help reduce any tensions there, such as limits on when a child can use the bathroom.

4. **Try to figure out what is stressing your child.** Meet with other family members and try to think of a stressful event that may have occurred 1 or 2 days before the frequency began. Also ask school or day care staff for ideas. Talk about your ideas with your child and try to help him overcome the stress. Common stressful events are
   - Death in the family
   - Accident or other life-threatening event
   - Tension in the marriage
   - A sick parent or sibling
   - School entry or a new school
   - Too much concern about staying dry at night
   - Wetting himself in the presence of peers

5. **Ignore the symptom of frequency.** When your child is using the toilet frequently, don't comment on it. Comments remind him that the symptom is worrying you. Stop keeping any record of amount or frequency of urination. Do not collect any urine samples or measure volumes. Don't ask your child about his symptom or watch him urinate. Do not have your child do bladder-stretching exercises. Your child does not need to tell you when he has urinated; you will have a general impression about whether he is getting better or staying the same.

   Be sure that none of your child's caretakers or teachers is punishing or criticizing him about this symptom.

   Stop all family conversation about the frequency. The less said about it, the less anxious your child will be about it. If your child brings up the topic, reassure him that he will gradually get better.

6. **Avoid bubble bath and other irritants.** Bubble bath can cause frequent urination in children, especially girls. Bubble bath can irritate the opening of the urinary tract. Taking a bath in water that contains hair shampoo can also cause similar symptoms.

 CALL OUR OFFICE

During regular hours if
- The frequency of urination is not back to normal after you have followed these recommendations for 1 month.
- Your child begins to have pain or burning.
- Your child begins to wet himself during the day.
- Your child begins to drink excessive fluids.
- You have other questions or concerns.

 Instructions for Pediatric Patients, **2nd Edition,** ©1999 by WB Saunders Company.
Written by Barton D. Schmitt, MD, pediatrician and author of *Your Child's Health,* Bantam Books, a book for parents.

DEFINITION

A child who passes bowel movements (BMs) into her underwear has a problem called soiling or encopresis. Many children who are soiling small amounts several times a day are severely constipated or blocked up (impacted). The soiling occurs because pieces of the large mass of hard stool in the rectum break loose at unexpected times. This is especially likely to happen when your child is running or jumping. The soiling is not deliberate. The impaction is usually too wide to pass spontaneously, and the child can't control the leakage until the blockage is removed.

There are many reasons why children become constipated—high milk diet, genetic differences, avoiding bowel movements because they cause pain, or holding back BMs (stool holding) as a way of resisting toilet training. The possibility of physical causes requires a complete examination by your child's physician.

TREATMENT OF SOILING WITH CONSTIPATION IN CHILDREN WHO WON'T SIT ON THE TOILET

1. **First use enemas to remove the impaction.** Start with a Fleet's hyperphosphate enema. The dose is 1 ounce for every 20 pounds of your child's weight. For example, a 30-pound child should receive 1½ ounces of hyperphosphate enema. Don't give any child more than 4 ounces of the enema.

    Have your child try to hold the enema back for 5 minutes. Then insist that she sit on the toilet for release of the enema.

    Give a second hyperphosphate enema 1 or 2 hours after the first one. A third hyperphosphate enema can be given 12 to 24 hours later if you think your child is still impacted. Signs that your child is still impacted include continued soiling or a lump that can be felt in the lower abdomen.

    Before giving the enemas, give your child one to two glasses of water to drink because the enemas may cause some dehydration.

    If you don't know how to give an enema, ask someone in your physician's office. Once an impaction is cleared, enemas are no longer necessary. Your child's constipation can be treated entirely with oral medicines. Continuous use of enemas irritates the rectum and can cause your child to hold back BMs.

2. **Use stool softeners to keep the bowel movements soft.** Stool softeners make the stool softer and easier to pass. Unlike laxatives, they do not cause any bowel contractions or pressure. Some commonly prescribed stool softeners are mineral oil, Kondremul, Metamucil, Mitrolan, Citrucel, Maltsupex, Petrogalar, and fiber wafers. Your child must take stool softeners for at least 3 months to prevent another impaction. By then, your child's intestines will be able to contract and empty normally again.

If you use mineral oil, keep it in the refrigerator because it tastes best cold. Have your child take it with fruit juice to disguise the flavor or follow it with something tasty. Give your child a vitamin pill each day at about noon while she is on the mineral oil.

Your child's stool softener is _____.

The dose is _____ each morning and _____ each evening. Increase the dose gradually until your child is having two or three soft bowel movements each day.

3. **Use laxatives to keep the rectum empty if stool softeners aren't effective.** Laxatives (or bowel stimulants) cause the large intestine to contract, squeezing the stool toward the rectum. Commonly used laxatives are Senokot, Fletcher's Castoria, milk of magnesia (MOM), Haley's M-O, and Dulcolax. Don't worry that your child will become dependent on the laxatives (i.e., that the bowels won't move well without them). The most important goal is keeping the rectum empty. Children can always be gradually withdrawn from laxatives, even after 6 months of using them.

Your child's laxative is _____.

The dose is _____ given with dinner or _____. If your child goes 48 hours without a BM, give _____.

4. **Encourage your child to eat a nonconstipating diet.** Have your child eat plenty of fruits and vegetables every day (raw ones are best). Some examples are figs, dates, raisins, peaches, pears, apricots, celery, cabbage, and corn.

    Bran is an excellent natural laxative because it has a high fiber content. Have your child eat bran daily by including such foods as the new "natural" cereals, bran flakes, bran muffins, or whole wheat bread in her diet. Popcorn, nuts, shredded wheat, oatmeal, brown rice, lima beans, navy beans, chili beans, and peas are also good sources of fiber. Only milk products (milk, cheese, yogurt, ice cream) and cooked carrots have been proven to be constipating. Your child should limit her intake of milk products to 2 glasses or the equivalent per day. Encourage lots of fruit juices because they increase bowel movements.

5. **Transfer all responsibility to your child about using the toilet.** Your child will decide to use the toilet only after she realizes that she has nothing left to resist. Have one last talk with her about the subject. Tell your child that her body makes "poop" every day and it belongs to her. Explain that her "poop" wants to go in the toilet and her job is to help the "poop" come out. To help her

Instructions for Pediatric Patients, 2nd Edition, ©1999 by WB Saunders Company.
Written by Barton D. Schmitt, MD, pediatrician and author of *Your Child's Health,* Bantam Books, a book for parents.

function independently, put her in loose-fitting underwear or training pants (not diapers or pull-ups). Tell your child you're sorry you punished her for not using the toilet, forced her to sit on the toilet, or reminded her so much. Tell her from now on she doesn't need any help from you or other people. Then stop all talk about the subject. When your child stops receiving attention for not using the toilet, she will eventually decide to use it to gain some attention.

6. **Stop all reminders about using the toilet.** Let your child decide when she needs to go to the bathroom. She should not be reminded to go to the bathroom nor asked if she needs to go. Your child knows what it feels like when she has to "poop" and where the bathroom is. Reminders are a form of pressure, and pressure doesn't work. She should not be made to sit on the toilet against her will because this will give her a negative attitude about the whole process. Don't accompany your child into the bathroom or stand with her by the potty chair. Your child needs to get the feeling of success that comes from doing it on her own and then finding you to tell you what she did.

7. **Give incentives for bowel movements in the toilet.** If your child has a bowel movement in the toilet, give her immediate positive feedback, such as praise and a hug. This positive response should occur every time your child uses the toilet. Special incentives, such as favorite sweets or video time, can be invaluable for helping a child change a bad habit. For using the toilet, err on the side of rewarding generously; for example, you might give your child 20 M&Ms. If you want a breakthrough—that is, use of the toilet for the first time—make your child an offer she can't refuse. One of your main jobs is to find the right incentive. The potency of incentives is increased by reducing baseline access to them. Perhaps you'll let her watch a new video she has been talking about. A grab bag containing a variety of treats is also a powerful motivator.

8. **Give stars for using the toilet.** Get a calendar for your child and hang it where she sees it all the time. Place a star on it every time she uses the toilet. Keep this record of progress until your child has gone 1 month without any accidents. Bring the calendar to your visits with your child's physician.

9. **Make the potty chair convenient.** Be sure to keep the potty chair in the room she usually plays in. This gives your child a convenient *visual* reminder about her options whenever she feels the need to urinate or defecate.

Give a pleasant verbal reminder only if she is clearly having an urge to go and is holding back. You can say "The poop wants to come out and go in the toilet. The poop needs your help." Tell your child that you want sitting on the potty to be lots of fun. What would she like to do? Then let your child decide how she wishes to respond to the pressure in her rectum.

10. **Use diapers and pull-ups as little as possible.** We want your child to look forward to releasing bowel movements, rather than holding back. If your child refuses to sit on the toilet, having bowel movements in diapers is better than stool holding. Therefore, permit her access to diapers. However, don't let your child wear diapers all day. Keep your child in loose-fitting underwear or training pants, so that she has to decide each time she has an urge to pass a BM whether to use the toilet or to come to you for a diaper. To help her make the right choice, offer major incentives (e.g., a trip to a favorite restaurant or ice cream store) for BMs in the toilet. Offer minor incentives (e.g., candy) for BMs in the diaper. (*Note:* Being in underwear will give her an incentive to maintain bladder control and stay dry.)

11. **If your child is complaining about abdominal pain, clarify how to make it go away.** Tell her: "The poop wants to come out"; "The poop needs your help"; "It won't hurt"; "Holding back is a bad idea." Offer to help her sit in a basin of warm water to relax the anal sphincter. If she refuses, tell her "I can't help you. You have to help yourself." Then ignore your child or put her in time-out. Tell her to come back after the poop is out. Do not give positive attention for holding-back behavior.

12. **Help your child change her clothes if she soils herself.** Don't ignore soiling. As soon as you notice that your child has messy pants, clean her up immediately. The main role you have in this new program is to enforce the rule "we can't walk around with messy pants." Make changing pants a neutral, quick interaction. If your child is soiled, she will probably need your help with cleanup, but keep her involved. If your child refuses to let you change her, ground her until she is ready.

13. **Respond gently to accidents.** The responses to soiling listed below will only delay successful training and may cause emotional problems:

- Threatening or lecturing your child
- Forcing your child to sit on the potty chair
- Punishing or scolding your child for accidents
- Keeping your child in soiled pants
- Giving frequent reminders
- Allowing siblings to tease your child

 CALL OUR OFFICE

During regular hours if
- You think your child is blocked up again.
- Your child's bowel movements continue to hurt.
- You have other questions or concerns.

Instructions for Pediatric Patients, **2nd Edition,** ©1999 by **WB Saunders Company.**
Written by Barton D. Schmitt, MD, pediatrician and author of *Your Child's Health,* Bantam Books, a book for parents.

DEFINITION

Masturbation is self-stimulation of the genitals for pleasure and self-comfort. Children may rub themselves with a hand or other object. Masturbation is more than the normal inspection of the genitals commonly observed in 2-year-olds during baths. During masturbation, a child usually appears dazed, flushed, and preoccupied. A child may masturbate as often as several times each day or just once per week. Masturbation occurs more commonly when a child is sleepy, bored, watching television, or under stress.

Cause

Occasional masturbation is a normal behavior of many toddlers and preschoolers. Up to one third of children in this age group discover masturbation while exploring their bodies. Often they continue to masturbate simply because it feels good. Some children masturbate frequently because they are unhappy about something, such as having their pacifier taken away. Others are reacting to punishment or pressure to stop masturbation completely.

Masturbation has no medical causes. Irritation in the genital area causes pain or itching; it does not cause masturbation.

Expected Course

Once your child discovers masturbation, he will seldom stop doing it completely. Your child may not do it as often if any associated power struggles or unhappiness is remedied. By 5 or 6 years of age most children can learn some discretion and will masturbate only in private. Masturbation becomes almost universal at puberty in response to the normal surges in hormones and sexual drive.

Common Misconceptions

Masturbation does not cause any physical injury or harm to the body. It is not abnormal or excessive unless it is deliberately done in public places after 5 or 6 years of age. It does not mean your child will be oversexed, promiscuous, or sexually deviant. Only if adults overreact to a child's masturbation and make it seem dirty or wicked will it cause emotional harm, such as guilt and sexual hang-ups.

COMING TO TERMS WITH MASTURBATION IN PRESCHOOLERS

1. **Set realistic goals.** It is impossible to eliminate masturbation. Accept the fact that your child has learned about it and enjoys it. All that you can control is where he does it. A reasonable goal is to permit it only in the bedroom and bathroom. You might say to your child, "It's okay to do that in your bedroom when you're tired." If you completely ignore the masturbation, no matter where it's done, your child will think he can do it freely in any setting.

2. **Ignore masturbation at naptime and bedtime.** Leave your child alone at these times and do not keep checking on him. Do not forbid your child from lying on the abdomen and do not ask if his hands are between the legs.

3. **Distract or discipline your child for masturbation at other times.** First, try to distract your child with a toy or activity. If this fails, explain to your child: "I know that rubbing your body feels good, but you can't do that around other people. It's okay to do it in your room or the bathroom but not in the rest of the house." By the time children are 4 or 5 years old, they become sensitive to other people's feelings and understand that they should masturbate only when they are alone. Younger children may have to be sent to their rooms to masturbate.

4. **Discuss this approach with your child's day care or preschool staff.** Ask your child's caregiver or teacher to respond to your child's masturbation by first trying to distract the child. If this doesn't work, they should catch the child's attention with comments such as "We need to have you join us now." Masturbation should be tolerated at school only at nap time.

5. **Increase physical contact with your child.** Some children will masturbate less if they receive extra hugging and cuddling throughout the day. Try to be sure that your child receives at least 1 hour every day of special time together and physical affection from you.

6. **Avoid these common mistakes.** The most common mistake that parents make is to try to eliminate masturbation completely. This leads to a power struggle that the parents inevitably lose. Children should not be physically punished for masturbation, nor yelled at or lectured about it. Do not label masturbation as bad, dirty, evil, or sinful, and do not tie your child's hands or use any kind of restraints. All of these approaches lead only to resistance and possibly to sexual inhibitions later.

 ## CALL OUR OFFICE

During regular hours if
- Your child continues to masturbate when other people are around.
- You suspect that your child has been taught to masturbate by someone.
- You child tries to masturbate others.
- You feel your child is unhappy.
- You cannot accept any masturbation by your child.
- This approach does not bring improvement within 1 month.
- You have other questions or concerns.

Instructions for Pediatric Patients, 2nd Edition, ©1999 by WB Saunders Company.

Written by Barton D. Schmitt, MD, pediatrician and author of *Your Child's Health,* Bantam Books, a book for parents.

189

By 4 years of age, most children develop a healthy sexual curiosity. They ask a variety of questions and need honest, brief answers. If they don't ask sexual questions by 5 years of age, it is your job to bring up this subject. If you don't they may acquire a lot of misinformation from their schoolmates.

PROMOTING GOOD SEX EDUCATION

- Teach the differences in anatomy and the proper names for body parts. This is easy to do during baths with siblings or friends.
- Teach about pregnancy and where babies come from. The easiest way is to get a pregnant friend to volunteer and have your child feel her baby moving about.
- Explain the birth process. Tell your child that the baby comes out through a special passage called the vagina. Help her understand the process by seeing the birth of some puppies or kittens.
- Also, explain sexual intercourse. Many parents who discuss everything else keep postponing this topic. Get past this hurdle by reading your child some picture books on sex education. If you cover these topics by 5 years of age, your child will find it easy to ask you more about them as she grows older.

NORMAL SEXUAL PLAY

A common part of normal sexual development between 3 and 5 years of age is for children to get undressed together and look at each other's genitals. This is their attempt to learn about sexual differences. There's no reason why you can't turn this discovery into a positive one.

- After your child's friends have gone home, read her a book about sex education. Help your child talk about how boys' and girls' bodies differ.
- Tell your child that genitals are private. That's why we wear clothes. Clarify some basic rules: It's acceptable to see other people's genitals but not to touch them or stare at them. It's not acceptable to deliberately show someone your genitals.
- In the future, supervise the play a little more closely. If the children occasionally expose their bodies to each other, just ignore it. But if it seems to be happening more frequently, tell the children it's not polite and has to stop. If this doesn't get your mes-

sage across, give them a 5-minute time-out in separate rooms or send them home for the day, but don't give any major punishment or act horrified.
- It's up to parents to put the brakes on undressing games. If you don't, they usually escalate into touching and poking, but keep your response low-key.

NUDITY AND YOUR CHILD

Feelings about nudity vary from family to family. Exposure to nudity with siblings or the parent of the same sex is fine and continues indefinitely (e.g., in locker rooms), but nudity with the parent or sibling of the opposite sex probably should be phased out between 4 and 5 years of age. Some reasons for this are the following:

- Your child will soon be entering school, and nudity is clearly not accepted there.
- Most families in our society practice modesty, so a child who is interested in looking at other people's bodies can get into trouble.
- It is more comfortable for children to learn genital anatomy from siblings and age-mates than from seeing their parents nude.

If you are in agreement with these comments, then between 4 and 5 years of age begin to teach a respect for privacy.

- Stop any showering and bathing with your children (especially of the opposite sex).
- Close the bathroom door when you use the toilet.
- Close the bedroom door when you get dressed and suggest they do the same.

Wasn't that easy?

 ## CALL OUR OFFICE

During regular hours if
- Your child won't stop touching other children's genitals.
- Your child won't stop exposing his or her genitals.
- Your child has an excessive interest in sex or nudity.
- You have other questions or concerns.

Instructions for Pediatric Patients, 2nd Edition, ©1999 by WB Saunders Company.
Written by Barton D. Schmitt, MD, pediatrician and author of *Your Child's Health*, Bantam Books, a book for parents.

DEFINITION

- Rapid, repeated muscle twitches (also called habit spasms), such as eye blinking, facial grimacing, forehead wrinkling, head jerking, or shoulder shrugging
- Most tics last only 1 second.
- Increase with stress
- Decrease with relaxation and disappear during sleep
- Occur in 20% of children and are three times more frequent in boys than in girls
- Occur most often in children 6 to 10 years old

Causes

Most motor tics are due to inherited biochemical differences, not emotional problems. Flurries of tics, however, reflect the spilling over of emotional tension and indicate that your child is under pressure. All tics are involuntary, not deliberate. Children who have tics are usually normal, bright, and sensitive. Tics are more severe in children who are shy or overly self-conscious. Tics can be worsened by critical parents who nag, press a child for achievement beyond his ability, or draw negative comparisons with siblings.

Expected Course

If tics are ignored, they usually disappear in 2 months to 1 year. If extra effort is made to help your child relax, they usually improve more quickly. Even if the tics are not ignored and a child continues to feel stress or pressure, the tics usually improve or clear spontaneously during adolescence. Approximately 3% of children with tics develop incapacitating tics if they are not handled appropriately.

HOW TO HELP YOUR CHILD WITH TICS

1. **Help your child to relax in general.** Tics are a barometer of inner tension. Make sure your child has free time and fun time every day. If your child is overscheduled with activities, try to lighten the commitments. If your child is unduly self-critical, praise him more and remind him to be a good friend to himself.
2. **Identify and remove specific environmental stresses.** Whenever your child has a flurry of tics, write in a diary the date, time, and preceding event. From this diary, you should be able to identify when your child feels pressure. (**Note:** Your child should not know that you are keeping this diary.) In general, criticize your child less about grades, music lessons, sports, keeping his room clean, table manners, and so forth. Avoid stimulant medications (such as decongestants), which can lower the threshold for tics.
3. **Ignore tics when they occur.** When your child is having tics, don't call his attention to them. Reminders imply that they are bothering you. If your child becomes worried about the tics, then every time they occur, the child will react with tension rather than acceptance. The tension in turn will trigger more tics. Don't allow siblings or others to tease your child about the tics. Be sure that relatives, friends, and teachers also ignore the tics. When tics occur, people should focus on reducing any pressure they may be causing your child.
4. **Don't talk about tics when they are not occurring.** Stop all family conversation about tics. The less said about them, the less your child will be apprehensive of them. If your child brings up the subject, say something reassuring, such as "Eventually your face muscles will learn to relax and the tics will go away."
5. **Avoid any punishment for tics.** Some parents have the mistaken idea that tics are a bad habit that can be broken. This idea is absolutely false. If a child is made to practice "controlling tics" in front of a mirror, he will realize only that he cannot control them and they will become worse. Any facial exercises or massage should be discontinued because it only draws undue attention to the problem.

 CALL OUR OFFICE

During regular hours if
- The tics interfere with friendships or studies at school.
- The tics involve sounds, words, or profanity.
- The tics involve coughing.
- The tics involve parts of the body other than the head, face, or shoulders.
- The tics become frequent (more than 10 each day).
- The tics have lasted for more than a year.
- The tics are not better after trying this program for 1 month.
- You have other questions or concerns.

STUTTERING VERSUS NORMAL DYSFLUENCY

DEFINITIONS
Characteristics of Normal Dysfluency and Dysarthria

"Normal dysfluency" and "pseudostuttering" are the terms used to describe the normal repetition of sounds or syllables children make when they are learning to speak between 18 months and 5 years of age. "Normal dysarthria" and "mispronunciation" are the terms used to describe the incorrect pronunciation of many children as they learn to speak; sounds are substituted or left out, so that some words become hard to identify.

Characteristics of True Stuttering (Stammering)

- Repetitions of sounds, syllables, or short words
- Hesitations and pauses in speech
- Absence of smooth speech flow
- More frequent when child is tired, excited, or stressed
- Fear of talking
- Four times more likely in boys than in girls

Causes of Dysfluency, Dysarthria, and True Stuttering

Normal dysfluency occurs because the mind is able to think of words faster than the tongue can produce them. The cause of normal dysarthria is usually genetic. In most cases, true stuttering develops when a child with normal dysfluency or dysarthria is pressured to improve and in the process becomes sensitive to her inadequacies. Soon thereafter the child begins to anticipate speaking poorly and struggles to correct it. The child becomes tense when she speaks, and the more she attempts to control her speech, the worse it becomes (a vicious cycle). The repetitions become multiple, rather than single. Temporary stuttering can occur at any age if a person becomes overly critical and fearful of her own speech. Although it is normal for us to be aware of what we are saying, how we are saying it is normally subconscious. Genetic factors also play a role in stuttering.

Incidence

Normal dysfluency occurs in 90% of children, in contrast to true stuttering, which occurs in only 1% of children. Approximately 70% of children pronounce words clearly from the onset of speech; however, the other 30% of children between the ages of 1 and 4 years have normal dysarthria and say many words that are unintelligible to their parents and others.

Expected Course of Dysfluency, Dysarthria, and True Stuttering

Normal dysfluency lasts for approximately 2 or 3 months if handled correctly. Unlike normal dysfluency, normal dysarthria is not a brief phase but instead shows very gradual improvement over several years as development unfolds. The speech of 90% of the children who have dysarthria becomes completely understandable by 4 years of age, and the speech of 96% is understandable by 5 or 6 years of age. Without treatment, true stuttering will become worse and persist in adulthood.

HELPING YOUR CHILD COPE WITH NORMAL DYSFLUENCY AND DYSARTHRIA

The following recommendations should prevent progression to true stuttering in these children.

1. **Encourage conversation.** Sit down and talk with your child at least once each day. Keep the subject matter pleasant and enjoyable. Avoid asking for verbal performance or reciting. Make speaking fun.
2. **Help your child relax when stuttering occurs.** Mild stuttering that's not causing your child any discomfort should be ignored. When your child is having trouble speaking, however, say something reassuring such as "Don't worry, I can understand you." If your child asks you about her stuttering, reassure her that "Your speech will get easier and someday the stuttering will be gone."
3. **Don't correct your child's speech.** Avoid expressing any disapproval, such as by saying, "Stop that stuttering" or "Think before you speak." Remember that this is your child's normal speech for her age and is not controllable. Do not try to improve your child's grammar or pronunciation. Also, avoid praise for good speech because it implies that your child's previous speech wasn't up to standard.
4. **Don't interrupt your child's speech.** Give your child ample time to finish what she is saying. Don't complete sentences for her. Try to pause 2 seconds between the end of your child's sentence and the start of yours. Don't allow siblings to interrupt one another.
5. **Don't ask your child to repeat herself or start over.** If possible, guess at the message. Listen very closely when your child is speaking. Only if you don't understand a comment that appears to be important should you ask your child to restate it.
6. **Don't ask your child to practice a certain word or sound.** This just makes the child more self-conscious about her speech.
7. **Don't ask your child to slow down when she speaks.** Try to convey to your child that you have plenty of time and are not in a hurry. Model a relaxed rate of speech. A rushed type of speech is a temporary phase that can't be changed by orders from the parent.
8. **Don't label your child a stutterer.** Labels tend to become self-fulfilling prophecies. Don't discuss your child's speech problems in her presence.

Instructions for Pediatric Patients, 2nd Edition, ©1999 by WB Saunders Company.
Written by Barton D. Schmitt, MD, pediatrician and author of *Your Child's Health,* Bantam Books, a book for parents.

9. **Ask other adults not to correct your child's speech.** Share these guidelines with babysitters, teachers, relatives, neighbors, and visitors. Don't allow siblings to tease or imitate your child's stuttering.

10. **Help your child to relax and feel accepted in general.** Try to increase the hours of fun and play your child has each day. Try to slow down the pace of your family life. Avoid situations that seem to bring on stuttering. If there are any areas in which you have been applying strict discipline, back off.

 ## CALL OUR OFFICE

During regular hours for a referral to a speech therapist if
- Your child is over 5 years of age.
- Your child has true stuttering.

- Your child has associated facial grimacing or tics.
- Your child has become self-conscious or fearful about her speech.
- Your family has a history of stuttering in adulthood.
- Speech is also delayed (no words by 18 months or no sentences by 2½ years).
- Speech is totally unintelligible to others, and your child is over 2 years old.
- Speech is more than 50% unintelligible to others, and your child is over 3 years old.
- Speech is 10% unintelligible to others, and your child is over 4 years old.
- The dysfluency doesn't improve after trying this program for 2 months.
- You have other questions or concerns.

DEFINITION

A child who passes bowel movements (BMs) into his underwear has a problem called soiling or encopresis. Many children who are soiling small amounts several times a day are severely constipated or blocked up (impacted). The soiling occurs because pieces of the large mass of hard stool in the rectum break loose at unexpected times. This is especially likely to happen when your child is running or jumping. The soiling is not deliberate. The impaction is usually too wide to pass spontaneously, and the child can't control the leakage until the blockage is removed.

There are many reasons why children become constipated—high milk diet, genetic differences, avoiding bowel movements because they cause pain, or holding back BMs (stool holding) as a way of resisting toilet training. The possibility of physical causes requires a complete examination by your child's physician.

TREATMENT OF SOILING WITH CONSTIPATION FOR CHILDREN WHO WILL SIT ON THE TOILET

1. **First use enemas to remove the impaction.** Start with a Fleet's hyperphosphate enema. The dose is 1 ounce for every 20 pounds of your child's weight. For example, a 50-pound child should receive 2½ ounces of hyperphosphate enema. Don't give any child more than 4 ounces of the enema.

    Have your child try to hold the enema back for 5 minutes. Then insist that he sit on the toilet for release of the enema.

    Give a second hyperphosphate enema 1 or 2 hours after the first one. A third hyperphosphate enema can be given 12 to 24 hours later if you think your child is still impacted. Signs that your child is still impacted include continued soiling or a lump that can be felt in the lower abdomen.

    Before giving the enemas, give your child one to two glasses of water to drink because the enemas may cause some dehydration.

    If you want to make your own enemas, use normal saline. You can make normal saline by adding 2 teaspoons of table salt to a quart of warm water. Give 2 ounces of normal saline per year of your child's age. Don't give any child more than 16 ounces of saline enema.

    If you don't know how to give an enema, ask someone in your physician's office. Once an impaction is cleared, enemas are no longer necessary. Your child's constipation can be treated entirely with oral medicines. Continuous use of enemas irritates the rectum and can cause your child to hold back bowel movements.

2. **Use stool softeners to keep the bowel movements soft.** Stool softeners make the stool softer and easier to pass. Unlike laxatives, they do not cause any bowel contractions or pressure. Some commonly prescribed stool softeners are mineral oil, Kondremul, Metamucil, Mitrolan, Citrucel, Maltsupex, Petrogalar, and fiber wafers. Your child must take stool softeners for at least 3 months to prevent another impaction. By then, your child's intestines will be able to contract and empty normally again.

    If you use mineral oil, keep it in the refrigerator because it tastes best cold. Have your child take it with fruit juice to disguise the flavor or follow it with something tasty. Give your child a vitamin pill each day at about noon while he is on the mineral oil.

    Your child's stool softener is _____.

    The dose is _____ each morning and _____ each evening. Increase the dose gradually until your child is having two or three soft bowel movements each day.

3. **Use laxatives to keep the rectum empty if stool softeners aren't effective.** Laxatives (or bowel stimulants) cause the large intestine to contract, squeezing the stool toward the rectum. Commonly used laxatives are Senokot, Fletcher's Castoria, milk of magnesia (MOM), Haley's M-O, and Dulcolax. Don't worry that your child will become dependent on the laxatives (i.e., that the bowels won't move well without them). The most important goal is keeping the rectum empty. Children can always be gradually withdrawn from laxatives, even after 6 months of using them.

    Your child's laxative is _____.

    The dose is _____ given with dinner or _____. If your child goes 48 hours without a BM, give _____.

4. **Encourage your child to eat a nonconstipating diet.** Have your child eat plenty of fruits and vegetables every day (raw ones are best). Some examples are figs, dates, raisins, peaches, pears, apricots, celery, cabbage, and corn.

    Bran is an excellent natural laxative because it has a high fiber content. Have your child eat bran daily by including such foods as the new "natural" cereals, bran flakes, bran muffins, or whole wheat bread in his diet. Popcorn, nuts, shredded wheat, oatmeal, brown rice, lima beans, navy beans, chili beans, and peas are also good sources of fiber.

    Only milk products (milk, cheese, yogurt, ice cream) and cooked carrots have been proven to be constipating. Your child should limit his intake of milk products to 2 glasses or the equivalent per day. Encourage lots of fruit juices because they increase bowel movements. (**Exception:** Orange juice doesn't help.) However, don't pressure your

Instructions for Pediatric Patients, 2nd Edition, ©1999 by WB Saunders Company.
Written by Barton D. Schmitt, MD, pediatrician and author of *Your Child's Health*, Bantam Books, a book for parents.

child about diet; instead, offer choices and include your child in the decisions about what foods to eat.

5. **Encourage your child to sit on the toilet for 10 minutes after meals.** Your child should sit on the toilet until a bowel movement is passed, or at least for 10 minutes. Unless your child does this, the medicines will not work. Normally, children and adults know when their rectum is full because it is uncomfortable and causes some bowel contractions (the "defecation urge"). Children who have been impacted for a long time lose this sensation and need 2 to 4 weeks to get it back. During this time, your child must sit on the toilet even when he doesn't feel the need to go. The best time seems to be 20 or 30 minutes after a meal.

Your physician will try to get your child to promise to do this on his own, but he may need some help from you. Try a reminder sign. By all means, don't remind him more than two times a day or in a stern way because this will foster a negative attitude about the whole process. Never insist that he sit on the toilet if he is busy doing something else. Tell him you want sitting on the toilet to be fun and ask what would he like to do. Try to pick good times for gentle reminders and mention that "your doctor asked me to help you remember."

Other toileting tips for your child that are essential for success are:

• Push while sitting on the toilet. The bowel movement won't just fall out.
• Bend forward so the chest touches the upper legs. This position opens up the rectum. Bending forward and then relaxing a little may also help move stool downward.
• If your child's feet can't easily reach the floor, use a footstool to provide pushing leverage.

Your child should sit on the toilet more often: until he has a large bowel movement if he is cooperative and

• Any soiling occurs (soiling always means the rectum is very full).
• Your child feels blocked up.
• Your child has a stomachache or cramps.

6. **Clarify for your child how he can stay clean.**

• Stay unblocked and empty.
• Go poop every day.
• Take your medicine every day.
• If your poops aren't coming out like they should, sit on the toilet after every meal.

7. **Help your child respond to soiling (leakage).** If your child is on the correct medicines and sitting on the toilet, there shouldn't be any accidents. However, finding the correct treatment program may take several weeks. Also, some children will have recurrences of soiling (usually after 4 or 5 days without a BM). In such cases, handle soiling in the following way:

• Recognize soiling. Don't ignore soiling. As soon as you notice soiling by odor or behavior, remind your child to immediately clean himself.
• Clean the skin. Before your child sits on the toilet, suggest a 5-minute soak in the bathtub. At the least, your child's bottom needs cleaning off with a wet washcloth. Your child should be able to do most of this on his own. This may relax the anal sphincter and give your child the urge to go.
• Have your child sit on the toilet. After soaking in warm water, have your child sit on the toilet until a large bowel movement is passed, or at least 10 minutes out of every hour until it does. If stool is leaking out, the rectum is clearly full and should be emptied.
• Clean soiled clothes. First, scrape the underwear partially clean with a butter knife or spatula. Then rinse it out in the toilet. Finally, store the soiled underwear until the next washday in a conveniently located bucket of water with some bleach in it and a lid. You can encourage your child to help with this, but you will need to do most of it until he is 7 or 8 years old.
• Avoid punishment. Do not blame, criticize, or punish your child. In addition, do not allow siblings to tease him. Never put your child back into diapers.

8. **Ask the school staff for their help.** These children need ready access to the bathroom at school, especially if they are shy. Encourage your child not to be embarrassed about leaving the classroom to go to the bathroom. Your physician will send the school a note requesting unlimited privileges to go to the school bathroom any time your child wants to and without having to raise his hand. He should also be allowed to come in from outside recess. If the problem is significant, you might also temporarily supply the school with an extra set of clean underwear.

 ## CALL OUR OFFICE

During regular hours if
• Your child soils two or more times and sitting on the toilet doesn't help.
• You feel your child is blocked up again.
• Bowel movements continue to hurt.
• Your child won't take the medicines.
• Your child won't sit on the toilet.
• You have other questions or concerns.

SCHOOL PHOBIA OR REFUSAL

DEFINITION

- A child with school phobia is a child who misses considerable school because of vague physical symptoms. When she is not in school, she is at home; that is, she is not a truant.
- The symptoms are usually the type that people get when they are upset or worried, such as stomachaches, headaches, nausea, vomiting, diarrhea, tiredness, or dizziness. These physical symptoms mainly occur in the morning, and they worsen at the time of departure for school.
- Your child otherwise seems healthy and vigorous.
- School phobia is very common and affects at least 5% of elementary-school children and 2% of middle-school children.
- Often the symptoms begin in September or October.
- This diagnosis must be confirmed by a physician.

Causes

A school-phobic child is usually afraid of leaving home in general, rather than afraid of anything in particular at school. For example, she may experience homesickness when staying at a friend's house. Often the first test of a child's independence comes when she must attend school daily. Aside from poor attendance, these children usually are good students and well behaved at school. The parents are typically good parents who are conscientious and loving. Such parents are sometimes overly protective and close, and the child finds it difficult to separate from them (separation anxiety). She may lack the self-confidence that comes from handling life's normal stresses without her parents' help.

Sometimes a change of schools, a strict teacher, hard tests, a learning problem, or a bully may be seen as causes of the child's fear of going to school. However, such factors may be only part of the problem, and your child should still go to school while these problems are being resolved.

Expected Course

If daily school attendance is enforced, the problem of school phobia will improve dramatically in 1 or 2 weeks. On the other hand, if you do not require your child to attend school every day, the physical symptoms and the desire to stay home will become more frequent. The longer your child stays home, the harder it will be for her to return. Your child's future social life and education may be at stake.

HELPING YOUR CHILD OVERCOME SCHOOL PHOBIA

1. **Insist on an immediate return to school.** The best therapy for school phobia is to be in school every day. Fears are overcome by facing them as soon as possible. Daily school attendance will cause most of your child's physical symptoms to magically improve. They will become less severe and occur less often, and your child will eventually enjoy school again. At first, however, your child will test your determination to send her every day. You must make school attendance a non-negotiable, iron-clad rule. Be optimistic with your child and reassure her that she will feel better after she gets to school.

2. **Be extra firm on school mornings.** In the beginning, mornings may be a difficult time. You should never ask your child how she feels because it will encourage her to complain. If she is well enough to be up and around the house, she is well enough to go to school. If your child complains of physical symptoms, but they are her usual ones, she should be sent to school promptly with minimal discussion. If you are uncertain about your child's health, try to err on the side of sending her to school; if later the symptoms worsen, the school nurse can reevaluate your child's health.

   If your child is late, she should go to school anyway. When she misses the school bus, you should have a prearranged alternative plan of transportation. If your child wanders home on her own during lunch or recess, she should be sent back promptly. Sometimes a child may cry and scream, absolutely refusing to go to school. In that case, after talking with her about her worries, she has to be taken there. One parent may be better at enforcing this than the other. Sometimes a relative can take charge of the matter for a few days.

3. **Have your child see her physician on any morning she stays home.** If your child has a new physical symptom or seems quite sick, you will probably want her to stay home. If you are puzzled, your physician will usually be able to determine the cause of her sickness. Call the office as soon as it opens, and try to have your child seen that morning. If the symptom is caused by a disease, appropriate treatment can be started. If the symptom results from anxiety, your child should be back in school before noon. Working closely with your child's physician in this way can solve even the most difficult of school phobia problems. You should probably keep your child at home when she has any of the following symptoms:

   - Fever (over 100°F [37.8°C] orally)
   - Vomiting (more than once)
   - Frequent diarrhea
   - Frequent cough
   - Widespread rash
   - Earache
   - Toothache

   On the other hand, children with a sore throat, moderate cough, runny nose, or other cold symptoms but no fever can be sent to class. Children should not be kept home for "looking sick," "poor color," "circles under the eyes," or "tiredness."

4. **Ask the school staff for assistance.** Schools are usually very understanding about school phobia,

Instructions for Pediatric Patients, 2nd Edition, ©1999 by WB Saunders Company.
Written by Barton D. Schmitt, MD, pediatrician and author of *Your Child's Health,* Bantam Books, a book for parents.

once they are informed of the diagnosis, because this problem is such a common one. Ask the school nurse to let your child lie down for 5 to 15 minutes in her office and regroup, rather than being sent home if her symptoms occur in school. It is often helpful if you talk to your child's teacher about the situation.

If your child has special fears, such as reciting in class, the teacher will usually make special allowances.

5. **Talk with your child about school fears.** At a time other than a school morning, talk with your child about her problems. Encourage her to tell you exactly what upsets her. Ask her what is the worst possible thing that could happen to her at school or on the way to school. If there's a situation you can change, tell her you will work on it. If she's worried about the physical symptoms becoming worse at school, reassure her that she can lie down for a few minutes in the nurse's office as needed. After listening carefully, tell her you can appreciate how she feels, but it's still necessary to attend school while she's getting better.

6. **Help your child spend more time with her age-mates.** Outside of school, school-phobic children tend to prefer to be with their parents, play indoors, be alone in their rooms, and watch a lot of television. Many of them cannot stay overnight at a friend's home without developing overwhelming homesickness. They need encouragement to play more with their peers. This can be difficult for a parent who enjoys the child's company, but it is the best course of action in the long run. Encourage your child to join clubs and athletic teams (noncontact sports are usually preferred). Send her outside more or to other children's homes. Ask her friends to join your family for outings or for overnight stays. Help your child learn to stay overnight with relatives and friends. Send your child to a summer camp—it can be a turning point.

 ## CALL OUR OFFICE

During regular hours if
- The school phobia is not resolved in 2 weeks using this approach.
- The school phobia recurs.
- You think the cause of the symptoms may be physical rather than emotional.
- Your child continues to have other fears or separation problems.
- Your child is withdrawn in general or seems depressed.
- You have other questions or concerns.

ATTENTION DEFICIT DISORDER (SHORT ATTENTION SPAN)

DEFINITION

Attention deficit disorder (ADD) occurs in 3% to 5% of children, most of them boys. A normal attention span is 3 to 5 minutes per year of a child's age. A child in kindergarten needs a 15-minute attention span. First and second graders need a 20-minute span to do the work. (*Note:* The attention span while watching television doesn't count.) If you suspect that your child has a short attention span, ask another adult (a teacher or day care provider, for example) if she has observed this also. The following characteristics are common:

- A child hasn't learned to listen when someone talks, wait his turn, complete a task, or return to a task if interrupted. (*Caution:* These can be normal characteristics of children less than 3 or 4 years old.)
- Some children (80% of boys and 50% of girls) also have associated hyperactivity (increased motor activity) with symptoms of being restless, impulsive, and in a hurry. This is called attention deficit hyperactivity disorder, or ADHD.
- Some children (50%) also have an associated learning disability. The most common one is an auditory processing deficit (i.e., they have difficulty remembering complex verbal directions). However, the intelligence of most children with ADD is usually normal.

Similar Conditions

Disruptive children, children who don't mind, and aggressive children are sometimes included under the broad category of hyperactivity. These children should be looked on as children with behavior problems and approached with appropriate discipline techniques.

Causes

ADD is the most common developmental disability. "Developmental" means that the disability is caused by delayed brain development (immaturity). This delay results in poor self-control, requiring external controls by the parents for a longer period of time. Often this type of temperament and short attention span are hereditary. Minor brain damage has not been proven to cause ADD.

Expected Course

Children with developmental ADD can improve significantly if parents and teachers provide understanding and direction and preserve the children's self-esteem. When these children become adults, many of them have good attention spans but remain restless, have to keep busy, and, in a sense, have not entirely outgrown the problem. However, not only does society learn to tolerate such traits in adults, but in some settings the person with endless energy is prized.

GUIDELINES FOR LIVING WITH A CHILD HAVING A SHORT ATTENTION SPAN AND HYPERACTIVITY

ADD is a chronic condition that needs special parenting and school intervention. If your child seems to have a poor attention span and is over 3 years of age, these recommendations may assist you. Your main obligations involve organizing your child's home life and improving discipline. Only after your child's behavior has improved will you know for certain if your child also has ADD. If he does, specific interventions to help him learn to listen and complete tasks ("stretch" his attention span) can be initiated. Even though you can't be sure about ADD until your child is 3 or 4 years of age, you can detect and improve behavior problems after 8 months of age.

1. **Accept your child's limitations.** Accept the fact that your child is intrinsically active and energetic and possibly always will be. The hyperactivity is not intentional. Don't expect to eliminate the hyperactivity but merely to bring it under reasonable control. Any criticism or other attempt to change an energetic child into a quiet or model child will cause more harm than good. Nothing helps a hyperactive child more than having a tolerant, patient, low-keyed parent.

2. **Provide an outlet for the release of excess energy.** This energy can't be bottled up and stored. Daily outdoor activities such as running, sports, and long walks are good outlets. A fenced yard helps. In bad weather your child needs a recreational area where he can play as he pleases with minimal restrictions and supervision. A garage will suffice. Too many toys can cause him to be more easily distracted from playing with any one toy. The toys should be safe and relatively unbreakable. Encourage your child to play with one toy at a time.

3. **Keep your home well organized.** Household routines help the hyperactive child to accept order. Keep the times for wake-up, meals, chores, naps, and bed regular. Keep your environment relatively quiet to encourage thinking, listening, and reading at home. In general, leave the radio and television off. Predictable daily events help your child's responses become more predictable. ADD symptoms are made worse by sleep deprivation and hunger. Be sure your child has an early bedtime and a big breakfast on school days.

4. **Try not to let your child become fatigued.** When a hyperactive child becomes exhausted, his self-control often breaks down and the hyperactivity becomes worse. Try to have your child sleep or rest when he is fatigued. If he can't seem to "turn off his motor," hold and rock him in a rocking chair.

5. **Avoid taking your child to formal gatherings.** Except for special occasions, avoid places where

Instructions for Pediatric Patients, 2nd Edition, ©1999 by WB Saunders Company.
Written by Barton D. Schmitt, MD, pediatrician and author of *Your Child's Health*, Bantam Books, a book for parents.

hyperactivity would be extremely inappropriate and embarrassing (such as churches or restaurants). You also may wish to reduce the number of times your child goes with you to stores and supermarkets. After your child develops adequate self-control at home, he can gradually be introduced to these situations.

6. **Maintain firm discipline.** These children are unquestionably difficult to manage. They need more carefully planned discipline than the average child. Rules should be formulated mainly to prevent harm to your child and to others. Aggressive behavior, such as biting, hitting, and pushing, should be no more accepted in the hyperactive child than in the normal child. Try to eliminate such aggressive behaviors, but avoid unnecessary or unattainable rules; that is, don't expect your child to keep his hands and feet still. Hyperactive children tolerate fewer rules than the normal child. Enforce a few clear, consistent, important rules and add other rules at your child's pace. Avoid constant negative comments like "Don't do this" and "Stop that."

7. **Enforce rules with nonphysical punishment.** Physical punishment suggests to your child that physically aggressive behavior is acceptable. We want to teach hyperactive children to be less aggressive. Your child needs adult models of control and calmness. Use a friendly, matter-of-fact tone of voice to discipline your child. If you yell, your child will be quick to imitate you.

Punish your child for misbehavior immediately. When your child breaks a rule, isolate him in a chair or time-out room if a show of disapproval doesn't work. The time-out should last about 1 minute per year of your child's age. Without a time-out system, success is unlikely.

8. **Stretch your child's attention span.** Encouraging attentive (nonhyperactive) behavior is the key to preparing your child for school. Increased attention span and persistence with tasks can be taught at home. Don't wait until your child is of school age and expect the teacher to change him. By 5 years of age he needs at least a 15-minute attention span to perform adequately.

Set aside several brief periods each day to teach your child listening skills by reading to him. Start with picture books, and gradually progress to reading stories. Coloring pictures can be encouraged and praised. Teach games to your child, gradually increasing the difficulty by starting with building blocks and progressing to puzzles, dominoes, card games, and dice games. Matching pictures is an excellent way to build your child's memory and concentration span. Later, consequence games such as checkers or tic-tac-toe can be introduced. When your child becomes restless, stop and return to it later. Praise your child for attentive behavior. This process is invaluable in preparing your child for school.

9. **Buffer your child against any overreaction by neighbors.** Ask neighbors with whom your child has contact to be helpers. If your child is labeled by some adults as a "bad" kid, it is important that this image doesn't carry over into your home life. At home the attitude that must prevail is that your child is a good child with excess energy. It is extremely important that you not give up on him. Your child must always feel loved and accepted within the family. As long as a child has this acceptance, his self-esteem will survive.

10. **From time to time, get away from it all.** Periodic breaks help parents to tolerate hyperactive behavior. If just the father works outside the home, he should try to look after the child when he comes home, not only to give his wife a deserved break but also to understand better what she must contend with during the day. A babysitter one afternoon each week and an occasional evening out can provide much-needed breaks for an exhausted mother. Preschool is another helpful option. Parents need time to rejuvenate themselves so they can continue to meet their child's extra needs.

11. **Use special programs at school.** Try to start your child in preschool by 3 years of age to help him learn to organize his thoughts and develop his ability to focus. However, consider enrolling your child in kindergarten a year late (i.e., at 6 years old rather than 5) because the added maturity may help him fit in better with his classmates.

Once your child enters grade school, the school is responsible for providing appropriate programs for your child's ADD and any learning disability he might have. Some standard approaches used to help children with ADD are smaller class size, isolated study space, spaced learning techniques, and inclusion of the child in tasks such as erasing the blackboard (as outlets for excessive energy). Many of these children spend part of their day with a teacher specializing in learning disabilities who helps to improve their skills and confidence.

If you think your child has ADD and he has not been tested by the school's special education team, you can request an evaluation. Usually you can obtain the help your child needs with schoolwork by working with the school through parent-teacher conferences. Your main job is to continue to help your child improve his attention span and self-discipline, at home.

12. **Medications are sometimes helpful.** Stimulant drugs can improve a child's ability to concentrate. Discuss the use of drugs with your child's physician. In general, medications are not prescribed before school age. Medications without special education and home management programs have no long-term benefit. They need to be part of a broader program.

HOMEWORK AND SCHOOLWORK PROBLEMS (SCHOOL UNDERACHIEVERS)

DEFINITION

- Performs below her potential at school
- Has average or better intelligence, with no learning disabilities
- Doesn't finish schoolwork or homework
- "Forgets" to bring homework home
- "Forgets," loses, or doesn't turn in finished homework
- "Doesn't remember" what parents have taught
- Gets poor report card
- Doesn't want any help

Causes

Some children get into bad habits with their homework because they become preoccupied with television programs or video games. Some middle-school children become sidetracked by their hormones or by sports. Other children who find schoolwork difficult would simply rather play. If parents help these children to cut back other activities to reasonable amounts and count on the teacher to grade the child's efforts on schoolwork and homework, most of these children will improve. Motivation for good grades eventually comes from a desire to please the teacher and be admired by peers, enjoyment in knowing things, ability to see studying as a pathway to a future career, knowledge that the student needs a 3-point average to get into college, and the student's own self-reproach when she falls short of her goals.

When parents overrespond to this behavior and exert pressure for better performance, they can start a power struggle around schoolwork. "Forgetfulness" becomes a game. The child sees the parents' pressure as a threat to her independence. More pressure brings more resistance. Poor grades become the child's best way to prove that she is independent of her parents and that she can't be pushed. Good evidence for this is the child who does worse in the areas where she receives the most help. If parental interference with a child's schoolwork continues for several years, the child becomes a school "underachiever."

HELPING YOUR CHILD REGAIN RESPONSIBILITY FOR SCHOOLWORK

1. **Get out of the middle regarding homework.** Clarify that completing and turning in homework is between your child and the teacher. Remember that the purpose of homework is to teach your child to work on her own. Don't ask your child if she has any. Don't help with homework except at your child's request. Allow the school to apply natural consequences for poor performance. Walk away from any power struggles. Your child can learn the lesson of schoolwork accountability only through personal experience. If possible, apologize to your youngster, saying, for example, "After thinking about it, we have decided you are old enough to manage your own affairs. Schoolwork is your business and we will try to stay out of it. We are confident you will do what's best for you."

   The result of this "sink or swim" approach is that arguments will stop, but your child's schoolwork may temporarily worsen. Your child may throw caution to the winds to see if you really mean what you have said. This period of doing nothing but waiting for your child to find her own reason for doing well in school may be very agonizing. However, children need to learn from their mistakes. If you can avoid "rescuing" your child, her grades will show a dramatic upswing in anywhere from 2 to 9 months. This planned withdrawal of parental pressure is best done in the early grades, when marks are of minimal importance but the development of the child's own personal reason for learning is critical.

2. **Avoid reminders about schoolwork.** Repeatedly reminding your child about schoolwork promotes rebellion. So do criticizing, lecturing, and threatening your child. Pressure is different from parental interest and encouragement. If pressure works at all, it works only temporarily.

   We can never force children to learn or to be productive. Learning is a process of self-fulfillment. It is an area that belongs to the child and one that we as parents should try to stay out of, despite our yearnings for our children's success.

3. **Coordinate your plan with your child's teacher.** Schedule a parent-teacher conference. Discuss your views on schoolwork and homework responsibility. Tell your child's teacher that you want your child to be responsible to the teacher for homework. Clarify that you would prefer not to check or correct the work, because this has not been helpful in the past. Tell the teacher that you want to be supportive of the school and could do this best if she sent home a brief, weekly progress report. If the teacher thinks your youngster needs extra help, encourage her to suggest a tutoring program. In middle school, peer tutoring is often a powerful motivator.

4. **Limit television until schoolwork improves.** Although you can't make your child study, you can increase the potential study time. Eliminate all television and video game time on school nights. Explain to your child that these privileges will be reinstated after the teacher's weekly report confirms that all homework was handed in and the grades or overall quality of work is improving. Explain that you are doing this to help her better structure her time.

5. **Consider adding incentives for improved schoolwork.** Most children respond better to incentives than disincentives. Ask your youngster what she thinks would help. Some good incentives are taking your child to a favorite restaurant, amusement park, video arcade, sports event, or the movies. Sometimes earning "spending money" by work-

Instructions for Pediatric Patients, 2nd Edition, ©1999 by WB Saunders Company.
Written by Barton D. Schmitt, MD, pediatrician and author of *Your Child's Health*, Bantam Books, a book for parents.

ing hard on studies will interest your child. The payments can be made weekly based on the teacher's progress reports. A's, B's, and C's can receive a different cash value. What your child buys with this money should be her business (e.g., music or toys). Rewarding hard work is how the adult marketplace works.

6. **Consider removing other privileges for a fall-off in schoolwork.** You have already eliminated school-night television viewing because it obviously interferes with studying. If the school reports continue to be poor, you may need to eliminate all television and video games. Other privileges that may need to be temporarily limited should be those that matter to your child (e.g., telephone, bike, outside play, or visiting friends). If your teenager drives a car, this privilege may need to be curtailed until her grades are at least a 3-point (B) average. For youngsters who have fallen behind in their work, grounding (i.e., no peer contact) for 1 to 2 weeks may be required until they "catch up." Avoid severe punishment, however, because it will leave your youngster angry and resentful. Canceling something important (such as membership in Scouts or an athletic team) or taking away something they care about (such as a pet) because of poor marks is unfair and ineffective. Being part of a team is also good for motivation.

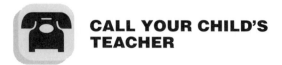

CALL YOUR CHILD'S TEACHER

For a conference if
- Your child's schoolwork and grades do not improve within 2 months.
- Homework is still an issue between you and your child after 2 months.
- You think your child has a learning problem that makes school difficult.

CALL OUR OFFICE

- If you think your child is preoccupied with some stresses in her life.
- If you think your child is depressed.
- If you have other questions or concerns.

Note: If these attempts to motivate your child fail, she may need an evaluation by a child psychologist or psychiatrist.

SCHOOLWORK RESPONSIBILITY: HOW TO INSTILL IT

DEFINITION

Taking responsibility for schoolwork helps children grow up to be responsible adults who keep their promises, meet deadlines, and succeed at their jobs. Responsible children finish schoolwork, homework, and long-term projects on time. They remember their assignments and turn in papers. They occasionally ask for help (e.g., with a spelling list) but usually like to think through their work by themselves.

HOW TO ENCOURAGE SCHOOLWORK RESPONSIBILITY

The following suggestions should help you cultivate the trait of responsibility in your child and avoid problems with schoolwork that may be difficult to correct later on.

1. **Encourage learning and responsibility in the preschool years.** Listen attentively to your child's conversation. Encourage him to think for himself. Take your child to the library and read to him regularly. Watch educational programs together and talk about them. Be a role model of someone who reads, finds learning exciting, enjoys problem solving, and likes to try new things.

2. **Show your child you are interested in his school performance.** Ask your child about his school day. Look at and comment positively on the graded papers your child brings home. Praise your child's strong points on his report card. Show interest in the books your child is reading. Help your child attend school regularly; don't keep him home for minor illnesses. Go to regular parent-teacher conferences and tell your child about them. If you feel discouraged, rather than conveying this to your child, schedule conference with his teacher.

3. **Support the school staff's recommendations.** Show respect for both the school system and the teacher, at least in your child's presence. Verbal attacks on the school may pit your child against the school and give him an excuse for not working. Even when you disagree with a school's policy, you should encourage your child to conform to school rules, just as he will need to conform to the broader rules of society.

4. **Make it clear that schoolwork is between your child and the teacher.** When your child begins school he should understand that homework, schoolwork, and marks are strictly between him and his teacher. The teacher should set goals for better school performance, not the parents. Your child must feel responsible for successes and failures in school. People take more pride in accomplishments if they feel fully responsible for them. Parents who feel responsible for their child's school performance open the door for the child to turn his responsibilities over to them. Occasionally, elementary-school teachers may ask you to review

basic facts with your child or see that your child completes work that was put off at school. When your child's teacher makes such requests, it's fine for you to help, but only as a temporary measure.

5. **Stay out of homework.** Asking if your child has homework, helping nightly, checking the finished homework, or drilling your child in areas of concern all convey to your child that you don't trust him. If you do your child's homework, your child will have less confidence that he can do it himself. If your child asks for help with homework, help with the particular problem only. Your help should focus on explaining the question, not on giving the answer. A good example of useful help is reading your child's spelling list to him while he writes the words, but then letting him check his own answers. A chief purpose of homework is to teach your child to work on his own.

6. **Avoid dictating a study time.** Assigning a set time for your child to do homework is unnecessary and looked on as pressure. The main thing parents can do is to provide a quiet setting with a desk, a comfortable chair, and good lighting. If any, the only rule should be "No television until homework is done." Accept your child's word that the work is done without checking. For long-term assignments, help your child organize his work the first few times if he seems overwhelmed. Help him estimate how many hours he thinks the project will take. Then help him write up a list of the days at home when he will work on the project.

7. **Provide home tutoring for special circumstances.** Occasionally, a teacher will request parental assistance when a child has lots of makeup work following a prolonged absence or transfer to a new school. If your child's teacher makes such a request, ask him to send home notes about what he wants you to help your child with (for instance, multiplication for 2 weeks). By using this approach you are still not taking primary responsibility for your child's schoolwork because the assignments and request for help come from the teacher. Provide this home instruction in a positive, helping way. As soon as your child has met the teacher's goal for improvement, remove yourself from the role of tutor. In this way you have provided temporary tutoring to help your child over an obstacle that the school staff does not have time or resources to deal with fully.

8. **Request special help for children with learning problems.** Some children have learning problems that interfere with learning some of the basic skills (e.g., reading). The comments so far have assumed that your child has no learning limitations. If a child with a reading disability slips too far behind, the child may lose confidence in his ability to do schoolwork. If you have concerns about your child's ability to learn, set up a conference with your child's teacher. At that time, inquire about an evaluation by your school's special education team.

Instructions for Pediatric Patients, 2nd Edition, ©1999 by **WB Saunders Company.**
Written by Barton D. Schmitt, MD, pediatrician and author of *Your Child's Health*, Bantam Books, a book for parents.

Home video games have swept the United States. Over 30% of American homes have a computerized game system hooked up to the television set. Over 500 different game cartridges are available. Video games are currently the most popular toy in the United States. Portable video games are the latest option. Every day more 6- to 16-year-olds become part of Nintendo mania.

VIDEO GAMES VERSUS TELEVISION

Compared to watching television, video games are a better form of entertainment. Video games are interactive. Your child's mind has to be turned on and working. The following are some potential benefits of the better games:

- Promote paying attention to details (e.g., to clues), memory, sequencing, and planning strategies
- Promote eye-hand (visual motor) coordination
- Improve visual perception (spatial awareness)
- Encourage use of imagination

DISADVANTAGES OF VIDEO GAMES

The drawbacks of video games are similar to the ones we see with television:

- Video games can dominate your child's leisure and study time. Video games can eliminate time needed to develop competence in sports, music, or art. If reading and homework are displaced, school performance can be affected.
- Video games can be a solitary activity, reducing social interactions with family and friends. Your youngster can become a junior hermit, interacting with friends only to pump them for pieces of information about hidden passages or secret trapdoors. Encourage playing video games with other children.
- Violent video games can teach an acceptance of violent behavior in real life.
- Overall, realize that your child is overdosing on video games if her grades have fallen, she doesn't finish her homework, she gets inadequate sleep, she doesn't play outdoors, she has become a loner, or she is preoccupied with karate chops or other aggressive behavior that is part of one of her video games.

TAKE A STAND ON VIDEO GAMES

Don't expect your youngster to limit the time allocated to this mesmerizing form of entertainment. Given her own way, she might play Nintendo every waking moment. You are responsible for protecting your child from harm. You must decide on rules that are appropriate for your child. If the rules are broken, the game (or control panel) needs to be put away for 1 or more days.

1. **Allow video games only after homework and chores are completed.** Access to video game time can even be presented as an incentive for finishing these tasks properly.

2. **Limit video game time.** Two hours each day or less is a reasonable goal. An alternative is to limit it to 1 hour on school nights and 2 or 3 hours per day on weekends. Some parents allow the system to be used only on weekends. If your child is doing poorly in school, temporarily eliminate video game time on school nights. Some parents have their children earn video game time by putting in equivalent time reading.

3. **Don't allow your child to postpone bedtime because she wants to finish a video game.** Remember that children who are allowed to stay up late are usually too tired the next day to remember what they are taught in school. Don't allow your child to have a video game set in her bedroom because this eliminates your control over the hours of play. When bedtime is drawing near, give your child a 10-minute warning.

4. **Encourage your children to settle their own disputes over using the video game.** When possible, stay out of disagreements, as long as they remain verbal. Children can't go through life having a referee to resolve their differences. If the argument becomes too loud, remove the control panel until your children work out a schedule.

5. **Help your child buy video games that are not excessively violent.** Encourage her to buy or rent sports, puzzle, maze, or adventure games. Avoid games that contain lots of murder, combat, and destruction. Since your child is an active participant in the mayhem on video games, research suggests that the games have a greater impact on her aggressive behavior than do violent television shows, in which she is strictly an observer. If your child borrows a video cartridge from a friend, have a rule that you have to approve its contents before she uses it.

6. **If you own a computer, take advantage of some of the educational games.** These tap the motivational power of the arcade games to help your child learn. They combine academics and entertainment. They also teach computer skills. If you have a choice, buy computer games rather than video games.

7. **Try to channel your child's leisure time into a variety of activities.** Video games are not bad for children. They can teach skills. They are more educational than television. Moreover, if you try to forbid video games, your child will play them at another child's home. So help your child learn to use them in moderation after the first weeks of normal infatuation have passed. Encourage more reading, music, hobbies, sports, and playing with friends.

TELEVISION: REDUCING THE NEGATIVE IMPACT

Television has a tremendous influence on how children view our world. Many youngsters spend more hours watching television from birth to 18 years of age than they spend in the classroom. The positive aspects of television viewing include seeing different lifestyles and cultures. Children today are entering school more knowledgeable than children before the era of television. In addition, television has great entertainment value. Although television can be a good teacher, many children watch it excessively and therefore experience some of the negative consequences described below.

HARMFUL ASPECTS OF TELEVISION

1. **Television displaces active types of recreation.** It decreases time spent playing with peers. A child has less time for self-directed daydreaming and thinking. Television takes away time for participating in sports, music, art, or other activities that require practice to achieve competence.
2. **Television interferes with conversation and discussion time.** It reduces social interactions with family and friends.
3. **Television discourages reading.** Reading requires much more thinking than television. Reading improves a youngster's vocabulary. A decrease in reading scores may be related to too much time in front of the television.
4. **Heavy television viewing (more than 4 hours per day) definitely reduces school performance.** This much television interferes with study, reading, and thinking time. If children do not get enough sleep because they are watching television, they will not be alert enough to learn well on the following day.
5. **Television discourages exercise.** An inactive lifestyle leads to poor physical fitness. If accompanied by frequent snacking, watching television may contribute to weight problems.
6. **Television violence can affect how a child feels toward life and other people.** Viewing excessive violence may cause a child to be overly fearful about personal safety and the future. Television violence may numb the sympathy a child normally feels toward victims of human suffering. Young children may be more aggressive in their play after seeing violent television shows.

PREVENTION OF TELEVISION ADDICTION

1. **Encourage active recreation.** Help your child become interested in sports, games, hobbies, and music. Occasionally turn off the television and take a walk or play a game with your child.
2. **Read to your children.** Begin reading to your child by 1 year of age and encourage him to read on his own as he becomes older. Some parents help children earn television or video game time

by spending an equivalent time reading. Help your child improve his conversational skills by spending more of your time talking with him.
3. **Limit television time to 2 hours per day or less.** An alternative is to limit television to 1 hour on school nights and 2 or 3 hours per day on weekends. You occasionally may want to allow extra viewing time for special programs.
4. **Don't use television as a distraction or a babysitter for preschool children.** Preschoolers' viewing should be limited to special television shows and videotapes that are produced for young children. Because the difference between fantasy and reality is not clear for this age group, regular television shows may cause fears.
5. **If your child is doing poorly in school, limit television time to ½ hour each day.** Make a rule that homework and chores must be finished before television is watched. If your child's favorite show is on before he can watch, try to record it for later viewing.
6. **Set a bedtime for your child that is not altered by television shows that interest your child.** Children who are allowed to stay up late to watch television are usually too tired the following day to remember what they are taught in school. By all means, don't permit your child to have a television set in his bedroom because this eliminates your control over television viewing.
7. **Turn off the television set during meals.** Family time is too precious to be squandered on television shows. In addition, don't have the television always on as a background sound in your house. If you don't like a quiet house, try to listen to music without lyrics.
8. **Teach critical viewing.** Turn the television on only for specific programs. Don't turn it on at random and scan for something interesting. Teach your child to look first in the program guide.
9. **Teach your child to turn off the television set at the end of a show.** If the television stays on, your child will probably become interested in the following show and then it will be more difficult for your child to stop watching.
10. **Encourage your child to watch some shows that are educational or teach human values.** Encourage watching documentaries or real-life dramas. Use programs about love, sex, family disputes, drinking, and drugs as a way to begin family discussions on these difficult topics.
11. **Forbid violent television shows.** This means you have to know what your child is watching and turn off the television set when you don't approve of the program. Develop separate lists of programs that are acceptable for older and younger kids to watch. Make your older children responsible for keeping the younger ones out of the television room at these times.
12. **Set a good example.** If you watch a lot of television, you can be sure your child will also. The types of programs you watch also send a clear message to your child.

Instructions for Pediatric Patients, 2nd Edition, ©1999 by WB Saunders Company.
Written by Barton D. Schmitt, MD, pediatrician and author of *Your Child's Health*, Bantam Books, a book for parents.

The following symptoms have all been reported in children after watching violent R-rated movies:

- Bedtime fears
- Recurrent nightmares
- Daytime flashbacks of something frightening
- Disruption of concentration and study
- A fearful view of the world

Since these movies were made to frighten teenagers and adults, this information should come as no surprise to you. Frequent exposures to violent material can also cause a child to become insensitive to human suffering. The impact of these movies on disturbed children may go a step further; some of them try to imitate the movies.

Causes

Most bad reactions are to R-rated movies containing horror, graphic violence, or sexual violence. The content of violent movies has changed over the last 10 years. Mutilation is the message. Thanks to improved special effects, we can now see the details of torture or brutality in slow, agonizing closeup.

The 12-year-and-under age group is most at risk for severe reactions. Most elementary-school children don't have the adult defense mechanisms needed to cope with these movies. They are most threatened by movie villains who seem real and play on their deepest fears (e.g., surprise attack, kidnapping, torture, or death). Children younger than 7 or 8 years old also think concretely. If it can happen on the screen, it could happen to them tonight.

Access to these violent movies has also changed. The uncut versions of violent movies are now readily available through cable television and video rentals. Parents say, "I didn't know he was watching that. I can't keep track of everything he sees." A popular party game in middle school involves renting a horror movie and seeing how much of it your friends can watch before becoming ill.

Most of the research done on the impact of violence on children has used television violence. This research shows that television affects children's behavior. No research review committee will ever approve a study in which children are exposed to R-rated movies. You don't have to be a psychiatrist to know that viewing graphic violence in movies (which is much more powerful than anything on television) is harmful to children. Yet some parents allow it.

Expected Course

Without treatment, these fears and preoccupations can last 1 to 6 months. With treatment, they usually improve over a few weeks.

PROTECTING YOUR CHILD FROM MOVIE VIOLENCE

1. **Understand the movie rating system.** Don't lump all R-rated movies together. The R rating means that children under 17 years old are not admitted without a parent. This rating is given for nudity, profanity, violence, *or* a combination of the above. Nudity, depending on the context, may be harmless. Profanity has become unavoidable, even on school playgrounds. It is the violence in the movie that has the disturbing impact on children. In fact, if one reads the ratings carefully, the degree of violence is also often listed (e.g., "graphic" violence or rape).

2. **Forbid all R-rated movies before 13 years of age.** Never allow a child who is younger than 13 years of age to see any R-rated film, no matter how liberal you may be about nudity and profanity. Between 13 and 17 years the maturity and sensitivity of your child must be carefully considered in deciding when she is ready to deal with some of these movies. Don't allow your child to see movies with personal or sexual violence (graphic violence) before 17 years of age. These movies are not a required part of life experiences at any age.

3. **Select your child's movies.** Don't let your child see a movie unless you know the rating and have read a review. Don't give in to her pressure to see something that is potentially harmful (that's an adult decision). Keep a list of movies of which you approve. Read reviews that look at films through the eyes of the child and note content that may upset children (e.g., cruelty to animals).

4. **Monitor what your child is watching on cable and network television.** Don't allow her to turn on the cable movie channel unless she has your permission to view a specific program. Even some of the edited versions of movies on network television can be too frightening for young children. Some young children who have viewed fires, tornadoes, earthquakes, warfare, or terrorism on the news have become worried about their personal safety.

5. **Warn your child about violent movies outside the home.** Protect your youngster from being unintentionally victimized by film violence. Be especially vigilant about slumber parties or Halloween parties. Tell your child to call you if the family she is visiting or a babysitter is showing any scary movies. Teach her to walk out of movies that make her scared or upset.

6. **Discuss any movie that upsets your child.** Respect your child's fears. Don't make fun of them. Help her to talk about what scared her. Help her gradually to come to grips with the situation.

7. **Practice prevention.** Protect your child's mental health from unnecessary fears. R-rated movies are never harmless for children in elementary school. Use the movie ratings and your common sense to choose age-appropriate movies for your child. Never let your child see anything that frightens you.

HELPING YOUR CHILD TO COPE WITH DIVORCE

More than 1 million children are affected by divorce each year. Our primary goal should be to minimize the emotional harm to these children. The main way to achieve this is to help the children to maintain a close and secure relationship with both parents. The following recommendations may be helpful.

1. **Reassure your children that both parents love them.** Make it clear that, although you are unhappy with each other and disagree about many things, the one subject you both completely agree on is how much you love your children. Demonstrate this love by spending time with your children. Preschoolers especially need lots of physical affection and cuddling from both parents.

2. **Keep constant as many aspects of your child's world as you can.** Try to keep your child in the same home or neighborhood. The fewer the changes, the better your child will cope with the stress of divorce. If this is impossible, at least try to keep your child in the same school with the same teachers, friends, and teams, even if only temporarily. Reassure your child that although your standard of living will decrease somewhat, you will continue to have the basic necessities of living (i.e., food, clothing, and shelter).

3. **Reassure your child that the noncustodial parent will visit.** Your child needs both parents. Young children are confused by divorce and fear that one parent may abandon them. Children need to know that they will have ongoing contact with both their father and their mother. Have a scheduled, predictable time for visiting. The custodial parent should strongly support the visiting schedule. One full day every 1 or 2 weeks is usually preferable to more frequent, brief (and rushed) visits. Try not to do too much in one day. If there is more than one child, all should spend equal time or the same time with the noncustodial parent to prevent feelings of favoritism. Your child will eagerly look forward to the visits, so the visiting parent must keep promises, be punctual, and remember birthdays and other special events. Both parents should work to make these visits pleasant. Allow your child to tell you that he had a good time during the visit with your ex-spouse.

    Provide your children with the telephone number of the noncustodial parent and encourage them to call at regular intervals.

4. **If the noncustodial parent becomes uninvolved, find substitutes.** Ask relatives or Big Brother or Big Sister volunteers to spend time with your son or daughter. Explain to your child, "Your Dad [or Mom] is not capable right now of being available for you. He [she] is sorting out his [her] own problems. There's not much we can do to change that." Help your child talk about disappointment and the sense of loss.

5. **Help your child talk about painful feelings.** At the time of separation and divorce, many children become anxious, depressed, and angry. They are frequently on the brink of tears, sleep poorly, have stomachaches, or don't do as well in school. To help your children get over these painful feelings, encourage them to talk about their feelings and respond with understanding and support. A divorce discussion group at school can help children feel less isolated and ashamed.

6. **Make sure that your children understand that they are not responsible for the divorce.** Children often feel guilty, believing that they somehow caused the divorce. Your children need reassurance that they did not in any way cause the divorce.

7. **Clarify that the divorce is final.** Some children hold on to the hope that they can somehow reunite the parents, and they pretend that the separation is temporary. Making it clear to children that the divorce is final can help them mourn their loss and move on to a more realistic adjustment to the divorce.

8. **Try to protect your child's positive feelings about both parents.** Try to mention the good points about the other parent. Don't be overly honest about negative feelings you have toward your ex-spouse. (You need to unload these feelings with another adult, not your children.) Devaluing or discrediting the other parent in your child's presence can reduce your child's personal self-esteem and create greater stress.

    Don't ask your child to take sides. A child does not need to have a single loyalty to one parent. Your child should be able to love both of you, even though you don't love each other.

9. **Maintain normal discipline in both households.** Children need consistent child-rearing practices. Overindulgence or too much leniency by either parent can make it more difficult for the other parent to get the child to behave. Constant competition for a child's love through special privileges or gifts leads to a spoiled child.

10. **Don't argue with your ex-spouse about your child in the child's presence.** Children are quite upset by seeing their parents fight. Most important, avoid any arguments regarding visiting, custody, or child support in your child's presence.

11. **Try to avoid custody disputes.** Your child badly needs a sense of stability. Challenge custody only if the custodial parent is causing obvious harm or repeated distress to your child. False accusations of physical or sexual abuse cause great emotional anguish for the child. If possible, don't split siblings unless they are adolescents and state a clear preference for living in a different setting.

Instructions for Pediatric Patients, 2nd Edition, ©1999 by WB Saunders Company.
Written by Barton D. Schmitt, MD, pediatrician and author of *Your Child's Health,* Bantam Books, a book for parents.

DEFINITION

The main task of adolescents in our culture is to become psychologically emancipated from their parents. The teenager must cast aside the dependent relationship of childhood. Before she can develop a new adult relationship with her parents, the adolescent must first distance herself from the way she related to them in the past. This process is characterized by a certain amount of intermittent normal rebellion, defiance, discontent, turmoil, restlessness, and ambivalence. Emotions usually run high. Mood swings are common. Under the best of circumstances, this adolescent rebellion continues for approximately 2 years; not uncommonly it lasts for 4 to 6 years.

DEALING WITH NORMAL ADOLESCENT REBELLION

The following guidelines may help you and your teenager through this difficult period.

1. **Treat your teenager as an adult friend.** By the time your child is 12 years old, start working on developing the kind of relationship you would like to have with your child when she is an adult. Treat your child the way you would like her to treat you when she is an adult. Your goal is mutual respect, support, and the ability to have fun together. Strive for relaxed, casual conversations during bicycling, hiking, shopping, playing catch, driving, cooking, and working and especially at mealtimes. Use praise and trust to help build her self-esteem. Recognize and validate your child's feelings by listening carefully and making nonjudgmental comments. Remember that listening doesn't mean you have to solve your teen's problems. The friendship model is the best basis for family functioning.

2. **Avoid criticism about "no-win" topics.** Most negative parent-adolescent relationships develop because the parents criticize their teenager too much. Much of the teen's objectionable behavior merely reflects conformity with the current tastes of her peer group. Peer-group immersion is one of the essential stages of adolescent development. Dressing, talking, and acting differently than adults help your child to feel independent from you.

   Try to avoid any criticism of your child's clothing, hairstyle, makeup, music, dance steps, friends (unless they're in trouble with the law), recreational interests, room decorations, use of free time, career choices, use of money, speech, posture, religion, and philosophy. Allowing your teen to rebel in these minor areas often prevents testing in major areas, such as experimentation with drugs, truancy, or stealing. Intervene and try to make a change only if your teenager's behavior is harmful or infringes on your rights (see section on house rules). Another common error is to criticize your teen's mood or attitude. A negative or lazy attitude can be changed only through good example and praise. The more you talk about these nontraditional behaviors, the longer they will last.

3. **Let society's rules and consequences teach responsibility outside the home.** Your teenager must learn from trial and error. As she experiments, she will learn to take responsibility for her decisions and actions. The parent should speak up only if the adolescent is going to do something dangerous or illegal. Otherwise, the parent must rely on the teen's own self-discipline, pressure from her peers to behave responsibly, and the lessons learned from the consequences of her actions.

   City curfew laws will help control late hours. A school's requirement for punctual school attendance will influence when your teen goes to bed at night. If she has trouble getting up in the morning, buy her an alarm clock. School grades will usually hold your teenager accountable for homework and other aspects of school performance. (It's not your job to check the homework.) If your teen has bad work habits, she will lose her job. If your teenager makes a poor choice of friends, she may find her confidences broken or that she gets into trouble. If she doesn't practice hard for a sport, she will be pressured by the team and coach to do better. If she misspends her allowance or earnings, she will run out of money before the end of the month. If her mood or attitude is negative, she will lose friends.

   If by chance your teenager asks you for advice about outside activities, try to describe the pros and cons in a brief, impartial way. Ask some questions to help her think about the main risks. Then wrap up your remarks with a comment such as, "Do what you think is best." Teenagers need plenty of opportunities to learn from their own mistakes before they leave home and have to solve problems without an ever-present support system.

4. **Clarify the house rules and consequences.** You have the right and the responsibility to make rules regarding your house and other possessions. Written rules cut down on misunderstandings. A teenager's preferences can be tolerated within her own room but they need not be imposed on the rest of the house. You can forbid loud music or incoming telephone calls after 10 PM that interfere with other people's concentration or sleep. You can forbid a television set in her room. While you should make your teen's friends feel welcome in your home, clarify the ground rules about parties or where snacks can be eaten. Your teen can be placed in charge of cleaning her room, washing her clothes, and ironing her clothes. You can insist on clean clothes and enough showers to prevent or overcome body odor. You must decide whether you will loan her your car, bicycle, camera, radio, television, clothes, and other possessions.

   Reasonable consequences for breaking house rules include loss of telephone, television, stereo, and car privileges. (Time-out is rarely useful in this age group, and physical punishment can escalate to a serious breakdown in your relationship.) If your teenager breaks something, she should repair it, pay for its repair or replacement, or work for you until the debt is paid off. If she makes a mess, she should clean it up. If your teen is doing poorly in school, you can restrict television time. You can also put a limit on telephone privileges and weeknights out. If your teen stays out too late or doesn't call you when she's delayed, you can ground her for a day or a weekend. In general, grounding for more than a few days is looked on as unfair and is hard to enforce.

5. **Use family conferences for negotiating house rules.** Some families find it helpful to have a brief meeting after dinner once each week. At this time your teenager can ask for changes in the house rules or bring up family issues that are causing problems. You can also bring up issues (such as your teen's demand to drive her too many places and your need for her help in arranging carpools). The family unit often functions better if the decision making is democratic. The objective of negotiation should be that both parties win. The atmosphere can be one of: "Nobody is at fault, but we have a problem. How can we solve it?"

6. **Give space to a teenager who is in a bad mood.** Generally when your teenager is in a bad mood, she won't want to talk about it with you. If teenagers want to discuss a problem with anybody, it is usually with a close friend. In general, it is advisable at such times to give your teen lots of space and privacy. This is a poor time to talk to your teenager about anything, pleasant or otherwise.

7. **Use "I" messages for rudeness.** Some talking back is normal. We want our teenagers to express their anger through talking and to challenge our opinions in a logical way. We need to listen. Expect your teenager to present her case passionately, even unreasonably. Let the small stuff go; it's only words. But don't accept disrespectful remarks, such as calling you a "jerk." Unlike a negative attitude, these mean remarks should not be ignored. You can respond with a comment like, "It really hurts me when you put me down or don't answer my question." Make your statement in as nonangry a way as possible. If your adolescent continues to make

angry, unpleasant remarks, leave the room. Don't get into a shouting match with your teenager because this is not a type of behavior that is acceptable in outside relationships. What you are trying to teach is that everyone has the right to disagree and even to express anger but that screaming and rude conversation are not allowed in your house. You can prevent some rude behavior by being a role model of politeness, constructive disagreement, and the ability to apologize.

 CALL OUR OFFICE

During regular hours if
- You think your teenager is depressed, suicidal, drinking, using illegal drugs, or going to run away.
- Your teenager is taking undue risks (e.g., reckless driving or unsafe sex).
- Your teenager has no close friends.
- Your teenager's school performance is declining markedly.
- Your teenager is skipping school frequently.
- Your teenager's outbursts of temper are destructive or violent.
- You feel your teenager's rebellion is excessive.
- Your family life is seriously disrupted by your teenager.
- You find yourself escalating the criticism and punishment.
- Your relationship with your teenager does not improve within 3 months after you begin using these approaches.
- You have other questions or concerns.

RECOMMENDED READING

Peter H. Buntman and E. M. Saris: How to Live with Your Teenager. Birch Tree Press, Pasadena, CA, 1990.
Lois Davitz and Joel Davitz: How to Live (Almost) Happily with a Teenager. Signet, New York, 1983.
Don Dinkmeyer and Gary D. McKay: Parenting Teenagers. American Guidance Service, Circle Pines, Minn., 1990.
D. E. Greydanus (Editor): AAP's Caring for Your Adolescent. Bantam Books, New York, 1991.
Kathleen McCoy and Charles Wibbelsman: Crisis-proof Your Teenager. Bantam Books, New York, 1991.

DEFINITION

"Enuresis" is the term used for the involuntary passage of urine during sleep. It is a very common problem affecting 40% of 3-year-olds, 10% of 6-year-olds, and 3% of 12-year-olds. We consider it normal until at least 6 years of age.

Causes

Most of these children have inherited small bladders, which cannot hold all the urine produced in a night. In addition, they are deep sleepers who don't awaken to the signal of a full bladder. The kidneys are normal. Physical causes are very rare, and your physician can easily detect them. Emotional problems do not cause enuresis, but can occur if the enuresis is mishandled.

Measuring your child's bladder size may help you understand how important it is for him to get up at night. Do this by having your child hold his urine as long as possible on at least three occasions. Each time have your child urinate into a container. Measure the amount of urine in ounces. The largest of the three measurements can be considered your child's bladder capacity. The normal capacity is 1 or more ounces per year of age. In a 6-year-old, a capacity of 5 ounces or less is small; a capacity of 6 to 8 ounces is normal and means that the bladder can hold a night's urine production until morning. Normal adult bladder size is 14 to 16 ounces.

Expected Course

Most children who wet the bed overcome the problem between 6 and 10 years of age. Even without treatment, all children eventually get over it. Therefore, treatments that might have harmful complications should not be used. On the other hand, treatments without side effects can be started as soon as your child has achieved complete daytime bladder control for 6 to 12 months.

HOME CARE FOR A CHILD OF ANY AGE WHO IS WETTING THE BED

1. **Encourage your child to get up to urinate during the night.** This advice is more important than any other. Tell your child at bedtime, "Try to get up when you have to pee."
2. **Improve access to the toilet.** Put a bright light in the bathroom. If the bathroom is at a distant location, try to put a portable toilet in your child's bedroom. Boys will do fine with a bucket.
3. **Encourage daytime fluids.** Encourage fluid during the day. The more fluids your child drinks, the more urine your child will produce, and more urine leads to larger bladders.
4. **Discourage evening fluids.** Discourage your child from drinking excessively during the 2 hours before bedtime. Give gentle reminders about this,

but don't worry about normal amounts. Avoid any drinks containing caffeine.
5. **Empty the bladder at bedtime.** Sometimes the parent needs to remind the child. Older children may respond better to a sign at their bedside or on their bathroom mirror.
6. **Take your child out of diapers or pull-ups.** Although this protective layer makes morning cleanup easier, it can interfere with motivation for getting up at night. Pull-ups or special absorbent underpants can be used selectively for camping or overnights at other people's homes. They should be used only if your child wants to use them and rarely should be permitted beyond age 8.
7. **Protect the bed from urine.** Odor becomes a problem if urine soaks into the mattress or blankets. Protect the mattress with a plastic mattress cover.
8. **Include your child in morning cleanup.** Including your child as a helper in stripping the bedclothes and putting them into the washing machine provides a natural disincentive for being wet. Older children can perform this task independently. Also, make sure that your child takes a shower each morning so that he does not smell of urine in school. The mattress can be protected with a plastic cover.
9. **Respond positively to dry nights.** Praise your child on mornings when he wakes up dry. A calendar with gold stars or "happy faces" for dry nights may also help.
10. **Respond gently to wet nights.** Your child does not like being wet. Most bed-wetters feel quite guilty and embarrassed about this problem. They need support and encouragement, not blame or punishment. Siblings should not be allowed to tease bed-wetters. Your home needs to be a safe haven for your child.

ADDITIONAL HOME CARE WHEN YOUR CHILD REACHES 6 YEARS OF AGE

Follow the previous recommendations in addition to the guidelines given below:

1. **Help your child understand his goal.** The key to becoming dry is to learn how to self-awaken every night and find the toilet. Getting up and urinating during the night can keep a person dry regardless of how small the bladder is or how much fluid he drinks. Help your child assume responsibility for doing this. Some children think that enuresis is the parent's problem to solve; they need to be reminded that "only you can solve this."
2. **Bedtime pep talk about self-awakening.** To help your child learn to awaken himself at night, encourage him to practice the following pep talk at bedtime.

• Lie on your bed with your eyes closed.

- Pretend it's the middle of the night.
- Pretend your bladder is full.
- Pretend you feel pressure.
- Pretend your bladder is trying to wake you up.
- Pretend your bladder is saying: "Get up before it's too late."
- Then run to the bathroom and empty your bladder.
- Remind yourself to get up like this during the night.

3. **Daytime practice of self-awakening.** Whenever you have an urge to urinate and you're home, go to your bedroom rather than the bathroom. Lie down and pretend you're sleeping. Tell yourself this is how your bladder feels during the night when it tries to awaken you. After a few minutes, go to the bathroom and urinate (just as you should at night).

4. **Parent-awakening.** If self-awakening fails, use parent-awakening to teach your child the correct goal: urinating into the toilet during the night. It makes much more sense than putting your child back into pull-ups and having him urinate in bed every night (the wrong goal). Your job is to wake your child up; his job is to locate the bathroom and use the toilet. You can awaken him at your bedtime. Try a hierarchy of prompts (the minimal one being the best), ranging from turning on a light, saying his name, touching him, shaking him or turning on an alarm clock. If your child is confused and very hard to awaken, try again in 20 minutes. Once he's awake, he needs to find the bathroom without any directions or guidance. When he awakens quickly to sound or touch for 7 consecutive nights, he's either cured or ready for an enuresis alarm.

5. **Encourage changing wet clothes during the night.** If your child wets at night, he should try to get up and change himself. First, if your child feels any urine leaking out, he should try to close the bladder's valve and stop the flow of urine. Second, he should hurry to the toilet to see if he has any urine left in his bladder. Third, he should change himself and put a dry towel over the wet part of the bed. This step can be made easier if dry pajamas and towels are always kept on a chair near the bed. The child who shows the motivation to carry out these steps is close to being able to awaken from the sensation of a full bladder.

ADDITIONAL INTERVENTION WHEN YOUR CHILD REACHES 8 YEARS OF AGE

Follow the previous recommendations. Talk with us about possibly using enuresis alarms or drugs as well, as described below.

Bed-Wetting Alarms

Alarms are used to teach a child to awaken when he needs to urinate during the night. They go off when they become wet. One type awakens you with a loud noise (buzzer), the other type with an annoying vibration. They have the highest cure rate (about 70%) of any available approach. They are the treatment of choice for any bed-wetter with a small bladder who can't otherwise train himself to awaken at night. The new transistorized alarms are small, lightweight, sensitive to a few drops of urine, not too expensive (about $50), and easy for a child to set up by himself. Some children as young as 5 years want to use them. Children using alarms still need to work on the self-awakening program. Request the special instruction sheet on bed-wetting alarms.

Alarm Clock

If your child is unable to awaken himself at night and you can't afford a bed-wetting alarm, teach him to use an alarm clock or clock radio. Set it for 3 or 4 hours after your child goes to bed. Put it beyond arm's reach. Encourage your child to practice responding to the alarm during the day while lying on the bed with eyes closed. Have your child set the alarm each night.

Drugs

Most bed-wetters need extra help with staying dry during slumber parties, camping trips, vacations, or other overnight stays. Some take an alarm clock with them and stay dry by awakening once at night. Some are helped by temporarily taking a drug at bedtime. One drug (given by nasal spray) decreases urine production at night and is quite safe. Another drug (taken as a pill) temporarily increases bladder capacity. It is safe at the correct dosage but dangerous if too much is taken or a younger sibling gets into it. If you do use a drug, be careful about the amount you use and where you store the drug, and be sure to keep the safety cap on the bottle. The drawback of these medicines is that when they are stopped, the bed-wetting usually returns. They do not cure bed-wetting. Therefore children on drugs for enuresis should also be using an alarm and learning to get up at night.

 CALL OUR OFFICE

During regular hours if
- Urination causes pain or burning.
- The urine stream is weak or dribbly.
- Your child also has daytime wetting.
- Your child also drinks excessive fluids.
- Bed-wetting is a new problem (your child used to be dry).
- Your child is over 12 years old.
- Your child is over 6 years of age and is not better after 3 months of using this treatment program.

Instructions for Pediatric Patients, 2nd Edition, ©1999 by WB Saunders Company.
Written by Barton D. Schmitt, MD, pediatrician and author of *Your Child's Health*, Bantam Books, a book for parents.

Almost all children and teens who wet the bed need to get up during the night to urinate. A bed-wetting (enuresis) alarm, which is activated by moisture, can help your child learn to awaken in time to go to the bathroom. The new models are lightweight and easy for the child to operate. Enuresis alarms can be used on any child from age 5 onward who wants to try one. On the other hand, they should never be imposed on a child at any age, even a teenager, if they don't want to use one.

DIRECTIONS FOR YOUR YOUNGSTER ON USING A BED-WETTING ALARM

1. **This is your alarm.** It can help you cure your bed-wetting if you use it correctly. Remember, the main purpose of the alarm is to help you get up during the night and use the toilet. The alarm won't work unless you listen for it carefully and respond to it quickly. Better yet, get up *before* the alarm goes off.

2. **Hook up the alarm system by yourself.** Trigger the buzzer a few times by touching the moisture sensors with a wet finger and practice going to the bathroom as you will do if it goes off during the night.

3. **Have a night-light or flashlight near your bed.** A light should be handy so it will be easy to see what you are doing when the alarm sounds. Turn on the night-light.

4. **Go through your self-awakening pep talk at bedtime.** Try to "beat the buzzer." Wake up when your bladder feels full but before any urine leaks out. If the buzzer does go off, try to wake up and stop urinating at the first moment that you think you hear the alarm (even if you think you are hearing it in a dream).

5. **When you hear the alarm.** As soon as you hear the alarm, close the valve to your bladder. Then jump out of bed and run to the bathroom.

6. **Use the toilet.** In the bathroom, empty your bladder to see how much urine you were able to hold back. Only after you have used the toilet, work on turning off the buzzer. Remove the metal strip from the little pocket in your underwear (if you have a Wet-Stop) or disconnect the clips (if you have a Nytone) and dry them off.

7. **Change to dry clothes.** Put on dry underwear and pajamas, and reconnect the alarm. Put a dry towel over the wet spot on your bed. Remind yourself to get up before the alarm buzzes next time and review your plan before going to sleep.

8. **Write on your calendar.** In the morning, write on your calendar "dry" (no alarm), "wet spot" (you got up after the alarm went off), or "wet" (you didn't get up).

9. **Use the alarm every night.** Use the alarm every night until you go 3 or 4 weeks without bed-wetting. This usually takes 2 to 3 months, so try to be persistent.

A SELF-AWAKENING PROGRAM FOR YOUR YOUNGSTER

While using the alarm, it's very important that you also practice the following self-awakening program at bedtime. You are trying to teach yourself to awaken during the night and to use the toilet when your bladder feels full. Until you learn how to do this, you won't be dry.

- Lie on your bed with your eyes closed.
- Pretend it's the middle of the night.
- Pretend your bladder is full.
- Pretend you feel the pressure.
- Pretend your bladder is trying to wake you up.
- Pretend your bladder is saying: "Get up before it's too late."
- Then run to the bathroom and empty your bladder.
- Remind yourself to get up like this during the night.

PARENTS' ROLE WITH BED-WETTING ALARMS

If your child doesn't awaken immediately to the sound of the buzzer, she needs your help. You may need to be involved every night for the first 2 to 3 weeks.

1. Go to your child's room as quickly as you can. Turn on the light and say loudly, "Get out of bed and stand up."

2. If that doesn't work, get your child to a sitting position and run a cold washcloth over her face to bring her out of her deep sleep.

3. Only after your child is standing, remind her to turn off the alarm. By all means, don't turn off the buzzer for her. Your child has to learn to carry out this step for herself.

4. Make sure your child is wide awake and walks into the bathroom before you leave her. If necessary, ask her questions to help awaken her.

5. Your goal is to help your child awaken immediately and get out of bed when the buzzer goes off. Phase out of your child's alarm program as soon as possible. Going to bed with the radio *off*, going to bed at a reasonable hour, and using a night-light can help your child respond faster to the alarm.

HOW TO ORDER ENURESIS ALARMS

Nytone Alarm: Nytone Medical Products, 2424 South 900 West, Salt Lake City, UT 84119 or call 801-973-4090

Nite Train'r Alarm: Koregon Enterprises, 9735 S.W. Sunshine Court, Suite 100, Beaverton, OR 97005 or call 800-544-4240

Wet-Stop Alarm: Palco Laboratories, 8030 Soquel Ave., Suite 104, Santa Cruz, CA 95062 or call 800-346-4488

Potty Pager (silent alarm): Ideas for Living, 1285 North Cedarbrook, Boulder, CO 80304 or call 800-497-6573

BED-WETTING: SELF-CARE FOR TEENS

DEFINITION

"Enuresis" (bed-wetting) is the term used for the involuntary passage of urine during sleep. It is a very common problem that affects 10% of 6-year-olds, 5% of 10-year-olds, 3% of 12-year-olds, and 1% of 18-year-olds.

Causes

Most teens with enuresis have inherited a small bladder, which cannot hold all the urine produced during a night. Measure your bladder size to see what you have to overcome. (Normal teen size is 12 to 16 ounces of urine.) In addition, most teens with enuresis are deep sleepers who don't awaken to the signal of a full bladder. If they did, they wouldn't be wet. Physical causes are very rare and your physician can easily detect them. Emotional problems do not cause enuresis, but they can occur if it is mishandled.

Expected Course

Even without treatment, all children eventually get over their bed-wetting, but it may take years. With treatment, you can become dry much sooner. Using the following suggestions, most teenagers can learn to use the toilet during the night.

HOME CARE FOR BED-WETTING

1. **Your goal is to wake up every night and use the toilet.** Teens with small bladders cannot stay dry unless they get up to urinate one or more times every night. Getting up can keep you dry regardless of how small your bladder is or how much you drink. You will not be cured completely until you learn how to do this.
2. **Decrease evening fluids.** Normal fluid intake is fine, but try not to drink excessive fluids during the 2 hours before bedtime. Especially avoid beverages that contain caffeine because caffeine increases urine production. (**Remember:** Everything you drink eventually becomes urine. During the day, however, drink all you want.)
3. **Empty your bladder at bedtime.** Start the night with an empty bladder. Put up a sign if you have trouble remembering to do this.
4. **Bedtime pep talk about self-awakening.** To help awaken yourself at night, practice the following routine at bedtime:

   - Lie on your bed with your eyes closed.
   - Pretend it's the middle of the night.
   - Pretend your bladder is full.
   - Pretend you feel the pressure.
   - Pretend your bladder is trying to wake you up.
   - Pretend your bladder is saying, "Get up before it's too late."
   - Then run to the bathroom and empty your bladder.
   - Remind yourself to get up like this during the night.

   - If you think of a better way to remind your brain to get you up every night, do it and you'll be dry.

5. **Daytime practice of self-awakening.** Whenever you have an urge to urinate and you're home, go to your bedroom rather than the bathroom. Lie down and pretend you're sleeping. Tell yourself this is how your bladder feels during the night when it tries to awaken you. After a few minutes, go to the bathroom and urinate (just as you should at night).
6. **Bed-wetting alarms.** Alarms are used to teach you to awaken when you need to urinate during the night. They go off when they become wet. One type awakens you with a loud noise (buzzer), the other type with an annoying vibration. They have the highest cure rate (about 70%) of any available approach. They are the treatment of choice for any bed-wetter with a small bladder who can't otherwise train himself to self-awaken at night. The new transistorized alarms are small, lightweight, sensitive to a few drops of urine, not too expensive (about $50), and easy for a teenager to set up by himself or herself. Teens using alarms still need to work on the self-awakening program. For further information, request the special instruction sheet, Bed-Wetting Alarms.
7. **Alarm clock.** If you are unable to awaken yourself at night and you can't afford a bed-wetting alarm, use an alarm clock or clock radio. Set it for 3 or 4 hours after you go to bed. Put it beyond your arm's reach. Practice responding to the alarm during the day while lying on the bed with your eyes closed. Set the alarm each night.
8. **Parent-awakening.** If self-awakening fails, don't give up hope. Ask your parent to help you learn how to awaken. Your parent's job is to wake you up; your job is to locate your bathroom and use the toilet. Your parent can awaken you at his or her bedtime. Your parent can try a hierarchy of prompts (the minimal one being the best), ranging from turning on a light, saying your name, touching you, shaking you, or turning on an alarm clock. If you are confused and very hard to awaken, your parent can try again in 20 minutes. Once you're awake, you need to find the bathroom without any directions or guidance. If you awaken quickly to sound or touch for 7 consecutive nights, you're either cured or ready for an enuresis alarm.
9. **Change wet clothes during the night.** If you are wet at night, try to get up and change yourself. First, if you feel any urine leaking out, try to close the bladder's valve and stop the flow of urine. Second, hurry to the toilet to see if you have any urine left in your bladder. Third, change yourself and put a dry towel over the wet part of the bed. (This step can be made easier if you always keep dry pajamas and towels on a chair near the bed.) If you are able to carry out these steps, you are

Instructions for Pediatric Patients, 2nd Edition, ©1999 by WB Saunders Company.
Written by Barton D. Schmitt, MD, pediatrician and author of *Your Child's Health,* Bantam Books, a book for parents.

close to being able to awaken from the sensation of a full bladder.

10. **Establish a morning routine for wet pajamas and wet bedding.** On wet mornings, rinse your pajamas and underwear in the sink until the odor is gone. To make sure you smell good, take a quick rinse in the shower. You can cut down on the laundry by placing a dry towel under your bottom each night. The towel can also be rinsed in the morning. If a wet bed is left open to the air, the wet sheets will usually be dry by noon. Because of odor, the sheets may need to be washed a few times each week.

11. **Medication.** Most bed-wetters need extra help with staying dry during slumber parties, camping trips, vacations, or other overnights. Some take an alarm clock with them and stay dry by awakening once at night. Some are helped by temporarily taking a drug at bedtime. One drug decreases urine production at night and is quite safe. Another temporarily increases bladder capacity. It is safe at the correct dosage, but dangerous if too much is taken or a younger sibling gets into it.

If you do use a medication, be careful about the amount you use and where you store the medicine, and be sure to keep the safety cap on the bottle. The drawback of these medicines is that when they are stopped, the bed-wetting usually returns. They do not cure bed-wetting. Therefore, teenagers using drugs for enuresis should also be using an alarm and learning to get up at night.

 CALL OUR OFFICE

During regular hours if
- Urination causes pain or burning.
- The stream of urine is weak or dribbly.
- You also have wetting during the daytime.
- Bed-wetting is a new problem (you used to stay dry).
- You are not better after 3 months of following this treatment program.

Index